Diseases of Donkeys and Mules

Editor

RAMIRO E. TORIBIO

VETERINARY CLINICS OF NORTH AMERICA: EQUINE PRACTICE

www.vetequine.theclinics.com

Consulting Editor
THOMAS J. DIVERS

December 2019 • Volume 35 • Number 3

ELSEVIER

1600 John F. Kennedy Boulevard • Suite 1800 • Philadelphia, Pennsylvania, 19103-2899

http://www.vetequine.theclinics.com

VETERINARY CLINICS OF NORTH AMERICA: EQUINE PRACTICE Volume 35, Number 3
December 2019 ISSN 0749-0739, ISBN-13: 978-0-323-70874-6

Editor: Colleen Dietzler
Developmental Editor: Donald Mumford

Veterinary Clinics of North America: Equine Practice (ISSN 0749-0739) is published in April, August, and December by Elsevier Inc., 360 Park Avenue South, New York, NY 10010-1710. Business and Editorial Offices: 1600 John F. Kennedy Blvd., Suite 1800, Philadelphia, PA 19103-2899. Subscription prices are $287.00 per year (domestic individuals), $557.00 per year (domestic institutions), $100.00 per year (domestic students/residents), $334.00 per year (Canadian individuals), $702.00 per year (Canadian institutions), $365.00 per year (international individuals), $702.00 per year (international institutions), and $180.00 per year (international and Canadian students/residents). To receive student/resident rate, orders must be accompanied by name of affiliated institution, date of term, and the signature of program/residency coordinator on institution letterhead. Orders will be billed at individual rate until proof of status is received. Foreign air speed delivery is included in all *Clinics* subscription prices. All prices are subject to change without notice. **POSTMASTER:** Send address changes to *Veterinary Clinics of North America: Equine Practice*, 3251 Riverport Lane, Maryland Heights, MO 63043. Customer Service (orders, claims, online, change of address): Elsevier Health Sciences Division, Subscription **Customer Service, 3251 Riverport Lane, Maryland Heights, MO 63043. Tel: 1-800-654-2452 (U.S. and Canada); 314-447-8871 (outside U.S. and Canada). Fax: 314-447-8029. E-mail: journalscustomerservice-usa@elsevier.com (for print support);** E-mail: **journalsonlinesupport-usa@elsevier.com (for online support).**

Reprints. For copies of 100 or more of articles in this publication, please contact the Commercial Reprints Department, Elsevier Inc., 360 Park Avenue South, New York, NY 10010-1710. Tel.: 212-633-3874; Fax: 212-633-3820; E-mail: reprints@elsevier.com.

Veterinary Clinics of North America: Equine Practice is covered in *MEDLINE/PubMed (Index Medicus), Excerpta Medica, Current Contents/Agriculture, Biology and Environmental Sciences,* and *ISI.*

Contributors

CONSULTING EDITOR

THOMAS J. DIVERS, DVM
Diplomate, American College of Veterinary Internal Medicine; Diplomate, American College of Veterinary Emergency and Critical Care; Steffen Professor of Veterinary Medicine, Department of Clinical Sciences, Section of Large Animal Medicine, Cornell University College of Veterinary Medicine, Ithaca, New York, USA

EDITOR

RAMIRO E. TORIBIO, DVM, MS, PhD
Diplomate, American College of Veterinary Internal Medicine; Professor, Equine Internal Medicine, Department of Veterinary Clinical Sciences, College of Veterinary Medicine, The Ohio State University, Columbus, Ohio, USA

AUTHORS

ELENA BARRIO, MVDr, Cert AVP, MRCVS
Veterinary Surgeon, The Veterinary Department, The Donkey Sanctuary, Sidmouth, Devon, United Kingdom; The Veterinary Hospital, Honiton, Devon, United Kingdom

ERICA BEHLING-KELLY, DVM, PhD
Diplomate, American College of Veterinary Pathologists; Associate Professor, Department of Population Medicine and Diagnostic Sciences, Animal Health Diagnostic Center, College of Veterinary Medicine, Cornell University, Ithaca, New York, USA

NICOLA BELL, BSc, MSc
Senior Researcher, Research Department, The Donkey Sanctuary, Sidmouth, Devon, United Kingdom

MARGARET M. BROSNAHAN, DVM, PhD
Diplomate, American College of Veterinary Internal Medicine, Large Animal Internal Medicine; Assistant Professor of Equine Medicine, College of Veterinary Medicine, Midwestern University, Glendale, Arizona, USA

FAITH A. BURDEN, BSc, PhD
Director of Research, Research Department, The Donkey Sanctuary, Sidmouth, Devon, United Kingdom

IGOR FEDERICO CANISSO, DVM, MSc, PhD
Diplomate, American College of Theriogenologists, Diplomate, European College of Animal Reproduction (Equine Reproduction); Assistant Professor of Theriogenology (Equine Reproduction), Department of Veterinary Clinical Medicine, College of Veterinary Medicine, University of Illinois Urbana-Champaign, Urbana, IL, USA

ERIC DAVIS, DVM, MS
Diplomate, American College of Veterinary Surgeons; Diplomate, American College of Veterinary Internal Medicine, Large Animal Internal Medicine; Veterinary Medicine & Epidemiology, UC Davis International Animal Welfare Training Institute, School of Veterinary Medicine, Davis, California, USA

ROBYN E. ELLERBROCK, DVM, PhD
Assistant Professor of Theriogenology, Department of Large Animal Medicine, College of Veterinary Medicine, University of Georgia, Athens, Georgia, USA

FRANCISCO JAVIER NAVAS GONZÁLEZ, DVM, MSc, PhD
AGR218 PAIDI Group, Department of Genetics, Faculty of Veterinary Sciences, University of Córdoba, Córdoba, Spain

ERIN L. GOODRICH, DVM
Diplomate, American College of Veterinary Preventive Medicine; Senior Extension Associate, Department of Population Medicine and Diagnostic Sciences, Animal Health Diagnostic Center, College of Veterinary Medicine, Cornell University, Ithaca, New York, USA

DEREK C. KNOTTENBELT, BVM&S, DVM&S, MRCVS
Diploma of the European College of Equine Internal Medicine, Diplomate, American College of Veterinary Internal Medicine, Director, Equine Medical Solutions, Kildean Business and Enterprise Hub, Stirling, Scotland

GEMMA LILLY, BAEDT, BSc (hons) EDS, BA (hons) ESBM
Equine Dental Technician, Research and Operational Support Department, The Donkey Sanctuary, Trow Offices, Sidmouth, Devon, England

NORA MATTHEWS, DVM
Diplomate, American College of Veterinary Anesthesia and Analgesia; Professor Emeritus, Texas A&M University, Freeville, New York, USA

AMY KATHERINE McLEAN, PhD, MSc
Equine Lecturer, Animal Science Department, UC Davis Animal Science, University of California Davis, Davis, California, USA

FRANCISCO J. MENDOZA, DVM, PhD, MSc
Diplomate, European College of Equine Internal Medicine; Department of Animal Medicine and Surgery, University of Cordoba, Campus Rabanales, Cordoba, Spain

JORDI MIRÓ, DVM, PhD
Professor of Animal Reproduction, Department of Animal Medicine and Surgery, Faculty of Veterinary Medicine, Autonomous University of Barcelona, Barcelona, Spain

DUCCIO PANZANI, DVM, PhD
Associate Professor of Veterinary Obstetrics and Gynecology, Department of Veterinary Science, University of Pisa, Pisa, Italy

ALEJANDRO PEREZ-ECIJA, DVM, PhD, MSc
Diplomate, European College of Veterinary Pathologists; Department of Animal Medicine and Surgery, University of Cordoba, Campus Rabanales, Cordoba, Spain

LUKE A. POORE, MSc, MA, Vet MB, Cert ES (Orth), MRCVS
Head of Clinical Veterinary Services, The Veterinary Department, The Donkey Sanctuary, Brookfield Farm, Devon, United Kingdom

KAREN J. RICKARDS, PhD, BVSc, MRCVS
Head of Veterinary Services, The Veterinary Department, The Donkey Sanctuary, Sidmouth, Devon, United Kingdom; The Veterinary Hospital, Honiton, Devon, United Kingdom

JOÃO B. RODRIGUES, DVM, PhD
Lead, Welfare Assessment, Research and Operational Support Department, The Donkey Sanctuary, Trow Offices, Sidmouth, Devon, United Kingdom; CIMO – Mountain Research Center, Polytechnic Institute of Bragança (ESA/IPB), Bragança, Portugal

REBEKAH J.E. SULLIVAN, BVSc (Hons), Cert AVP (EM), MRCVS
Veterinary Surgeon, The Veterinary Department, The Donkey Sanctuary, Sidmouth, Devon, United Kingdom; The Veterinary Hospital, Honiton, Devon, United Kingdom

ALEXANDRA K. THIEMANN, MA, VetMB, Cert EP, MSc, AFHEA, MRCVS
Senior Veterinary Surgeon -Education, The Veterinary Department, The Donkey Sanctuary, Brookfield Farm, Sidmouth, Devon, United Kingdom; The Veterinary Hospital, Honiton, Devon, United Kingdom

RAMIRO E. TORIBIO, DVM, MS, PhD
Diplomate, American College of Veterinary Internal Medicine; Professor of Equine Internal Medicine, Department of Veterinary Clinical Sciences, College of Veterinary Medicine, The Ohio State University, Columbus, Ohio, USA

JOHANNES P.A.M. VAN LOON, DVM, PhD
Diplomate, European College of Veterinary Anaesthesia and Analgesia; Department of Equine Sciences, Faculty of Veterinary Medicine, Utrecht University, Utrecht, The Netherlands

KAREN J. RICKARDS, PhD, BVSc, MRCVS
Head of Veterinary Services, The Veterinary Department, The Donkey Sanctuary, Sidmouth, Devon, United Kingdom; The Veterinary Hospital, Honiton, Devon, United Kingdom

JOÃO B. RODRIGUES, DVM, PhD
Lead Welfare Assessment Research and Operational Support Coordinator, The Donkey Sanctuary, Sidmouth, Devon, United Kingdom; CIMO - Mountain Research Center, Polytechnic Institute of Bragança (ESA/IPB), Bragança, Portugal

REBEKAH J.E. SULLIVAN, BVSc (Hons), Cert AVP (EM), MRCVS
Veterinary Surgeon, The Veterinary Department, The Donkey Sanctuary, Sidmouth, Devon, United Kingdom; The Veterinary Hospital, Honiton, Devon, United Kingdom

ALEXANDRA K. THIEMANN, MA, VetMB, Cert EP, MSc, AFHEA, MRCVS
Senior Veterinary Surgeon (Education), The Veterinary Department, The Donkey Sanctuary, Brookfield Farm, Sidmouth, Devon, United Kingdom; The Veterinary Hospital, Honiton, Devon, United Kingdom

RAMIRO E. TORIBIO, DVM, MS, PhD
Diplomate, American College of Veterinary Internal Medicine; Professor of Equine Internal Medicine, Department of Veterinary Clinical Sciences, College of Veterinary Medicine, The Ohio State University, Columbus, Ohio, USA

JOHANNES P.A.M. VAN LOON, DVM, PhD
Diplomate, European College of Veterinary Anaesthesia And Analgesia; Department of Equine Sciences, Faculty of Veterinary Medicine, Utrecht University, Utrecht, The Netherlands

Contents

interspecies breeding results in healthy, although infertile, hybrid offspring. Most notable among these are the horse–donkey hybrids, the mule and hinny. Donkeys presently are used for everything from companion animals to beasts of burden. Although closely related from an evolutionary stand-point, differences in anatomy and physiology preclude the assumption that they can be treated identically to the domestic horse. Veterinarians should be aware of these differences and adjust their practice accordingly.

about anesthesia and analgesia in donkeys and mules is important to more equine practitioners. This review highlights the current knowledge on various anesthetic and analgesic approaches in donkey and mules. The authors emphasize that there is still much information that is not available about donkeys and mules; in many circumstances, the clinician must use available equine information to treat the patient, while monitoring for differences in response.

Research and clinical understanding of equine dentistry has progressed in recent years; however, specific knowledge about donkey dentistry is lacking. This article intends to revise unique anatomic features of the head and oral cavity of donkeys, as well as how to correctly examine, diagnose, prevent, and/or treat dental pathology, allowing for a better comprehension of oral and dental disorders affecting these animals throughout their life. It also emphasizes that these disorders need to be taken into account when assessing the welfare of donkeys.

Clinical evaluation and preventative care in donkeys should follow similar guidelines as for horses. There are species-specific differences due to the desert-adapted physiology of the donkey. Donkeys are mainly used as pack animals, companions and for production of meat or milk – they may be kept well into old age. Diseases often present late or may go unrecognized leading to poor welfare and quality of life. Basic knowledge of nutrition, blood values, pharmacology and common disease recognition will help veterinarians improve the health and welfare of donkeys.

Donkeys suffer from the same respiratory diseases as horses; however, owing to their nonathletic nature many conditions can present in a more advanced state before becoming clinically apparent. Anatomically, their respiratory tract is similar to the horse, with certain species-specific differences that are important to be aware of. Often donkeys do not receive the same level of routine care as horses, so many are not vaccinated against respiratory pathogens such as influenza or herpesviruses. Donkeys can act as a reservoir for certain infectious and parasitic respiratory diseases and the interpretation of diagnostic tests needs to be carried out with caution.

 Video content accompanies this article at http://www.vetequine. theclinics.com.

Donkeys and mules often are misunderstood because of their behavioral differences compared with horses. Working with these animals requires more patience and ability to notice the slightest changes in behavior to diagnose disease. Mules and donkeys form strong bonds and trust with familiar people and other equids. Training mules and hinnies from an early age is key to modifying behavior and acceptance of unfamiliar people. Reproductive behavior is different from that of horses and requires more patience when collecting jacks. Practitioners working with mules and donkeys should take a methodological approach and get to know the animal before performing examinations.

Francisco J. Mendoza, Alejandro Perez-Ecija, and Ramiro E. Toribio

Donkeys and mules show several pharmacodynamic and pharmacokinetic idiosyncrasies that have to be fully considered by any clinician dealing with these species. Because they possess an increased metabolic rate and cellular water content compared with horses, higher doses (or shorter dosing intervals) are usually recommended for those drugs where pharmacologic studies have been performed. Nonetheless, owing to the lack of species-specific information, this assumption cannot be arbitrarily applied. Thus, when a drug protocol published for horses is extrapolated to a donkey or a mule, a close monitoring is required to detect any secondary effect or subdosing.

Igor Federico Canisso, Duccio Panzani, Jordi Miró, and Robyn E. Ellerbrock

Donkeys are nonseasonal, polyestrous, territorial, and nonharem breeders. Although there are many similarities between horses and donkeys, there are also reproductive features that differ, from the longer cervix in the jenny to spermatogenic efficiency in the jack. Mules display reproductive cyclic activity but are rarely fertile. Frozen donkey semen has high pregnancy rates in mares, but lower rates in jennies. This article reviews key aspects of donkey and mule reproductive physiology, reproductive medicine, and assisted reproductive techniques that are useful for practitioners offering assisted reproductive techniques, and also for practitioners with the occasional client with a basic reproductive question.

Alexandra K. Thiemann and Luke A. Poore

This article provides a review of hoof anatomy and care in donkeys and mules. Hoof disease is a major cause of poor welfare and mortality globally. Problems associated with hoof disease are discussed in the context of behavior, diet, treatment, and prevention. The most common conditions encountered are discussed, including laminitis, the overgrown unbalanced hoof, white line disease, flexural deformities, and other significant issues. Differences between donkey and horse hoof anatomy are described.

VETERINARY CLINICS OF NORTH AMERICA: EQUINE PRACTICE

FORTHCOMING ISSUES

April 2020
Clinical Pathology for the Equine Practitioner
Sally DeNotta and Tracy Stokol, *Editors*

August 2020
Equine Genetic Diseases
Carrie Finno, *Editor*

December 2020
Update on Equine Dentistry
Edward Earley, Robert Barrett, and Steven S. Galloway, *Editors*

RECENT ISSUES

August 2019
Controversies in Equine Medicine and Surgery
Robert J. MacKay, *Editor*

April 2019
Clinical Cardiology
Colin C. Schwarzwald and Katharyn J. Mitchell, *Editors*

December 2018
Wound Management in the Horse
Earl M. Gaughan, *Editor*

RELATED SERIES

Veterinary Clinics of North America: Food Animal Practice

THE CLINICS ARE NOW AVAILABLE ONLINE!
Access your subscription at:
www.theclinics.com

VETERINARY CLINICS OF NORTH AMERICA: EQUINE PRACTICE

RELATED SERIES

Preface

Dear Donkey and Mule: You Deserve More Appreciation and Better Medicine

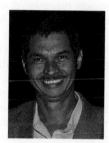

Ramiro E. Toribio, DVM, MS, PhD, DACVIM
Editor

I feel honored to be the guest editor of the first issue of the *Veterinary Clinics of North America: Equine Practice* devoted to donkeys and mules. I want to thank Dr Tom Divers as well as Don Mumford and Colleen Dietzler at Elsevier for inviting me to edit this issue, which will be a valuable resource for equine practitioners, residents, and veterinary medicine students. My special gratitude to the contributing authors for sharing their time and expertise: they are the ones who made it possible.

Those trying to find medical information on donkeys and mules have noticed that it is not readily available. Therefore, our goal was to cover common conditions of donkeys and mules in a single document. Due to space limitations, it was not possible to write about all diseases of donkeys and mules, for which I apologize.

The domestication of the donkey (*Equus africanus asinus*) occurred in Northern Africa approximately 6000 years ago. These are desert-adapted animals, and their ability to carry heavy loads through arid lands enabled human groups with agrarian life-styles to move farther, transforming ancient societies and states throughout Africa and Asia, with economic, cultural, religious, and territorial implications. It is important to note that the donkey and the mule also contributed to the development of countries such as the United States and the United Kingdom. The mule, in particular, played a major role in territorial protection and expansions, including wars. With industrialization, these animals became less relevant, even neglected.

To date, the donkey continues to have a positive impact in developing countries. The livelihood of many families in Africa depends on a single donkey, often making these animals their most prized asset. Their economic value comes from work, transportation, packing, and tourism, but also as a source of food. In contrast, in developed

Vet Clin Equine 35 (2019) xiii–xiv
https://doi.org/10.1016/j.cveq.2019.08.015
0749-0739/19/© 2019 Published by Elsevier Inc.

vetequine.theclinics.com

countries, donkeys and mules are mainly used for other purposes (recreation, tourism, hobby, shows, pets, companion, and onotherapy).

The donkey population in the world has been estimated at 44 million, which is substantial considering that there are around 58 million horses worldwide. Their resistance to harsh environmental conditions, efficient energy use, low maintenance cost, durability, ability to be used for multiple purposes, and apparent stoic nature have made donkeys in many underdeveloped countries more valuable than horses. It is ironic that these traits have also predisposed them to a number of diseases, but worse, rendered them victim of abuse and neglect.

Donkeys are afflicted with similar conditions as other equids; however, due to evolutionary anatomical and physiologic differences, the clinical signs, hematologic variables, and drug metabolism vary and should be taken into account when making a clinical assessment, making a diagnosis, implementing therapies, and also in making the prognosis. Otherwise, this could lead to misdiagnosis, inadequate treatment, unnecessary expenses, and worse, a negative outcome.

In recent years, there has been an increased global demand for donkey products, in particular, the skin, which is used in China to make a traditional medicine from donkey-hide gelatin (ejiao). This has also become a problem in many countries of Africa, Asia, and Latin America, where it has major connotations to not only animal welfare but also the worldwide donkey population. Another practice, although less common, is the slaughter of donkeys for their meat. This information is largely unknown to most people, including veterinarians.

The consumption of donkey milk is becoming more acceptable in developed countries, and it has been proposed as an alternative to bovine milk in infants with some allergic and inflammatory conditions. Donkey dairy farms are expanding in Europe, particularly in Italy, where these animals receive good care. Donkey milk is also used in the cosmetic industry.

From the previous points, it is evident that there is an increasing demand for veterinarians with donkey-specific knowledge, in both developing and developed countries, with underlying differences. In developing countries, the need is to provide medical care and support the welfare of a prized family asset, while in developed countries, veterinarians are expected to deliver routine and specialized veterinary care.

In conclusion, it is our goal with this issue of the *Veterinary Clinics of North America: Equine Practice* to provide valuable information on selected medical topics of donkeys and mules, but also to raise awareness on aspects of donkey welfare that are largely unknown.

Ramiro E. Toribio, DVM, MS, PhD
Department of Veterinary Clinical Sciences
College of Veterinary Medicine
The Ohio State University
601 Vernon Tharp Street
Columbus, OH 43210, USA

E-mail address:
toribio.1@osu.edu

Metabolic and Endocrine Disorders in Donkeys

Francisco J. Mendoza, DVM, PhD, MSc[a],*, Ramiro E. Toribio, DVM, MS, PhD[b],
Alejandro Perez-Ecija, DVM, PhD, MSc[a]

KEYWORDS

- Hyperlipemia • Metabolic syndrome • Parathyroid gland
- Pituitary pars intermedia dysfunction • Thyroid gland

KEY POINTS

- Endocrine and metabolic diseases are frequent in donkeys.
- Hyperlipemia is the most common metabolic disorder in donkeys.
- Because of their efficient energy use, obesity is frequent in donkeys, often associated with insulin dysregulation and endocrinopathic laminitis.
- Glucose and insulin dynamics differ between donkeys and horses.
- Basal adrenocorticotropic hormone and the thyrotropin-releasing hormone stimulation test are the preferred diagnostic methods for pituitary pars intermedia dysfunction in donkeys.

INTRODUCTION

The donkey (*Equus asinus*) continues to play major economic, social, and cultural roles in different regions of the world, mainly in developing countries. The economic value of donkeys as transport and traction animals in industrialized countries has practically disappeared. However, new uses, such as ecotourism, trekking, hippotherapy/ono-therapy, or simply as companion animals, are increasing. Donkeys are also used as a source of meat and milk, and milk byproducts are being used in the cosmetic indus-try.[1,2] Regrettably, the increasing demand for donkey hide gelatin from China to pro-duce ejiao has led to a major decline in the worldwide donkey population.

Because of the new purposes, donkey-specific and mule-specific knowledge as well as awareness of animal welfare are relevant to veterinarians. To date, more

Conflict of Interest: The authors have no financial or personal conflicts that could influence or bias the content of this publication.
[a] Department of Animal Medicine and Surgery, University of Cordoba, Campus Rabanales, Road Madrid-Cadiz km 396, Cordoba 14014, Spain; [b] Department of Veterinary Clinical Sci-ences, The Ohio State University, 601 Vernon Tharp Street, Columbus, OH 43210, USA
* Corresponding author. Department of Animal Medicine and Surgery, University of Cordoba, Campus Rabanales, Road Madrid-Cadiz km 396, Cordoba 14014, Spain.
E-mail address: fjmendoza@uco.es

donkeys are being admitted to veterinary hospitals or are receiving specialized care as a result of economic growth, cultural shifts, and programs to rescue almost extinct breeds. In addition, a species-specific approach is fundamental in donkeys, because extrapolating clinical data, diagnostic protocols, and treatments from horses can lead to misdiagnosis, unnecessary or inadequate treatments, and additional costs.[3–7]

A unique trait of donkeys compared with horses is their inherent energy efficiency and ability to accumulate adipose tissue, even when consuming poor-quality diets. These energy disposal features are likely a result of endocrine and metabolic adaptions to survive under harsh conditions. However, this efficiency has also increased the incidence of health problems (obesity, laminitis), in particular in developed countries, where food is abundant but the need to perform heavy work or physical activity is minimal. In addition, donkeys have longer life expectancy than horses, resulting in disproportionately high prevalence of endocrine and metabolic disorders. Donkeys are prone to dyslipidemias, insulin dysregulation (ID)/metabolic syndrome, pituitary pars intermedia dysfunction (PPID), and endocrinopathic laminitis.[8]

DYSLIPIDEMIAS

Dyslipidemia is an abnormal distribution of blood lipids, in particular cholesterol, phospholipids, and triglycerides. Hyperlipidemia, defined as high blood concentrations of triglycerides (hypertriglyceridemia), is the most common dyslipidemia in equids. Hyperlipemia refers to the clinical condition associated with increased triglyceride concentrations (hyperlipidemia).

Epidemiology

Dyslipidemia is more frequent in donkeys than in other equids. The high incidence of lipid disorders in these animals is likely related to their energy disposal efficiency, as previously mentioned. The incidence of hyperlipemia in mules is unknown but is anticipated to be higher than in horses.

Age seems to be a determinant for dyslipidemias, with higher prevalence in older animals. The age-related gradual loss of insulin sensitivity has been proposed to contribute to hyperlipidemia in donkeys.[9] There may be gender differences. Obesity and hyperlipidemia are more frequent in jennies than in jacks.[10] No breed predisposition has been established, but anecdotally they are higher in smaller breeds, with miniature donkeys showing the highest incidence (10%–20%).[11]

Predisposing factors for hyperlipemia include conditions leading to a negative energy balance (eg, anorexia, starving), increased energy demands (late pregnancy, lactation), and concurrent diseases (eg, stress, endotoxemia, parasitism, liver disease, gastrointestinal disease, laminitis). One study in 449 hyperlipemic donkeys found that most animals had a concurrent disease (72%), of which liver disease (19.4%) and colic (13.8%) were the most common.[12] Another study found that obesity, stress, and pregnancy were the most important risk factors for hyperlipemia.[13] This discrepancy is likely caused by the study population. Reported mortalities for hyperlipemia in donkeys vary from 48.5% to 80%.[12] These mortalities are similar to values reported for ponies and miniature horses.[14]

Pathophysiology

The scope of this article is not to provide an exhaustive description on the pathogenesis of hyperlipemia in donkeys but to cover important aspects of this condition. Physiologically, any increase in energy demands leads to activation of adipose triglyceride lipase and hormone-sensitive lipase to induce lipolysis and release of free fatty acids

(FFAs) into circulation. Lipolysis also occurs from pathologic processes that enhance lipase activity or suppress lipogenesis.[15]

In the liver, FFA are reesterified into triglycerides, to be rapidly released as very-low-density lipoprotein (VLDL) into systemic circulation (**Fig. 1**). In contrast with ruminants and cats, the liver of equids does not produce large quantities of ketone bodies when energy demands are high. Donkeys, small equids, and some equine breeds are very efficient at hepatic FFA esterification and VLDL release. If lipolysis persists and VLDL production exceeds peripheral VLDL uptake, triglyceride concentrations continue to increase, resulting in hyperlipidemia (hypertriglyceridemia), macroscopic lipemia (**Figs. 2** and **3**), hepatic fatty infiltration, and in severe cases liver rupture (see **Fig. 3**). As disease worsens, other organs (kidneys, pancreas, heart, intestine, skeletal muscle) are infiltrated by triglycerides, impairing their function.

Hormone-sensitive lipase activity is enhanced by catecholamines (epinephrine), glucocorticoids, adrenocorticotropic hormone (ACTH), growth hormone, glucagon, and proinflammatory cytokines (interleukin-6, tumor necrosis factor alpha), and inhibited by insulin (see **Fig. 1**).[16,17] Donkeys have a higher glucagon/insulin molar ratio compared with horses, suggesting that glucagon-driven lipolysis may contribute to their higher risk of hyperlipemia.[18] The link between glucagon and fat mobilization in dyslipemic donkeys, horses, and ponies remains to be investigated. However, high triglyceride concentrations are correlated with increased glucagon concentrations in critically ill foals (R. Toribio, personal communication).

Donkeys have lower low-density lipoprotein and cholesterol, slightly higher high-density lipoprotein, but similar VLDL concentrations compared with horses (F. Mendoza, 2019). This different lipoprotein profile in donkeys could potentially contribute to their higher risk of hyperlipemia. No effect of age or gender has been observed.

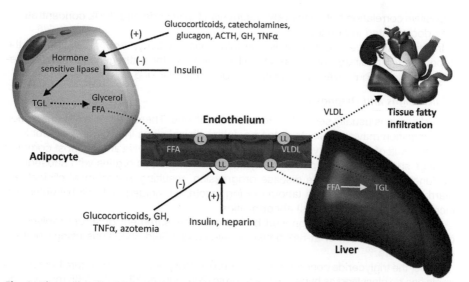

Fig. 1. The pathophysiology of hyperlipemia. Excessive lipolysis from increased lipolytic (glucocorticoids, adrenocorticotropic hormone [ACTH], growth hormone [GH], glucagon, and cytokines) or reduced lipogenic (insulin) factors results in the release of FFA into systemic circulation to be reesterified by the liver into triglycerides (TGL) that are released into circulation as VLDL. Glucocorticoids, GH, cytokines, and azotemia interfere with lipoprotein lipase (LL) activity to remove VLDLs from circulation. VLDL in high concentrations can infiltrate and impair organ function. TNFα, tumor necrosis factor alpha.

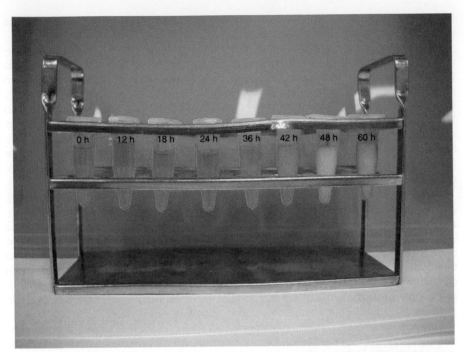

Fig. 2. Serial plasma samples collected from a donkey starved for 60 hours. Note the increasing plasma opacity consistent with increased triglyceride concentrations.

A positive correlation between body weight with triglyceride and VLDL concentrations was documented in donkeys.[19]

Insulin resistance, peripheral lipoprotein lipase activity, and activation of the hypothalamic-pituitary-adrenal axis may be relevant to the pathogenesis of hyperlipemia in donkeys, but investigations in this context are lacking.

Clinical Signs and Diagnosis

Hyperlipemia is usually secondary to other conditions. Therefore, delayed prevention or recognition may complicate outcome. Initial clinical signs in hyperlipemic donkeys are the result of the primary condition. Depression and anorexia are the most common findings specific to hyperlipemia. Fatty infiltration of various organs with subsequent dysfunction can exacerbate disease progression, resulting in additional clinical (eg, diarrhea, dysrhythmias) and laboratory (eg, azotemia, acidemia, hyperbilirubinemia, increased liver enzyme levels) abnormalities.

Hyperlipemia is easily diagnosed by routinely measurement of serum triglyceride concentrations in sick or at-risk donkeys, even under field conditions using point-of-care analyzers.[20]

Under the triglyceride concentration criteria used for ponies and miniature horses, animals can be classified as hypertriglyceridemic (200–500 mg/dL [2.26–5.65 mmol/L]; no evidence of tissue fatty infiltration) or lipemic/hyperlipemic (>500 mg/dL [5.65 mmol/L]; there could be fatty infiltration in various organs). Severe hyperlipemia is evident with triglyceride concentrations greater than 1000 mg/dL [11.3 mmol/L]. These cutoff values are arbitrary and perhaps should be higher considering that donkeys have greater resting triglyceride concentrations than other equids, with upper limits of 248 mg/dL (2.8 mmol/L) and 380 mg/dL (4.3 mmol/L) reported in healthy donkeys in 2 studies.[21]

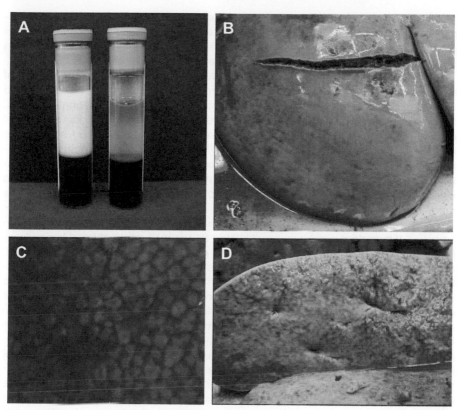

Fig. 3. Plasma and postmortem findings from a donkey with severe hyperlipemia. (*A*) Plasma was lipemic (*left*) compared with a healthy donkey (*right*). (*B*) This animal died acutely from severe hyperlipemia, hepatic lipidosis, and liver rupture. Fatty infiltration of hepatic lobules (*C*) and parenchyma (*D*) were evident.

Other laboratory parameters support the diagnosis of dyslipidemia (increased levels of cholesterol, VLDL, HDL, and nonesterified fatty acids), but they are rarely measured.[21] The association between leptin, triglyceride, and FFA concentrations has been evaluated in horses without conclusive results, although a leptin concentration greater than 5 ng/mL has been linked to hyperlipidemia.[22] Leptin concentrations have been determined in healthy donkeys (2.7 ± 0.3 ng/mL)[10] and, depending on the body condition score, values are similar to or higher than in horses.[23] Leptin information in dyslipemic donkeys is lacking; however, in other species, leptin is a lipolytic hormone.[24]

Serum sorbitol dehydrogenase, aspartate transaminase, gamma-glutamyltransferase, bile acids, creatinine, and blood urea nitrogen concentrations could be used as indicators of hepatic and renal function, and abnormalities could promote a more thorough evaluation to determine whether dysfunctions in these organs are the primary cause or secondary complications from hyperlipidemia.[9] Lipemic serum could interfere with several serum chemistry parameters and samples should be processed accordingly.

Treatment

The therapeutic principles for hyperlipemia in other equids apply to donkeys. The main goal is to halt fat mobilization, control the primary disease, reduce hepatic triglyceride synthesis, avoid stressful conditions, and restore a positive energy balance.[25] In pregnant animals, providing additional caloric intake should be considered, although it can predispose to other disorders (eg, ID). In extreme situations, pregnancy termination should be considered. In lactating animals, weaning is highly recommended.

Hyperlipemic donkeys should be encouraged to eat by offering a variety of high-caloric foodstuff (eg, honey, apples, carrots) that may stimulate hunger. Based on experience, oral honey (5–6 times a day) can stimulate appetite in some animals. Feeding via nasogastric tube should be considered in anorectic animals with normal gastrointestinal function. In more severe cases or in animals that do not tolerate enteral feeding, partial parenteral nutrition (PPN) without lipids could be implemented. Parental nutrition guidelines for horses and ponies are adequate for donkeys and mules,[26] but, considering that basal energy requirements in donkeys are lower than in horses,[27] starting PPN at lower resting energy requirements is recommended.

Parenteral nutrition has been used successfully to manage hyperlipemic donkeys.[25,28] If hypertriglyceridemia persists after 24 hours of treatment or if hyperglycemia develops, 0.1 IU/kg/h of intravenous (IV) regular insulin could be administered, together with close glucose monitoring to avoid hypoglycemia and/or to regulate insulin dosing. Insulin administration to these animals could potentially have deleterious effects, such as hyperinsulinism and secondary laminitis.[29] In donkeys with evidence of ID or endocrinopathic laminitis, insulin should not be used. The rationale for insulin administration is to suppress hormone-sensitive lipase and to increase lipoprotein lipase activity; however, its efficacy at the mechanistic level remains to be documented in horses, ponies, and donkeys. Regular heparin and low-molecular-weight heparin increase lipoprotein lipase activity in people and have been used in hyperlipemic donkeys.[9] However, there is no evidence that heparin increases lipoprotein lipase activity in equids, and, at least in hyperlipemic ponies, the activity of this enzyme is maximal.[30] In addition, heparin increases the risk of bleeding in animals with hepatic dysfunction. Protamine zinc insulin (40–60 IU, intramuscularly) and heparin sulfate (25,000 IU, IV) have been used in hyperlipemic donkeys.[25]

Triglyceride and glucose monitoring are important during treatment of hyperlipemic donkeys. Addressing the primary problem is central to success; however, hyperlipemia often ends up being a more serious problem than the initial inciting cause.

ENDOCRINE DISORDERS

Common endocrine disorders in donkeys include obesity, ID (donkey metabolic syndrome), and PPID.[8,31,32]

Donkey Metabolic Syndrome

Donkey metabolic syndrome (DMS) shares key features with equine metabolic syndrome (EMS), including obesity, ID, and endocrinopathic laminitis (Figs. 4 and 5). Similar to horses and ponies, not every obese donkey has ID and lean animals can be affected. However, the endocrine criteria to diagnose DMS/ID in donkeys differs from those for horses, and additional interspecific differences are likely to be identified in the near future.

Epidemiology

DMS is a recently recognized condition that seems to be highly prevalent in donkeys of different breeds in developed countries or where food is readily available. As a proportion, metabolic syndrome seems to be more prevalent in donkeys than in horses. However, the importance of this problem in the asinine population remains

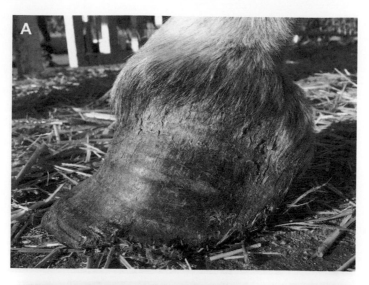

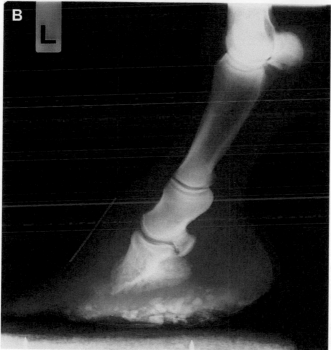

Fig. 4. A 10-year-old Andalusian jack with chronic bilateral forelimb laminitis diagnosed with metabolic syndrome. (*A*) Left forelimb showing long hoof and growth rings typical of chronic laminitis. (*B*) Lateral digital radiography showing bone remodeling, rotation, and sinking of the third phalanx.

to be evaluated. DMS occurs in different breeds, and a breed predisposition has not been documented, likely from the lack of epidemiologic studies. The incidence of DMS is higher in middle-aged to old animals. In relation to gender, jennies are more prone.[8,10]

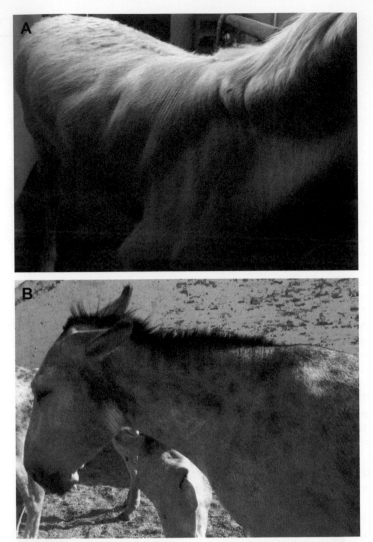

Fig. 5. Obesity in donkeys. (*A*) Note the fat distribution along the side, dorsum, and nuchal ligament (body condition score of 9 out of 9; neck score of 4 out of 4). (*B*) Andalusian jenny with a 4 out of 4 neck score (cresty neck).

Pathophysiology

Studies on the pathogenesis of DMS are lacking, but it can be speculated that the principles of EMS apply to donkeys. Donkeys are considered easy keepers, with lower energy requirements than horses.[27] They are more energy efficient than horses and access to calorie-rich diets, including high-quality grass, grain, or feed concentrates, easily leads to obesity and associated complications. As previously mentioned, donkey obesity is more common in developed countries, mainly from easy food access and reduced physical activity.

Obesity is a chronic proinflammatory state associated with excessive production of proinflammatory cytokines from adipose tissue–resident macrophages.[33] Inflammatory mediators and prolonged hyperinsulinemia disrupt lamellar cell function, which together with excessive body weight contributes to endocrinopathic laminitis development. Insulin concentrations are often increased in obese donkeys; however, a clear association between hyperinsulinemia and laminitis in these animals remains to be established. Proinflammatory cytokines interfere with insulin receptor signaling in peripheral tissues (skeletal muscle, adipose tissue, endothelium), reducing insulin sensitivity, which interferes with glucose uptake, promotes fat mobilization (peripheral ID), and alters endothelial integrity. In addition, these cytokines reduce insulin signaling in the liver (hepatic ID), which is worsened by hepatic fatty infiltration (steatosis). Tissue fatty infiltration can induce organ dysfunction (lipotoxicity).

Based on information generated in ponies, adipocyte factors (adipokines) such as leptin and adiponectin may contribute to the pathogenesis of ID and endocrinopathic laminitis.[34]

Leptin is considered the hormone of satiety and energy expenditure. It has endocrine and metabolic functions in different body systems. Leptin concentrations reflect energy reserves and, through actions in the central nervous system, adjust caloric intake and energy disposal. Leptin decreases insulin secretion, reduces hepatic glucose production, increases hepatic insulin extraction, and promotes insulin sensitivity, which all combine to reduce glycemia, insulinemia, and insulin resistance. The effect of leptin on pancreatic β cells to reduce insulin secretion is known as the adipoinsular axis, whose main function is perhaps to reduce adipogenesis. Leptin also has essential reproductive functions. Reduced leptin signaling (resistance) could alter various endocrine systems, with health consequences.

Leptin resistance has been proposed to play a role in the pathogenesis of EMS and may be important in the development of DMS.[35] Donkeys with high body condition scores (BCSs) and neck scores have higher plasma leptin concentrations.[10] Jennies with similar BCS to jacks have higher leptin concentrations. Leptin concentrations are also higher in older compared with young donkeys.[10] These results suggest that leptin resistance may contribute to conditions such as hyperlipemia, ID, and endocrinopathic laminitis in donkeys. An increase in plasma leptin concentration was observed at 240 minutes in healthy donkeys after IV glucose-insulin administration.[18] In addition, a season effect has been observed, with higher concentrations in the spring.[36]

Adiponectin increases insulin sensitivity, glucose uptake, fatty acid oxidation, and energy consumption, and protects against inflammation. Adiponectin concentrations are associated with fat mass in humans and horses.[37,38] In horses, adiponectin is negatively correlated with BCS and insulin concentrations,[39] but in donkeys no association between BCS or neck scores and adiponectin concentrations was observed.[10] To date, studies on the association between adiponectin, insulin sensitivity, and laminitis in donkeys are lacking.[40]

A series of studies have been performed in recent years to describe energy-regulating hormones in healthy donkeys,[10,18] and it seems that old jennies are more prone to obesity and ID than males.[10,41]

Clinical signs

Obesity and laminitis are the main clinical signs observed in donkeys with DMS. Clinical signs reported in horses, such as hypertension, reproductive disturbances, diabetes mellitus, and pancreatic insufficiency, have not been documented in donkeys.[42] However, according to the authors' experience, obese jennies have reproductive problems similar to obese mares.[43]

Diagnosis

- Laminitis

  A description on the diagnostic methods of laminitis is not within the scope of this review; however, hoof anatomy differs between donkeys and horses, with different radiology findings and measurements.[44]

- Obesity

  In donkeys, obesity is assessed using the BCS and the neck score. Because donkeys and horses have differences in fat distribution and neck morphology, species-specific protocols should be used. A donkey-specific BCS system has been developed, ranging from 1 to 9 (<3, under-weight; 4–6, optimal condition; >7, overweight).[45] Similar to horses,[46] a donkey-specific neck score was developed, ranging from 0 (thin neck without palpable crest) to 4 (thick neck, rounded and gross cresty) **(Fig. 6)**.[10] Published formulas to estimate body weight in horses do not apply to donkeys. The Donkey Sanctuary has developed formulas to estimate body weight in adult donkeys and in donkeys less than 2 years of age.

- ID

  Starving glucose and insulin concentrations, as well as dynamic tests, are the main methods used in the diagnosis of ID in donkeys. Factors that could interfere with the diagnosis of ID diagnosis include stress, starving time, carbohydrate-rich diets, physical activity, pain, transport, endocrinopathies (PPID), concomitant diseases, and α2-adrenoreceptor agonists. Starving insulin concentration is the main test used for ID diagnosis in horses, with a cutoff value of greater than 50 µIU/mL suggesting insulin insensitivity.[47] An insulin cutoff value to diagnose ID in donkeys is not available and 20 µIU/mL has been proposed.[48]

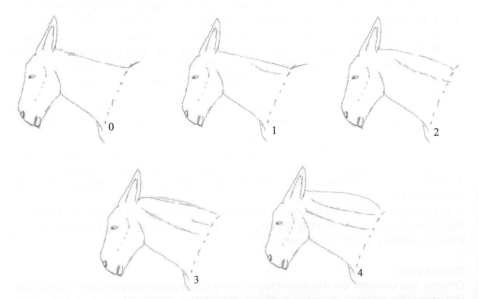

Fig. 6. Neck score system in donkeys. Grading from 0 (thin) to 4 (cresty neck). (*From* Mendoza FJ, Estepa JC, Gonzalez-De Cara CA, et al. Energy-related parameters and their association with age, gender, and morphometric measurements in healthy donkeys. Vet J 2015;204:201-207; with permission.)

Commercial immunoassays used to measure insulin concentrations in horses and ponies, including radioimmunoassays (DIASource, Millipore, Tecan, MP Biomedicals), enzyme-linked immunoassays (Mercodia, MP Biomedicals), and chemiluminescent assays (Immulite, Siemens), also work for donkey insulin. Similar to equine insulin, a limitation with these assays is the lack of a gold standard. Therefore, extrapolating insulin values between laboratories or assays can be misleading.

Similar to horses,[33] glucose, insulin ratios, and proxies are not recommended to diagnose ID in donkeys because of their practicality, limited information, and the influence of several factors that could cause erroneous diagnoses. Reference values for these ratios and proxies are available for healthy donkeys.[49] Compared with horses,[50,51] a higher modified insulin-to-glucose ratio (MIRG) was seen in donkeys, which could indicate a higher β-cell function. MIRG and the reciprocal of the square root of insulin have been described in obese and laminitic donkeys.[41] Insulin/glucagon (I:G) and glucagon/insulin (G:I) molar ratios have been characterized in healthy donkeys, showing that donkeys have higher G:I than horses, which could be another explanation for their prompt ability to mobilize fat in response to stress and energy demands.[18]

Dynamic tests should be considered when baseline insulin results are inconclusive or in incipient cases.[47] Dynamic protocols have been developed for donkeys,[32,49,52] showing differences with horses for the IV glucose tolerance test (IVGTT), the combined glucose-insulin test (CGIT), and the oral glucose tolerance test (OGTT).[42,53–55] Of clinical relevance, the glucose curves for the IVGTT and CGIT in donkeys are right shifted compared with horses.[49] For dynamic testing in donkeys, it is recommended to provide a flake of hay the night before to reduce stress and the risk of hyperlipemia. Dynamic tests are summarized in **Table 1**. The OGTT using corn syrup has not been evaluated in donkeys. However, this is the recommended test to diagnose ID in horses.[47]

The IV insulin tolerance test and frequently sampled IV glucose tolerance test (FSIGTT) have also been evaluated in healthy and obese donkeys.[56] FSIGTT results were comparable with those in horses with similar BCS.[57]

Table 1
Summarized recommendations for dynamic testing in donkeys with metabolic syndrome

Test	IVGTT	CGIT	OGTT
Protocol	Leave 1 flake of hay the night before		
	Collect baseline blood sample for starving glucose and insulin determination in the morning[a,b]		
	Administer a bolus of 50% dextrose (300 mg/kg, IV)	Administer a bolus of 50% dextrose (150 mg/kg, IV) followed by regular insulin[c] (0.1 IU/kg, IV)[3]	Administer dextrose (1 g/kg in a 20% solution) via nasogastric tube
	Second blood sample at 150–180 min	Second blood sample at 60–75 min	Second blood sample at 300–360 min
Interpretation	ID if blood glucose level is above baseline at 150–180 min[d]	ID if blood glucose level is above baseline at 60–75 min[d]	ID if blood glucose level is above baseline at 300–360 min[d]

The oral sugar test using corn syrup has not been evaluated in donkeys or mules.
[a] Check with reference laboratory on the preferred blood tube for insulin measurement. Oxalate fluoride tubes are recommended for glucose.
[b] Perform test in the morning to avoid prolonged starving.
[c] Crystalline rapid-action insulin.
[d] Insulin cutoff value for this test has not been validated for ID diagnosis in donkeys.

Leptin and adiponectin cutoff values for donkeys with evidence of ID and endocrinopathic laminitis have not been reported.

Treatment

Therapeutic approaches for DMS have not been established and clinicians rely on protocols for EMS. It is important to emphasize that interspecies phenotypic and endocrine differences should be taken into consideration.

In order to promote weight loss, caloric restrictions and increased physical activity are central to success. Because of their ability to subsist on poor-quality feedstuffs, dietary management should rely on low-quality hay (<10% nonstructural carbohydrates), eliminating grain, concentrates, and access to carbohydrate-rich pastures. Commercially available diets to manage ID and obesity in horses may not be appropriate for donkeys.

Whenever possible, and depending on the level of laminar disease, access to a paddock to promote physical activity is indicated. Long stays in paddocks are more appropriate than quick walks, which can be counterproductive. Grazing should be avoided early morning, after rainfall, and when grass is expected to be rich in soluble carbohydrates. Grazing muzzles could be used with caution in obese animals, although some clinicians do not recommend their use in donkeys because of their eating habits, curious behavior, and risk of hyperlipemia. Considering their gregarious behavior, the presence of other animals (donkeys, horses, goats) is recommended to reduce stress and promote physical activity. Weight loss in donkeys should be promoted slowly to avoid metabolic complications. A 1% to 2% body weight loss per month is a reasonable goal, although this is arbitrary and specific weight-loss protocols have not been developed. Weight loss in donkeys may be a very slow process.

Levothyroxine sodium is indicated for horses with EMS to promote weight loss and increase insulin sensitivity, particularly in laminitic animals. Levothyroxine sodium has not been evaluated in donkeys, and its safety and effective dose are unknown. The authors have used this drug in donkeys at equine doses (0.05 to 0.1 mg/Kg by mouth every 24 hours) without complications.

The pharmacology of metformin has not been investigated in donkeys, but it has been used at a dose of 15 to 30 mg/kg by mouth every 12 hours.[8,58] Thiazolidinediones (pioglitazone) and sulfonylureas (glyburide) have not been evaluated in donkeys.

Pituitary Pars Intermedia Dysfunction

It is suspected that PPID is frequent in geriatric donkeys; however, to the authors' knowledge, no epidemiologic studies have been performed. Because of the high prevalence of endocrinopathies in elderly equids and considering the longevity of asinine animals, these suspicions are valid.

Epidemiology

Although 15% to 20% of horses more than 15 years old develop PPID, its prevalence in donkeys remains to be elucidated. Some investigators suggest that it is lower than in horses.[59,60] Breed and gender do not seem to be risk factors.

Pathophysiology

There is no reason to believe that the pathogenesis of PPID in donkeys and mules is different than in horses and ponies, but no mechanistic studies have been reported.[61] It can be speculated that it results from loss of inhibitory control of the melanotropes in the pituitary pars intermedia from degenerative damage to the hypothalamic dopaminergic neurons. This loss of control leads to increased synthesis of proopiomelanocortin and subsequent release of cleavage products, including ACTH and α-melanocyte–stimulating hormone.[62,63]

Clinical signs

Clinical signs are similar between donkeys, horses, and ponies, with hypertrichosis being common. It is important to consider that some donkey breeds have long hair coats. Clinical signs such as lethargy could be overlooked because of their calm behavior. Laminitis (chronic laminitis) is a consistent finding in donkeys with PPID. Polyuria is rarely seen.

Disturbances described in horses with PPID, such as hyperhidrosis, ID, abnormal fat distribution (supraorbital deposits), muscle wasting, reproductive problems, predisposition to infections, endoparasitism, and orthopedic problems, also occur in donkeys.[62,64]

Information on PPID in mules is lacking.

Diagnosis

Baseline ACTH concentrations and the thyrotropin-releasing hormone (TRH)–stimulation test are the main diagnostic tests for PPID diagnosis in donkeys. ACTH concentrations in healthy donkeys are higher than in healthy horses.[41,65] This difference is relevant because extrapolating hypothalamic-pituitary-adrenal axis data from horses to donkeys could lead to misdiagnosis of PPID in healthy donkeys. Similar to horses,[66] donkeys show seasonal variations in ACTH concentrations that should be taken into consideration when measuring baseline ACTH concentrations or performing the TRH-stimulation test.[67] Compared to horses and ponies, donkeys have higher ACTH concentrations in the fall (A. Durham, personal communication). Basal cortisol concentrations are similar in healthy donkeys and horses.[65] Whether cortisol values are affected by season, as reported in horses, remains to be determined in donkeys. Hypercortisolemia is a rare finding in donkeys with PPID,[68] as is also the case for horses,[63] and its determination is not recommended for PPID diagnosis.

ACTH is not very stable at room temperature, so blood samples should be collected in ethylenediaminetetraacetic acid tubes, processed rapidly, and shipped on ice. The ACTH chemiluminescent immunoassay (Immulite, Siemens) works well for donkey and horse ACTH.[68,69] Samples for PPID diagnosis should not be taken from animals exercising, with acute laminitis or any other source of pain or stress, or that have received α2-adrenoreceptor agonists on the day of collection.

Dynamic testing is recommended in early-state disease or when basal ACTH concentrations are inconclusive.[62] Dynamic tests for PPID diagnosis were recently validated in donkeys,[68] showing that equine PPID diagnostic guidelines also apply to this species. The authors do not recommend the dexamethasone-suppression test and the combined dexamethasone-TRH test because of a high number of false-negative results.[60,61] The TRH-stimulation test provided the best results in donkeys with a confirmed diagnosis of PPID.[68] A donkey is considered PPID positive if plasma ACTH concentrations are higher than 110 pg/mL 10 minutes after injecting 1 mg of TRH intravenously.[68] The dose of TRH does not seem to influence the pituitary response in horses,[70,71] but this question has not been investigated in donkeys.

Treatment

Pergolide, a dopamine D2 receptor agonist, is the drug of choice to treat PPID in horses. Although pergolide pharmacology has not been studied in donkeys, it has been used successfully to treat donkeys with PPID at a dose of 0.25 to 0.5 mg/250 kg (0.001–0.002 mg/kg) by mouth every 24 hours.[8,32,60,61] During early therapy it is recommended to monitor animals because anorexia is a potential side effect of this drug in horses. In animals with severe anorexia, pergolide dose should be reduced or discontinued. Bromocriptine, another dopamine D2 receptor agonist, and cyproheptadine, a 5-HT receptor antagonist, have not been evaluated in this species.[72]

Annual measurement of basal ACTH determinations is indicated in donkeys under treatment to readjust dose.

There is no justification at this point to recommend the use of 3β-hydroxysteroid dehydrogenase inhibitors such as trilostane because hypercortisolemia is rare in donkeys and horses with PPID.[60,61,73]

Thyroid Gland Diseases

Information on thyroid diseases in donkeys is lacking, which is not surprising considering that thyroid disorders are also infrequent in other equids. Histologic lesions related to hypothyroidism have been observed in donkeys,[74] although thyroid hormone concentrations were not measured in these animals. Studies on the physiology of the hypothalamic-pituitary-thyroid axis in donkeys are scarce, but will be valuable to advance donkey and comparative endocrinology.

Donkeys have higher plasma free triiodothyronine (fT3) and total triiodothyronine (tT3), free thyroxine (fT4) and total thyroxine (tT4), and reverse T3 (rT3) concentrations than values reported for horses.[5,75,76] Because values can vary depending on the laboratory technique,[77–80] clinicians should use reference values from that particular laboratory. No gender differences for thyroid hormones have been documented in donkeys. Similar to horses,[81,82] young donkeys have higher fT4, tT4, and rT3 concentrations,[5] which could be related to the role of thyroid hormones in growth, development, and tissue differentiation.

Drugs such as phenylbutazone, dexamethasone, and sulfonamides reduce thyroid hormone concentrations in several species by competing with transporting proteins and/or inhibiting thyroid peroxidase.[76,83,84] The effect of these drugs on asinine thyroid function has not been investigated. However, clinicians should be aware of this information to avoid the misdiagnosis of hypothyroidism. Dynamic tests (TRH-stimulation test, TSH-stimulation test, T3-suppression test) to assess thyroid function in donkeys have not been evaluated.

Parathyroid Gland Diseases

Disorders of the parathyroid gland are rare in equids. Serum total calcium, total magnesium, and phosphorus concentrations in donkeys are within the reference range of values reported for horses.[85] However, one study found higher ionized calcium, complexed magnesium, and calcitriol concentrations, but lower parathyroid hormone and protein-bound magnesium concentrations in donkeys compared with horses.[85]

Nutritional secondary hyperparathyroidism may be seen in donkeys consuming diets with high phosphorus content, but more often occurs with the ingestion of oxalate-rich plants (R. Toribio, personal communication). Clinical signs (lameness, facial swelling, upper airway stridor, and neurologic signs), diagnosis, and treatment are similar to those in horses.[86]

REFERENCES

1. Martini M, Altomonte I, Salari F, et al. Monitoring nutritional quality of Amiata donkey milk: effects of lactation and productive season. J Dairy Sci 2014;97:6819–22.

2. Gonzalez-De Cara CA, Perez-Ecija A, Aguilera-Aguilera R, et al. Temperament test for donkeys to be used in assisted therapy. Appl Anim Behav Sci 2017; 186:64–71.

3. Burden F, Thiemann A. Donkeys are different. J Equine Vet Sci 2015;35:376–82.
4. Mendoza FJ, Perez-Ecija RA, Monreal L, et al. Coagulation profiles of healthy Andalusian donkeys are different than those of healthy horses. J Vet Intern Med 2011;25:967–70.
5. Mendoza FJ, Perez-Ecija RA, Toribio RE, et al. Thyroid hormone concentrations differ between donkeys and horses. Equine Vet J 2013;45:214–8.
6. Mendoza FJ, Toribio RE, Perez-Ecija A. Donkey internal medicine - part ii: cardio-vascular, respiratory, neurologic, urinary, ophthalmic, dermatology, and musculo-skeletal disorders. J Equine Vet Sci 2018;65:86–97.
7. Perez-Ecija A, Mendoza FJ. Characterisation of clotting factors, anticoagulant protein activities and viscoelastic analysis in healthy donkeys. Equine Vet J 2017;49:734–8.
8. Mendoza FJ, Toribio RE, Perez-Ecija A. Donkey internal medicine - Part I: meta-bolic, endocrine, and alimentary tract disturbances. J Equine Vet Sci 2018;65: 66–74.
9. Waitt LH, Cebra CK. Characterization of hypertriglyceridemia and response to treatment with insulin in horses, ponies, and donkeys: 44 cases (1995-2005). J Am Vet Med Assoc 2009;234:915–9.
10. Mendoza FJ, Estepa JC, Gonzalez-De Cara CA, et al. Energy-related parameters and their association with age, gender, and morphometric measurements in healthy donkeys. Vet J 2015;204:201–7.
11. Watson T. Equine hyperlipemia. In: Watson T, editor. Metabolic and endocrine problems of the horse. London: WB Saunders; 1998. p. 23–40.
12. Burden FA, Du Toit N, Hazell-Smith E, et al. Hyperlipemia in a population of aged donkeys: description, prevalence, and potential risk factors. J Vet Intern Med 2011;25:1420–5.
13. Reid SW, Mohammed HO. Survival analysis approach to risk factors associated with hyperlipemia in donkeys. J Am Vet Med Assoc 1996;209:1449–52.
14. McKenzie HC. Equine hyperlipidemias. Vet Clin North Am Equine Pract 2011;27: 59–72.
15. Divers TJ, Barton MH. Disorders of the liver. In: Reed SM, Bayly WM, Sellon DC, editors. Equine internal medicine. 4th edition. St. Louis (MO): Elsevier; 2018. p. 939–75.
16. Frank N, Sojka JE, Latour MA. Effects of hypothyroidism and withholding of feed on plasma lipid concentrations, concentration and composition of very-low-density lipoprotein, and plasma lipase activity in horses. Am J Vet Res 2003; 64:823–8.
17. Harrison A, Rickards K. Hyperlipaemia in donkeys. UK-Vet Equine 2018;2:154–7.
18. Mendoza FJ, Gonzalez-Cara CA, Aguilera-Aguilera R, et al. Effect of intravenous glucose and combined glucose-insulin challenges on energy-regulating hor-mones concentrations in donkeys. Vet J 2018;240:40–6.
19. Watson TD, Packard CJ, Shepherd J, et al. An investigation of the relationships between body condition and plasma lipid and lipoprotein concentrations in 24 donkeys. Vet Rec 1990;127:498–500.
20. Williams A, Peachey LE, Christley RM. Assessment of a point-of-care test for measurement of blood triglyceride levels for rapid detection of equid hypertrigly-ceridaemia. Equine Vet Educ 2012;24:520–8.
21. Burden FA, Hazell-Smith E, Mulugeta G, et al. Reference intervals for biochemical and haematological parameters in mature domestic donkeys (Equus asinus) in the UK. Equine Vet Educ 2016;28:134–9.

22. Kedzierski W, Kusy R, Kowalik S. Plasma leptin level in hyperlipidemic mares and their newborn foals. Reprod Domest Anim 2011;46:275–80.

23. Gordon ME, McKeever KH, Betros CL, et al. Plasma leptin, ghrelin and adiponectin concentrations in young fit racehorses versus mature unfit standardbreds. Vet J 2007;173:91–100.

24. Harris RBS. Direct and indirect effects of leptin on adipocyte metabolism. Biochim Biophys Acta 2014;1842:414–23.

25. Tarrant JM, Campbell TM, Parry BW. Hyperlipaemia in a donkey. Aust Vet J 1998; 76:466–9.

26. Durham AE, Thiemann AK. Nutritional management of hyperlipaemia. Equine Vet Educ 2015;27:482–8.

27. Martin-Rosset W. Donkey nutrition and feeding: nutrient requirements and recommended allowances - a review and prospect. J Equine Vet Sci 2018;65:75–85.

28. Durham AE. Clinical application of parenteral nutrition in the treatment of five ponies and one donkey with hyperlipaemia. Vet Rec 2006;158:159–64.

29. Asplin KE, Sillence MN, Pollitt CC, et al. Induction of laminitis by prolonged hyperinsulinaemia in clinically normal ponies. Vet J 2007;174:530–5.

30. Watson TDG, Burns L, Packard CJ, et al. Effects of pregnancy and lactation on plasma-lipid and lipoprotein concentrations, lipoprotein composition and postheparin lipase activities in Shetland pony mares. J Reprod Fertil 1993;97:563–8.

31. Frank N. Equine metabolic syndrome. J Equine Vet Sci 2009;29:259–67.

32. Mendoza FJ, Toribio RE, Perez-Ecija A. Aspects of clinical relevance in donkeys. In: Reed SM, Bayly WM, Sellon DC, editors. Equine internal medicine. 4th edition. St. Louis (MO): Elsevier; 2018. p. 1513–24.

33. Morgan R, Keen J, McGowan C. Equine metabolic syndrome. Vet Rec 2015;177: 173–9.

34. Carter RA, Treiber KH, Geor RJ, et al. Prediction of incipient pasture-associated laminitis from hyperinsulinaemia, hyperleptinaemia and generalised and localised obesity in a cohort of ponies. Equine Vet J 2009;41:171–8.

35. Frank N, Tadros EM. Insulin dysregulation. Equine Vet J 2014;46:103–12.

36. Cebulj-Kadunc N, Skibin A, Kosec M. Long-term leptin fluctuations in female donkeys. Equine Vet J 2015;47:731–5.

37. Wooldridge AA, Edwards HG, Plaisance EP, et al. Evaluation of high-molecular weight adiponectin in horses. Am J Vet Res 2012;73:1230–40.

38. Balsan GA, Vieira JL, Oliveira AM, et al. Relationship between adiponectin, obesity and insulin resistance. Revi Assoc Med Bras (1992) 2015;61:72–80.

39. Yadav A, Kataria MA, Saini V, et al. Role of leptin and adiponectin in insulin resistance. Clin Chim Acta 2013;417:80–4.

40. Kearns CF, McKeever KH, Roegner V, et al. Adiponectin and leptin are related to fat mass in horses. Vet J 2006;172:460–5.

41. Du Toit N, Trawford AF. Determination of serum insulin and insulin resistance in clinically normal donkeys and donkeys with a history of laminitis (obese and non-obese). In: American College of Veterinary Internal Medicine Forum. Anaheim, CA, June 9-12, 2010. p. 779.

42. Frank N. Equine metabolic syndrome. Vet Clin North Am Equine Pract 2011;27: 73–92.

43. Vick MM, Sessions DR, Murphy BA, et al. Obesity is associated with altered metabolic and reproductive activity in the mare: effects of metformin on insulin sensitivity and reproductive cyclicity. Reprod Fertil Dev 2006;18:609–17.

44. Collins SN, Dyson SJ, Murray RC, et al. Development of a quantitative multivariable radiographic method to evaluate anatomic changes associated with laminitis in the forefeet of donkeys. Am J Vet Res 2012;73:1207–18.
45. Pearson RA, Ouassat M. Estimation of live weight. In: Pearson RA, Ouassat M, editors. A guide to live weight estimation and body condition scoring of donkeys. 1st edition. Glasgow (Scotland): Thomson Colour Printers; 2000. p. 1–21.
46. Carter RA, Geor RJ, Staniar WB, et al. Apparent adiposity assessed by standardised scoring systems and morphometric measurements in horses and ponies. Vet J 2009;179:204–10.
47. Frank N, Bailey S, Bertin FR, et al. Recommendations for the diagnosis and treatment of Equine Metabolic Syndrome (EMS). Equine Endocrinol Group; 2018.
48. Du Toit n, Trawford AF, Keen J. Insulin and ACTH values in donkeys with and without laminitis in the UK. In: 49th British Equine Veterinary Association Congress. Birmingham, England, September 8-11, 2010.
49. Mendoza FJ, Aguilera-Aguilera R, Gonzalez-De Cara CA, et al. Characterization of the intravenous glucose tolerance test and the combined glucose-insulin test in donkeys. Vet J 2015;206:371–6.
50. Treiber KH, Kronfeld DS, Hess TM, et al. Use of proxies and reference quintiles obtained from minimal model analysis for determination of insulin sensitivity and pancreatic beta-cell responsiveness in horses. Am J Vet Res 2005;66:2114–21.
51. Borer KE, Bailey SR, Menzies-Gow NJ, et al. Use of proxy measurements of insulin sensitivity and insulin secretory response to distinguish between normal and previously laminitic ponies. Equine Vet J 2012;44:444–8.
52. June V, Soderholm V, Hintz HF, et al. Glucose-tolerance in the horse, pony and donkey. J Equine Vet Sci 1992;12:103–5.
53. Eiler II, Frank N, Andrews FM, et al. Physiologic assessment of blood glucose homeostasis via combined intravenous glucose and insulin testing in horses. Am J Vet Res 2005;66:1598–604.
54. Funk RA, Wooldridge AA, Stewart AJ, et al. Seasonal changes in the combined glucose-insulin tolerance test in normal aged horses. J Vet Intern Med 2012;26:1035–41.
55. Bertin FR, Sojka-Kritchevsky JE. Comparison of a 2-step insulin-response test to conventional insulin-sensitivity testing in horses. Domest Anim Endocrinol 2013;44:19–25.
56. Forhead AJ, Dobson H. Plasma glucose and cortisol responses to exogenous insulin in fasted donkeys. Res Vet Sci 1997;62:265–9.
57. McLean AK, Nielsen BD, Yokoyama M, et al. Insulin resistance in standard donkeys (Equus asinus) of three body conditions-thin, moderate, and obese. J Equine Vet Sci 2009;29:406–7.
58. Burden F. Practical feeding and condition scoring for donkeys and mules. Equine Vet Educ 2012;24:589–96.
59. Cox R, Burden F, Proudman CJ, et al. Demographics, management and health of donkeys in the UK. Vet Rec 2010;166:552–6.
60. Sprayson T. The care of the geriatric donkey. In: Duncan JL, Hadrill D, editors. The professional handbook of the donkey. 4th edition. Wiltshire (England): Whitted Books; 2008. p. 239–354.
61. Twickel S, Bartmann CP, Gehlen H. PPID and EMS in donkeys and mules - are there differences to horses? Pferdeheilkunde 2017;33:573–84.
62. McFarlane D. Equine pituitary pars intermedia dysfunction. Vet Clin North Am Equine Pract 2011;27:93–113.

63. McFarlane D. Pathophysiology and clinical features of pituitary pars intermedia dysfunction. Equine Vet Educ 2014;26:592–8.
64. Schwarz B, Anen C. Eselmedizin - Basiswissen. Cont Vet Educ 2014;3:1–36.
65. Dugat SL, Taylor TS, Matthews NS, et al. Values for triglycerides, insulin, cortisol, and ACTH in a herd of normal donkeys. J Equine Vet Sci 2010;30:141–4.
66. Copas VE, Durham AE. Circannual variation in plasma adrenocorticotropic hormone concentrations in the UK in normal horses and ponies, and those with pituitary pars intermedia dysfunction. Equine Vet J 2012;44:440–3.
67. Du Toit N, Shaw DJ, Keen J. Adrenocorticotropic hormone in domestic donkeys - reference values, seasonality and association with laminitis. In: 50th British Equine Veterinary Association Congress. Liverpool, England, September 7-10, 2011.
68. Mejia-Pereira S, Perez-Ecija A, Buchanan BR, et al. Evaluation of dynamic testing for pituitary pars intermedia dysfunction diagnosis in donkeys. Equine Vet J 2018; 51(4):481–8.
69. Banse HE, Schultz N, McCue M, et al. Comparison of two methods for measurement of equine adrenocorticotropin. J Vet Diagn Invest 2018;30:233–7.
70. Chapman AM, Ainsworth S, Keowen ML, et al. Adrenocorticotropin hormone response to varying dosages of thyrotropin releasing hormone in normal horses. Coral Gables (FL): Equine Endocrinology Summit; 2017.
71. Stallenberger L, Failing K, Fey K. ACTH responses after application of two TRH doses in healthy horses. Coral Gables (FL): Equine Endocrinology Summit; 2017.
72. Durham AE. Therapeutics for equine endocrine disorders. Vet Clin North Am Equine Pract 2017;33:127–39.
73. McGowan C. Diagnostic and management protocols for equine's syndrome. Practice 2003;25:586–92.
74. Stephen JO, Baptiste KE, Townsend HG. Clinical and pathologic findings in donkeys with hypothermia: 10 cases (1988-1998). J Am Vet Med Assoc 2000;216: 725–9.
75. Chen CL, Riley AM. Serum thyroxine and triiodothyronine concentrations in neonatal foals and mature horses. Am J Vet Res 1981;42:1415–7.
76. Abraham G, Allersmeier M, Schusser GF, et al. Serum thyroid hormone, insulin, glucose, triglycerides and protein concentrations in normal horses: association with topical dexamethasone usage. Vet J 2011;188:307–12.
77. Bugalia NS, Sharma S, Garg SL, et al. Plasma thyroid hormones concentrations in donkey stallions (Equus caballus). Indian J Anim Sci 2000;70:471–2.
78. Fazio E, Medica P, Cravana C, et al. Total and free iodothyronines profile in the donkey (Equus asinus) over a 12-month period. Acta Vet BRNO 2012;81:239–44.
79. Fazio E, Medica P, Cravana C, et al. Total and free iodothyronine changes in response to transport of Equidae (Equus asinus and Equus caballus). Vet Ital 2017;53:55–60.
80. Todini L, Salimei E, Malfatti A, et al. Thyroid hormones in donkey blood and milk: correlations with milk yield and environmental temperatures. Ital J Anim Sci 2015; 14:6.
81. Malinowski K, Christensen RA, Hafs HD, et al. Age and breed differences in thyroid hormones, insulin-like growth factor (IGF)-I and IGF binding proteins in female horses. J Anim Sci 1996;74:1936–42.
82. Panzani S, Comin A, Galeati G, et al. How type of parturition and health status influence hormonal and metabolic profiles in newborn foals. Theriogenology 2012;77:1167–77.

83. Ramirez S, Wolfsheimer KJ, Moore RM, et al. Duration of effects of phenylbuta-zone on serum total thyroxine and free thyroxine concentrations in horses. J Vet Intern Med 1997;11:371–4.
84. Rothschild CM, Hines MT, Breuhaus B, et al. Effects of trimethoprim-sulfadiazine on thyroid function of horses. J Vet Intern Med 2004;18:370–3.
85. Lopez I, Estepa JC, Mendoza FJ, et al. Serum concentrations of calcium, phos-phorus, magnesium and calciotropic hormones in donkeys. Am J Vet Res 2006; 67:1333–6.
86. Sasaki N, Shimoda T, Sato M, et al. Improvement of dietary total calcium to inor-ganic phosphorus ratio prevents progressive nutritional secondary hyperparathy-roidism in ponies and donkeys. J Equine Sci 2005;16:79–83.

Gastrointestinal Disorders of Donkeys and Mules

Alexandra K. Thiemann, MA, VetMB, Cert EP, MSc, AFHEA, MRCVS[a,b,*],
Rebekah J.E. Sullivan, BVSc (Hons), Cert AVP (EM), MRCVS[a,b]

KEYWORDS

- Donkey • Mule • Colic • Gastrointestinal • Parasite • Colitis • Hyperlipemia
- Behavior

KEY POINTS

- Donkeys with colic frequently show milder clinical signs than horses, despite the potential severity of the pathologic condition. Major presenting signs include dullness, inappetence, self-isolation, and recumbency.
- Hyperlipemia is a frequent finding in donkeys with colic. Triglyceride concentrations should be measured regularly in inappetent animals and treatment instituted. The presence of hyperlipemia reduces the prognosis.
- It is possible to perform a rectal examination in most donkeys; it is preferable to use spasmolytics before rectal examination. Ultrasound evaluation is useful if rectal examination is not possible and can be an adjunct to those cases whereby rectal examination alone has not been diagnostic.
- The presence of dental disease and parasitism increases the risk of colic; donkeys and mules should be included in routine preventative dental care and anthelmintic use.
- Because of their unique physiology, donkeys differ in their response to dehydration and drug metabolism compared with horses. Hematological and biochemical reference ranges are available for donkeys and mules.

INTRODUCTION

Donkeys are kept as companions or used as working or production animals, whereas mules are mainly used for working purposes. Gastrointestinal diseases are common in these animals worldwide. Awareness of their stoic behavior is paramount when interpreting the severity of clinical signs. Donkeys are desert-adapted animals with unique physiology and metabolism compared with horses. Knowledge of their particular behaviors and physiology is the key to successful handling and management of gastrointestinal disease.

Disclosure Statement: None.
a Education, The Veterinary Department, The Donkey Sanctuary, Sidmouth, Devon, EX10 0NU, UK; b The Veterinary Hospital, Brookfield, Honiton, Devon EX14 9SU, UK
* Corresponding author. The Veterinary Hospital, Brookfield, Honiton, Devon EX14 9SU, UK.
E-mail address: alex.thiemann@thedonkeysanctuary.org.uk

CLINICAL EXAMINATION

For many clinicians, the challenge when dealing with donkeys and mules is recognizing behavioral differences compared with horses. Donkeys have a highly developed prey species behavior and can mask low- to moderate-grade and chronic pain.[1] Common clinical signs in association with gastrointestinal disease include dullness, behavior changes, lack of appetite or sham eating, recumbency, head and neck held below withers height, ears less mobile or backwards/sideways pointing and unresponsive to stimuli, self-isolation away from companions, and weight loss in chronic disease.

Donkeys show signs of acute colic, such as flank watching, kicking the abdomen, lying down, and rolling, which are less evident than in horses (**Fig. 1**). Mules show pain response characteristics of both parent species, being less evident than in horses, but more overt than in donkeys. Their physiologic parameters fall between the donkey and horse.

In the United Kingdom and United States, donkeys and mules are mainly considered companion animals and often reach advanced age, whereas in developing countries, these animals are used for work in agriculture, transport, pulling, and tourism, often lack owner and veterinary care, and have a shorter lifespan.[2]

The significance is that donkeys, and to a lesser extent, mules, often present with signs of gastrointestinal disease later than horses, tend to be more systemically ill when signs are noted, and often are afflicted with multiple comorbidities.

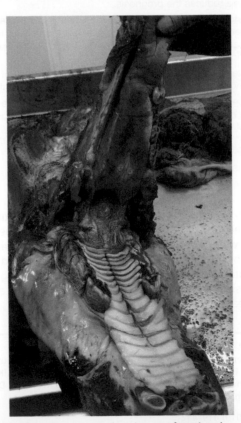

Fig. 1. Postmortem view of donkey mouth showing nonfunctional molar arcades leading to impaction.

In addition to a complete history, a clinical examination should be performed in donkeys and mules with gastrointestinal disease. This clinical examination should include an assessment of mentation, general health and body condition, rectal temperature, pulse and respiration, evaluation of mucous membrane color and moisture (hydration status), auscultation of all quadrants for increased or decreased intestinal sounds, a rectal examination, nasogastric intubation in animals with abdominal pain, fecal evaluation for consistency, presence of endoparasites, and poorly digested foodstuffs. In animals with diarrhea, frequency, estimated volume, consistency, and appearance of feces, full dental examination with a mouth speculum, and development of a list of differentials that could lead to abdominal pain and dullness are recommended.

Normal parameters for adult donkeys include a rectal temperature of 36.5°C to 37.8°C (97.7°F to 100°F), a heart rate of 36 to 52 beats/min, a respiration rate of 20 breaths/min (range 12–28), and moist mucous membranes with a capillary refill time of less than 2 seconds. Interpretation of digital pulses in donkeys can be challenging. General points to consider are as follows:

- Because of their pair bonding behavior, donkeys being transported for evaluation ideally should be accompanied by a bonded animal to reduce stress.
- Preventative care (anthelmintic use, dental care, regular vaccination) is often inadequate, in particular, in developing countries.
- Weight loss may be the only indicator of chronic gastrointestinal disease in donkeys and mules.
- Because of the large colon enhanced water absorption capacity, diarrhea is rarely seen with acute or chronic gastrointestinal disease, including colitis.
- Rectal examination should be performed in all, except in miniature animals. Intravenous spasmolytics (hyoscine/scopolamine) at standard equine doses facilitate rectal examination. In unhandled donkeys and mules where rectal examination may be dangerous, heavy sedation and the use of stocks are indicated. Mules may require between one-third to one-half extra dose of sedatives compared with a similarly sized pony or horse.
- If rectal examination is not possible, information about the nature of the feces and hydration status is useful.
- Hyperlipemia is frequent in colicky and dull donkeys and can worsen the prognosis, and triglyceride measurement is indicated in these animals.
- As donkeys evolved in dry and arid environments with limited water access, they can better tolerate dehydration and hemoconcentration than horses.
- Transabdominal ultrasonography may be challenging in obese animals. Clipping their thick coat is recommended to facilitate image acquisition.
- Abdominocentesis can be unrewarding in donkeys because of significant fat deposits on the linea alba; a teat cannula or catheter may be indicated, preferably after ultrasound evaluation.
- A foal- or pony-sized tube can be used for evaluation of gastric reflux and nasogastric therapy.
- In countries where rabies is endemic, the possibility of infection with this zoonosis must be considered, in particular when performing oral or rectal examination.
- Donkeys without tetanus prophylaxis are susceptible to this condition and develop signs similar to other equids.

ANATOMY AND PHYSIOLOGY

The donkey and mule have some anatomic differences from horses that are relevant to management and treatment. The head is larger in proportion to body size and supported ventrally by the strong cutaneous coli muscle. This muscle is highly developed in donkeys and can obscure the jugular vein in the midneck region, making jugular venipuncture more challenging. Donkeys have a narrower mandible and accentuated mandibular curve of Spee, which can lead to dental overcrowding, with rostral and caudal enamel overgrowths.

Recognition and treatment of dental problems are critical in the management and prevention of many gastrointestinal disorders (**Fig. 2**). See João B. Rodrigues and Gemma Lilly's article, "Dental Disorders of Donkeys," in this issue.

Donkeys have narrow nasal meati; hence, for nasogastric intubation, it is better to use a foal- or pony-sized tube with adequate lubrication and restraint to reduce the risk of hemorrhage.

The stomach of a 180-kg donkey can accommodate approximately 3 L of fluid. The length of the small intestine is around 6 m per 100 kg (vs 5 m for the horse); the transverse colon is short (10 cm), and the small colon is approximately 1 m. Other aspects of the internal anatomy of donkeys and mules are comparable to the horse.[3]

The spinal cord in the donkey terminates at the second sacral vertebra, and the dura may extend to the second coccygeal vertebrae. Epidural injections are best done in the second intercoccygeal space at an angle of 30° to the horizontal, 1 space further back and at a shallower angle than in the horse because of the lack of musculature over the rump and tail head.[4] Correct placement of the epidural injection is relevant to manage conditions such as rectal prolapse, reproductive manipulation, or orthopedic pain.

The donkey, and to a lesser extent the mule, is highly efficient in water compartmentalization and conservation; it is reported that they can lose 20% to 30% of body weight and recover faster once fluid is provided. Plasma volume is maintained even with 20% dehydration. Under normal conditions, they have a lower urinary output than horses when water is unrestricted.[5] These studies were done on a limited number of heat-adapted animals and should be viewed with caution when assessing companion donkeys in temperate climates.

Donkeys may show few clinical and hematologic signs of volume depletion until 12% to 15% dehydration is reached. Skin tenting is an unreliable sign of fluid loss in donkeys and mules (see Erin L. Goodrich and Erica Behling-Kelly's article, "Clinical Pathology of Donkeys and Mules"; and Elena Barrio and colleagues' article, "Clinical Evaluation and Preventative Care in Donkeys," in this issue). The hindgut acts as a water reservoir similar to the forestomach in ruminants; donkeys have an

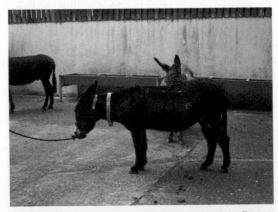

Fig. 2. Typical presentation of donkey with impaction of pelvic flexure showing dullness, head down, and ears back.

enhanced cecal capacity for fluid retention when faced with dehydration, which is evident by the scant diarrhea with colitis.

Donkeys and mules have a slower gut transit time than horses and digest fiber more efficiently. Per body weight, they require less dry matter and energy intake than resting and working horses.[6] Clinically, this is reflected by their ability to gain weight easily and develop large fat deposits on the neck, back, rump, around internal organs, and along the linea alba.

The donkey intestinal microbiome has not been extensively evaluated, but one can assume that there are differences with the horse and pony. Dysbiosis from different conditions (diet, antimicrobials, stress) can be a complication or potential cause of gastrointestinal disease.

EPIDEMIOLOGY AND RISK FACTORS

The risk factors for gastrointestinal disease in donkeys and mules are similar to those in horses, influenced by the management and environment in which they are kept. In donkeys and mules in arid regions and marginal communities with poor access to preventative care, colic may occur because of inadequate water access, fibrous or indigestible feed provision, poor dentition, foreign object ingestion (eg, plastic bags), or heavy endoparasitism (**Fig. 3**). Parasites such as *Strongylus vulgaris* have higher prevalence in developing countries because of poor management and minimal access to anthelmintics. Ingestion of moldy feed or excess seasonal lush grass can result in tympanic colic, whereas grazing low in poor grasslands may contribute to sand colic.[7]

Donkey studies in the United Kingdom have identified impaction colic as having high morbidity and mortality.[8] The pelvic flexure was the main site of impaction, but mortality was higher for cecal impactions. Colic impaction is also frequent with dental disease and aging. Multiple diastemata, painful periodontal disease, absent molars, and loss of masticatory function increase the incidence of colic. This can be reduced by dietary modifications, including a short chop, high-fiber feed, and provision of regular high-quality dental care. Note that diastemata and periodontal disease are not necessarily confined to geriatric patients, and younger animals should also have regular dental examinations.

Musculoskeletal disorders have also been associated with colic in geriatric donkeys, mainly due to reduced physical activity and water intake. In the United Kingdom, donkeys bedded on paper or cardboard have higher rates of impaction colic, because they regard the bedding as a fiber source and ingest large quantities. Donkeys are

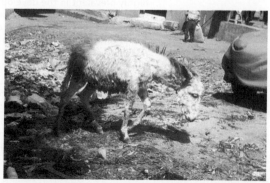

Fig. 3. Donkey browsing on inappropriate plastic, which can lead to obstructive colic.

natural browsers on a wide range of feedstuffs, and this exploratory behavior, while advantageous in some environments, can cause problems.

Hyperlipemia can be a cause or consequence of gastrointestinal disease. It can induce ileus, hepatic failure, and gastric ulceration, whereas colic, enteritis, colitis, peritonitis, inappetence, and anorexia often lead to hyperlipemia.

Other causes of colic (eg, grass sickness, neoplasia, enteroliths, peritonitis) have been reported in a small number of donkeys and mules with similar signs and treatments to horses.

The etiology and epidemiology of colitis in donkeys have not been fully elucidated, but is likely influenced by geography and management. In the United Kingdom, individual cases and outbreaks of diarrhea have been documented, with parasites, infectious agents, and husbandry changes proposed as the main causes.

ROLE OF PARASITES

An extensive discussion of donkey parasitology is provided elsewhere.[7,9] Relevant gastrointestinal parasites are listed in **Table 1**.

Table 1
Gastrointestinal parasites of donkeys

Organ	Parasites	Comments
Stomach	Gasterophilus spp Habronema spp Draschia megastoma	Their significance in relation to gastric ulcer syndrome is unclear. May be more relevant in working animals with malnutrition
Small intestine	Parascaris equorum	Adult donkeys do not seem to share the level of immunity demonstrated by horses and ponies, particularly in the case of immunocompromised working donkeys. Foals and heavily infested adult donkeys are at risk of ileal impaction and intestinal rupture in extreme cases
Ileocecal junction	Anoplocephala perfoliata	Rarely found among the UK herd at The Donkey Sanctuary, but higher infestation is found in working donkeys. Clinical signs of heavy burdens are similar to horses
Large intestine	Strongyle spp	S vulgaris and other large strongyles are rarely found in donkeys in developed countries owing to management and anthelmintic use, but are highly prevalent in the developing world and should be a differential for chronic and acute colic Cyathostomins (small strongyles) are common in both nonworking and working donkey populations. Encysted cyathostomes are a major cause of acute and chronic disease in the United Kingdom
Liver	F hepatica	Liver fluke is emerging as a potential cause of liver pathologic condition in the United Kingdom
Rectum	Oxyuris equi	Pinworm infestations appear to be on the increase in areas of the United Kingdom and perhaps in other countries and may be a significant cause of perianal discomfort
	Gasterophilus spp	Heavy infestations are associated with rectal prolapse in working donkey populations

GASTRIC PATHOLOGIC CONDITION
Gastric Ulceration

Gastric ulcers have been identified during endoscopic evaluation[10] and at postmortem examination,[11] confirming that donkeys are at risk of this pathologic condition. Donkeys with gastric ulcer syndrome (DGUS) do not usually exhibit the clinical signs displayed by horses with equine gastric ulcer syndrome, likely because of their stoic nature. For example, 1 study of 39 donkeys without symptomatic evidence of gastric disease found lesions in the squamous gastric mucosa in 49% of animals, whereas only 2.6% had glandular disease.[10] Postmortem data from The Donkey Sanctuary identified that most chronic gastric ulcers were located in the squamous area adjacent to the margo plicatus, whereas chronic active or acute ulcers affected both the glandular and the squamous part of the stomach in few animals (G. Paraschiou, personal communication, 2018). These findings are similar to those reported in Italy.[10]

Acute gastric ulcers are rarely documented in donkeys, but this may be a reflection of infrequent diagnostics rather than true pathologic condition. Concerns related to stress and risk of hyperlipemia from prolonged fasting for gastroscopic evaluation are valid. However, in 1 study where donkeys were fasted for 15 hours before the procedure, no adverse metabolic effects were noted.[10] It is the authors' opinion that donkeys undergoing gastroscopy should have triglyceride concentrations measured before fasting and after the procedure. If hyperlipidemia is identified, intravenous dextrose or oral administration of glucose or sugar-rich drenches is recommended to prevent clinical hyperlipemia.

Suggested risk factors for DGUS include high starch diets, chronic stress, hyperlipemia, long-term corticosteroid and nonsteroidal anti-inflammatory drug (NSAID) use. Prophylactic use of omeprazole is recommended when there are concerns.

Prophylaxis and treatment protocols for squamous and glandular ulcers with omeprazole have been extrapolated from horses. Pharmacologic information on injectable omeprazole is lacking in donkeys.

Other

Gastrointestinal transit time is longer in donkeys compared with horses and ponies, and there is suspicion that this could be in part due to delay gastric emptying, may have clinical relevance when planning gastroscopy as previously discussed or when withholding food for diagnostic testing purposes.

Gastric impaction occurs sporadically, primary or secondary to other conditions (liver disease, strictures, ileus). Gastric foreign bodies are more common in working donkeys because of their scavenging habits (eg, plastic bag ingestion). Affected donkeys are usually dull and inappetent and may display varying degrees of abdominal pain. Fecal output may be reduced. Diagnosis may be tentatively made on ultrasound examination; where ultrasound is not available, diagnosis may be made based on the presence of reflux or a marked discomfort on administration of enteral fluids.

Treatment of suspected gastric impaction is as for other equids.

SMALL INTESTINE

Pathologic condition of the small intestine is similar to horses, although there appears to be a reduced incidence of strangulating lipomas. Small intestinal pathologic condition may be harder to identify in donkeys because of limitations in rectal examination.

Equine grass sickness is rarely reported in donkeys, but should be kept as a differential diagnosis of weight loss, inappetence, and ileus in the United Kingdom.[12] Lack of clinical recognition may be the main reason for its apparent low incidence. Diagnosis and management are similar to other equids.

Ultrasonographic abdominal examination is recommended whereby acute or chronic small intestinal lesions are suspected from clinical signs or the results of other diagnostic tests.

The oral glucose absorption test may be used in donkeys suspected of small intestinal malabsorption, but careful consideration of the risks of prolonged food withholding should be made.

CECUM/COLONS/RECTUM

Impaction Colic

One of the most common causes of colic in donkeys and mules is pelvic flexure impaction from poorly masticated feedstuffs or foreign bodies (eg, plastic bags), followed by impactions of the transverse colon and cecum. Typically, these animals present with dullness but will continue to eat until the impaction is severe, when they show signs of abdominal pain or stand apart from the herd. There may be reduced intestinal motility.

Because of the delay in presentation for evaluation, there may be secondary hyperlipemia, which contributes to their higher mortality compared with large colon impaction in horses.

Transabdominal ultrasonography can be helpful in patients too small for rectal examination and can be also used to measure intestinal wall thickness and edema.

Impactions due to dehydrated feces or fibrous material can be managed via enteral fluids and osmotic laxatives (eg, magnesium sulfate or sodium sulfate), whereas impactions due to plastic bags or foreign matter may respond better to mineral oil as a nonosmotic lubricant.

Nutritional support via nasogastric or intravenous routes, and small amounts of grass or short chop, can be used to stimulate appetite and encourage gastrointestinal motility, but also to prevent hyperlipemia.

In dehydrated working donkeys and mules, NSAIDs should be administered at half the indicated dose to reduce the risk of renal toxicity.

Geriatric donkeys with dental disease, especially with absent molars, are more prone to large colon impaction and require short chop diets and grazing to reduce risk.

Colitis

Typhlitis and colitis in donkeys can be challenging to diagnose. Animals could be found dead from peracute colitis, whereas most cases show signs of intestinal inflammation and systemic inflammatory response syndrome, including dullness, fever, and occasionally diarrhea. Ventral edema and weight loss are common findings in chronic cases associated with protein-losing enteropathy and hypoalbuminemia.[13] As with colitis in other equids, achieving a definite diagnosis can be challenging, but may be linked to emerging cyathostomins and infectious agents (**Fig. 4**). Salmonella spp and Clostridium spp are occasionally isolated. Information on coronavirus and gastrointestinal disease in donkeys is limited. Feed contamination with mycotoxins has been implicated. Rapid dietary changes that alter the microbiota could be an aggravating or risk factor. Again, hyperlipemia is a frequent finding in donkeys with colitis. Therapeutic protocols for colitis in donkeys and mules are similar to horses.

Rectal Injuries

Rectal prolapse is seen more commonly in working donkeys, where exhaustion and parasitism are common. It has been associated with Gasterophilus nasalis in

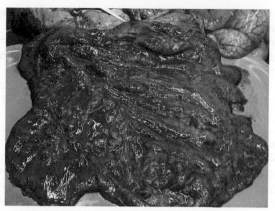

Fig. 4. Severe inflammation of colon: colitis, postmortem specimen.

Ethiopia, which causes irritation and constant straining when present on the rectal mucosa.[14] Rectal prolapse has been reported secondary to rectal tumors and penetrating injuries (**Fig. 5**). Rectal prolapse from acute colitis is unusual compared with horses. Treatment will depend on the size of prolapsed tissue and the severity of the damage. Simple cases can respond to osmotic reduction using sugar and lubrication to replace the prolapse, combined with anti-inflammatory drugs (see **Fig. 5**). Animals with severe lesions or that do not respond to medical management may require a purse-string suture or surgical resection. Sedation, epidural anesthesia, and local anaesthetics are required. The purse-string suture using thick suture material or sterile umbilical tape is often successful. The string must be loose

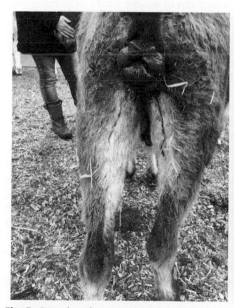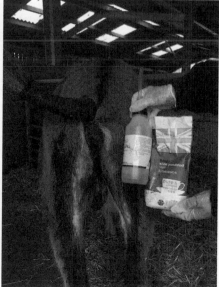

Fig. 5. Rectal prolapse in a donkey before (*left*) and after osmotic reduction using sugar and lubrication (*right*).

enough to allow defecation and should be removed within 72 hours. Depending on the inciting cause, a soft diet or a laxative may be helpful.

Rectal tears are a serious complication of rectal examination, and antispasmodic drugs with good restraint are recommended for rectal examination. Rectal tears have been reported when stallions attempt to cover geldings.

LIVER
Background

Liver disease has major morbidity and mortality in the UK donkey population. Clinical signs are often insidious, and liver pathologic condition may only be found because of investigation into other diseases. Clinical signs of liver disease include colic (dysmotility, gastric impaction), weight loss, fever, depression, photosensitization and other skin diseases, icterus, and neurologic signs (including behavioral changes). Weight loss is the most consistent finding but is not pathognomonic. Hepatic disease is frequently subclinical and often detected based on serum biochemistry evaluation. Liver dysfunction from excessive fat infiltration from a negative energy balance, stress, or insulin insensitivity may occur with severe hyperlipemia. Liver disease has been found in donkeys with elevated adreno cortico trophic hormone (ACTH) and assumed poorly controlled pars pituitary intermedia disorder (PPID), but firm data on any association are lacking at present.

Diagnosis and Treatments

Evaluation of serum chemistry should be an early diagnostic step to investigate liver function. Reference values for liver specific parameters are available in Erin L. Goodrich and Erica Behling-Kelly's article, "Clinical Pathology of Donkeys and Mules," in this issue.

Ultrasonography is useful to assess size, echogenicity, architecture, and the presence of focal or diffuse lesions, if there is suspicion of severe acute or chronic liver pathologic condition. A biopsy may provide the most meaningful diagnostic and prognostic information. There is no validated hepatic histopathology scoring system for donkeys, and the grading system for horses is the one used.[15] Hemosiderin accumulation is a common histopathological finding in donkey hepatic tissue, but its significance is unknown. It is important to note that liver biopsy carries risks, in particular, bleeding, which can be exacerbated from hepatic disease.

It is highly indicated to have another donkey available as a companion, but also as a potential blood donor. Close monitoring for signs of colic and bleeding for the next 24 hours after the procedure is recommended.

Treatment of liver pathologic condition will be dictated by the clinical and diagnostic findings. Liver fibrosis is frequently found in the UK donkey population. Use of corticosteroids and nutritional management are the mainstays of therapy. Repeat biopsies would be ideal to monitor response to treatment, but it is often impractical, costly, or hard to justify. Serial blood evaluation of markers of liver disease and function may be the most practical method. In animals with minor serum abnormalities of liver function, monthly chemistry evaluations are indicated.

Pyrrolizidine alkaloid toxicity has been documented in donkeys, with similar histopathological findings and prognosis as horses.

Antimicrobials should be reserved for cases where there is evidence of a bacterial hepatitis or cholangiohepatitis.

Hydatid cysts are occasionally found as an incidental finding on ultrasound examination. Treatment or monitoring is advised as for other equines.

The incidence of liver fluke (*Fasciola hepatica*) is increasing among the UK donkey population. This parasite should be considered in donkeys inhabiting wetter environments where the presence of lymnaeid intermediate hosts (*Lymnaea* spp; *Galba* spp) has been documented.

Flukes may increase liver enzymes because of pathologic condition of the bile ducts. Some animals will present with weight loss and marked elevation in liver enzymes from severe cholangiohepatitis.

Treatment of all animals in the herd is advised. There are no licensed fluke treatments for donkeys, and therapy is prescribed using the cascade system. The Donkey Sanctuary uses triclabendazole (18 mg/kg orally) with follow-up fecal egg analysis 14 to 28 days after treatment to assess efficacy. When triclabendazole is ineffective, closantel (20 mg/kg orally) may be considered, keeping in mind that it is only effective against adult flukes and redosing is required 8 to 10 weeks later. Closantel can cause anorexia, ataxia, and blindness if overdosed. Fencing off wet, marshy environments is advised to reduce exposure, and cattle or sheep screened and treated for liver flukes if they graze the same pasture as donkeys.

PANCREATITIS

Measurement of amylase and lipase activities in dull donkeys with nonspecific abdominal pain may be suggestive of pancreatitis, but a definitive diagnosis is rare, and very few cases have been confirmed at postmortem examination. Many veterinary laboratories do not measure amylase and lipase as routine tests, and results should be interpreted with caution. In horses, migrating *Strongylus* spp and *Parascaris* spp larvae have been proposed as a potential etiology,[16] but their role in donkey pancreatic disease remains to be determined. Hyperlipemia may further the risk of pancreatitis in donkeys.

SURGICAL CONSIDERATIONS AND PHARMACOLOGY

Indications for surgery in donkeys are similar to those in horses, with the caveat that their demeanor and physiology may mask deteriorating parameters. Pain level and dehydration are harder to assess in donkeys. Before embarking on exploratory laparotomy, a thorough clinical examination is recommended to ascertain that factors that could compromise a successful outcome (eg, dental disease, malnutrition, laminitis, osteoarthritis) are taken into consideration. Again, routine rectal examination and nasogastric intubation should be performed when feasible. Blood and peritoneal fluid lactate values can be used in a similar way as for horses. Normal blood and peritoneal fluid lactate values for donkeys have not been established; however, rising lactate concentrations suggest the presence of a surgical lesion or the presence of bacteria in the peritoneal fluid.

Success rates for abdominal surgery in donkeys tend to be lower than values reported for horses[17] for several reasons, including lack of medical and surgical experience with the species, presentation at an advanced stage of disease, delayed referral due to reduced veterinary experience, lack of knowledge regarding appropriate analgesia and donkey-specific pharmacology, and finances.

Hospital stall accommodation may need to be adapted for the donkey; stall doors that are too high to permit visibility may need to be replaced with a hurdle or gate. It is vital that the clinician has knowledge of how to estimate and measure donkey weight and condition score before giving any medications.[18]

Few drugs are licensed for use in donkeys and must be selected on the basis of the legislation of each country. In the United Kingdom, prescribing guidance to avoid animal suffering where no approved drug is available is based on the cascade system, whereas in the United States, the Animal Medicinal Drug Use Clarification Act permits the extralabel use of certain approved animal drugs under some conditions.

It is important to mention that for several drugs, there are pharmacologic differences between donkeys and mules with horses, and clinicians should use caution when extrapolating doses (see Francisco J. Mendoza and colleagues' article, "Clinical Pharmacology in Donkeys and Mules," in this issue).[19]

It is essential to monitor the response to analgesia given for gastrointestinal pain and be prepared to dose at more frequent intervals. Phenylbutazone and flunixin meglumine can be given twice daily at standard equine doses.[19] Multimodal pain relief using opioids and other drugs should be considered, as for other equines. Further information on sedation and general anesthesia in donkeys is described elsewhere (see Nora Matthews and Johannes P.A.M. van Loon article's, "Anesthesia, Sedation and Pain Management of Donkeys and Mules," in this issue).[20]

Abdominal surgery increases the risk of hyperlipemia, and preemptive measures to prevent and manage this complication should be in place. Postoperative food withholding should be weighed against the risk of hyperlipemia and other complications. Triglycerides should be monitored regularly, and parenteral support may be required to maintain normal levels (see Francisco J. Mendoza and colleagues' article, "Metabolic and Endocrine Disorders in Donkeys," in this issue).[21]

Postsurgical monitoring is essential to reduce stress. In donkeys that require prolonged stall rest, enrichment methods may be necessary. The following link provides information on enrichment for donkeys (https://www.thedonkeysanctuary.org.uk/what-we-do/knowledge-and-advice/for-owners/environment-enrichment).

FLUID THERAPY

There are no known published guidelines on fluid therapy for donkeys and mules, and recommendations are based on equine principles, taking into consideration that there are differences in body water partitioning.

Enteral fluid therapy is suitable for gastrointestinal disorders,[22] such as large colon impaction and mild dehydration, as long as there is no gastric distension or ileus, and when resources are limited. Nasogastric intubation might be the only option for working donkeys.

Commercially available isotonic fluids should be the first option before considering homemade recipes. Supplementation with dextrose should be done in most cases. For enteral fluids, do not exceed 3 L of fluid for a 180-kg donkey. The frequency of enteral fluid administration will depend on the metabolic status, the animal response to therapy, and feasibility. An indwelling nasogastric tube may be a more practical method for intermittent or continuous fluid administration.

Enteral fluids should not be used in animals in which reduced intestinal perfusion is suspected.

Intravenous fluid therapy is indicated in animals with evidence of volume depletion, when electrolyte and metabolic abnormalities are present, for those in which enteral fluid therapy is not an option, or in surgical cases. The approach follows the equine guidelines. When administering as a bolus, be aware that the advised crystalloid rate of 20 to 40 mL/kg over 1 to 2 hours[22] equates to 3.6 to 7.2 L for a 180-kg donkey. In animals with colitis, high intravenous fluid rates have been associated with mural edema and a poorer prognosis (A. Thiemann, personal communication). To reduce complications from overhydration, it is recommended to monitor urine output, respiratory rate, peripheral edema, and body weight. A full discussion of intravenous fluid therapy is beyond the scope of this article, and the reader is referred to equine fluid therapy reviews.[23]

Use of rectal fluids has been investigated,[24] but, in general, has been considered impractical and risky.

SUMMARY

Gastrointestinal disorders are common in donkeys and mules. Knowledge of these conditions, including their etiology, pathophysiology, and epidemiology can assist in their successful diagnosis and management. Awareness of donkey- and mule-specific behavior, anatomy, and physiology will improve the prognosis. Adequate pain management to reduce stress and understanding metabolic complications from gastrointestinal disease are essential for success.

REFERENCES

1. Ashley FH, Waterman-Pearson AE, Whay HR. Behavioural assessment of pain in horses and donkeys: application to clinical practice and future studies. Equine Vet J 2005;37(6):565–75.
2. Burns CC, Dennison TL, Whay HR. Relationships between behaviour and health in working horses, donkeys and mules in developing countries. Appl Anim Behav Sci 2010;126:109–18.
3. Jerbi H, Rejeb A, Erdogan S, et al. Anatomical and morphometric study of gastro-intestinal tract of donkey (Equus africanus asinus). J Morphol Sci 2014;31(1): 18–22.
4. Evans L, Crane M. Sedation, anaesthesia and analgesia. In: Evans L, Crane M, editors. Clinical companion of the donkey. 1st edition. Leicestershire: Troubador Publishing Ltd; 2018. p. 225.
5. Yousef MK, Dill DB, Mayes MG. Shifts in body fluid during dehydration in the burro, Equus asinus. J Appl Physiol 1970;29(3):345–9.
6. Pearson RA, Merritt JB. Intake, digestion and gastrointestinal transit time in resting donkeys and ponies and exercised donkeys given ad libitum hay and straw diets. Equine Vet J 1991;23(5):339–43.
7. Thiemann AK, Rickards KJ, Getachew M, et al. Colic in the donkey. In: Blikslager AT, White NA II, Moore JN, et al, editors. The equine acute abdomen. 3rd edition. Hoboken (NJ): John Wiley and Sons Inc; 2017. p. 469–87.
8. Cox R, Proudman CJ, Trawford AF, et al. Epidemiology of impaction colic in don-keys in the UK. BMC Vet Res 2007;3:1–11.
9. Matthews JB, Burden FA. Common helminth infections of donkeys and their con-trol in temperate regions. Equine Vet Educ 2013;25:461–7.
10. Sgorbini M, Bonelli F, Papini R, et al. Equine gastric ulcer syndrome in adult don-keys: investigation on prevalence, anatomical distribution and severity. Equine Vet J 2018;30(4):206–10.
11. Burden FA, Gallagher J, Thiemann AK, et al. Necropsy survey of gastric ulcers in a population of aged donkeys: prevalence, lesion description and risk factors. Animal 2009;3(2):287–93.
12. Mellor NE, Bladon B, Foote AK, et al. Successful treatment of chronic grass sick-ness in a donkey. Equine Vet Educ 2013;25(12):628–32.
13. McGorum BC, Pirie RS. Asinine typhlocolitis; 'scouring' the literature for diag-nostic and aetiological clues. Equine Vet Educ 2010;22(2):58–9.

14. Getachew AM, Innocent G, Trawford AF, et al. Gasterophilosis: a major cause of rectal prolapse in working donkeys in Ethiopia. Trop Anim Health Prod 2012b;44: 757–62.
15. Durham AE, Smith KC, Newton JR, et al. Development and application of a scoring system for prognostic evaluation of equine liver biopsies. Equine Vet J 2003;35(6):534–40.
16. Edery N, Rosenbaum A, Busnach A, et al. Acute pancreatitis in a horse–a case report. Israel J Vet Med 2015;70(1):49–52.
17. Merridale-Punter MS, Parker RA, Prutton JSW, et al. Outcome following exploratory laparotomy in 24 donkeys: a retrospective multicentre study. BEVA Conference Proceedings 2017. Liverpool, United Kingdom, 13–16 September, 2017.
18. Evans L, Crane M. Appendix 2, body weight estimator. In: Clinical companion of the donkey. 1st edition. Leicestershire: Troubador Publishing Ltd; 2018. p. 257.
19. Grosenbaugh DA, Reinmeyer CR, Figueiredo DA. Pharmacology and therapeutics in donkeys. Equine Vet Educ 2011;23(10):523–30.
20. Matthews N, van Loon JPAM. Anaesthesia and analgesia of the donkey and mule. Equine Vet Educ 2013;25(1):47–51.
21. Durham AE, Thiemann AK. Nutritional management of hyperlipaemia. Equine Vet Educ 2015;27(9):482–8.
22. Fielding LC. Practical fluid therapy and treatment modalities for field conditions for horses and foals with gastrointestinal problems. Vet Clin North Am Equine Pract 2018;34(1):155–68.
23. Fielding LC. Crystalloid and colloid therapy. Vet Clin North Am Equine Pract 2014; 30(2):415–25.
24. Khan A, Hallowell G, Underwood C, et al. Evaluation of the rectal route of fluid administration in horses. ECEIM conference proceedings, Helsinki 2016. J Vet Intern Med 2017;31(2):604–18.

Clinical Pathology of Donkeys and Mules

Erin L. Goodrich, DVM[a],*, Erica Behling-Kelly, DVM, PhD[b]

KEYWORDS

- Donkey • Mule • Hinny • Equid • Clinical pathology • Hemogram • Chemistry

KEY POINTS

- For several reasons, the generation of appropriate reference intervals for donkeys is challenging, and reliance on values established for closely related donkey breeds or horses can result in erroneous diagnoses.
- Sample collection, handling, and storage are essential components to obtaining accurate clinical pathology results.
- Many of the publications involving the generation of clinical pathology values for donkeys and/or their hybrids are limited by breed, numerical, or geographic constraints.
- In light of the challenges and constraints, the literature involving clinical pathology of donkeys and mules has been thoroughly reviewed and presented in this article.
- Use of clinical pathology literature relevant to the horse may lead to erroneous interpretation of laboratory data obtained for a donkey.

INTRODUCTION

The interpretation and thus diagnostic utility of clinical pathology data in evaluating the health of donkeys and their hybrids are confounded by a plethora of preanalytical and analytical variables that are often beyond the clinician's control. In this article, the authors outline the most significant of these obstacles and provide potential means to work around them when assessing these unique animals. They also highlight key areas, such as testing for metabolic disease and coagulation testing, whereby nuanced use of laboratory data and an understanding of these obstacles can help avoid potentially dangerous misdiagnoses.

Disclosure Statement: E.L. Goodrich: employee of Animal Health Diagnostic Center. E. Behling-Kelly: employee of Animal Health Diagnostic Center.
^a Department of Population Medicine and Diagnostic Sciences, Animal Health Diagnostic Center, College of Veterinary Medicine, Cornell University, A1-212 AHDC, 240 Farrier Road, Ithaca, NY 14853, USA; ^b Department of Population Medicine and Diagnostic Sciences, Animal Health Diagnostic Center, College of Veterinary Medicine, Cornell University, S1-062 Schurman Hall, Tower Road, Ithaca, NY 14853, USA
* Corresponding author.
E-mail address: elg25@cornell.edu

Vet Clin Equine 35 (2019) 433–455
https://doi.org/10.1016/j.cveq.2019.08.002
0749-0739/19/© 2019 Elsevier Inc. All rights reserved.

REFERENCE INTERVALS

The interpretation of clinical pathology data requires knowledge or assessment of what is considered normal, or associated with health, in the animal of interest. Most often, this relies on the use of population-based reference intervals (RIs). The number of donkey breeds, low numbers of animals within some of the breeds, and the harsh nature of the environments donkeys have acclimated to pose challenges to the generation of appropriate RIs and thus the interpretation of their clinical pathology data. Often clinicians may be forced to rely on published RIs applicable to a closely related donkey breed or even the horse. This can unfortunately lead to erroneous diagnoses. For example, the reported ranges of serum cholesterol concentration in Indian and Poitou donkeys are approximately half that of the horse.[1] Thus, use of a horse RI could potentially lead to a misdiagnosis of hypocholesterolemia in a healthy donkey, or overlooking what should be recognized as a hypercholesterolemia in a sick donkey. In a recent study comparing RIs for non-Thoroughbred horses to a large group of donkeys in the United Kingdom, intervals for 0 out of 15 hematological and only 4 of 20 biochemical analytes evaluated were transferable.[2]

The authors briefly discuss some donkey-specific RI data available in the literature as well as the most crucial aspects of RI generation as they pertain to this unique animal. For a more detailed discussion of RIs, the authors refer readers to the American Society of Veterinary Clinical Pathology (ASVCP) guidelines.[3] Although the use of best practices should always be the goal, the authors also attempt to provide some user-friendly suggestions when best practices are simply not an option.

According to the ASVCP guidelines, studies to generate RIs de novo by nonparametric methods with a 90% confidence interval should consist of 120 animals within the population of interest.[3] For some breeds of donkeys, this number is not practically attainable. The Catalonian donkey is among the most endangered of the donkey breeds worldwide, and its population has dipped to less than 500 individuals on more than 1 occasion.[4] Folch and colleagues[5] published RIs for the Catalonian donkey in 1998.[5] Their study consisted of 98 animals, which was a significant proportion of the total population. The investigators also partitioned the data to evaluate the impact of age, sex, and management practices. Donkeys in this study were subdivided into 2 major age groups: young (<3 years of age) and adult (≥3 years of age) animals. Although partitioning is only recommended if there are at least 40 individuals in each subgroup, exceptions to this numerical constraint might be necessary when there are very clear biological reasons to do so. Donkeys are notoriously long lived, and several published studies have documented an influence of advanced age on clinical pathology data and disease prevalence in the donkey.[6,7] However, given that the captive donkey can approach a lifespan of 50 years, the appropriate cutoff to use for "older" donkeys remains a point of debate.

There are several published RI studies involving donkey breeds that are of questionable utility in terms of RIs owing to numerical constraints, but they hold subjective value for the clinician. For example, in a study of 30 healthy donkeys, Zakari and colleagues[8] demonstrated differences in hematological data between foals and adults that varied directionally with the season. Many studies evaluating clinical pathology parameters in the endangered Martina Franca donkey have included fewer than 20 individual animals.[9,10]

If the number of individuals within the population of interest, or availability of laboratory resources, is limiting, one could consider transference of an established RI rather than a suboptimal generation of a de novo interval. Transference allows for a mathematical means to address bias in the data. Although facilitating interpretation of data using fewer animals, there are constraints to RI transference that may also be challenging in the donkey world. The population of interest should share most demographic attributes and the preanalytical factors in the laboratory that generated the interval with those in the laboratory seeking to adopt their intervals. Ideally, transference studies should include at least 20 individuals, and 2 or fewer results are permitted to fall outside the established RI if it is to be transferred to the new laboratory. RI studies should provide detailed information regarding testing methods and analyzers, and when forced to use an RI from a different laboratory than the one that generated the interval, one can peruse the literature for known variances. For example, the Bromocresol Green and Bromocresol Purple methods to measure albumin produces divergent results across species and clinical conditions.[11–14] If clinicians must use an RI generated in a laboratory using 1 method to interpret data generated in a laboratory using the other method, consultation with the literature and/or a clinical pathologist may be prudent. Differences in the environment, preanalytical factors, and what is known about analytical variables between laboratories should be considered when practicality mandates a side-by-side comparison of intervals provided in literature to evaluate data from the donkey (**Table 1**).

In what could be the most extensive data set available, Burden and colleagues[6] examined 138 donkeys residing in a sanctuary in the United Kingdom. Perhaps the most clinically relevant finding in comparing their data to previously published intervals generated from both the horse and the donkey was documented significant decline in the upper limit of serum triglyceride (TG) concentrations from 4.3 mmol/L (380 mg/dL) to 2.8 mmol/L (248 mg/dL). The investigators raised the possibility that management practices may have contributed to this decline. This reiterates the recommendation from the ASVCP that RIs be reevaluated approximately every 3 to 5 years.

PREANALYTICAL CONSIDERATIONS

Although not specific to donkeys, preanalytical variables can have profound effects on the results that are generated by laboratory tests. Preanalytical factors affecting hematologic values account for 50% to 75% of the errors seen in human clinical pathology testing.[13] That percentage is likely even higher in veterinary medicine, and in particular, when dealing with species like donkeys, whereby the samples are often collected in remote locations, without a laboratory nearby for prompt processing, from patients who may be exceedingly stressed by transport or handling. These preanalytical factors can be divided into biological and nonbiological components. Some biological components include species, breed, age, environment (geographic location), handling (stress), physical activity, nutrition (caloric intake, fasting), body condition, physiologic state (pregnancy, lactation, sedation, and so forth), diseases, and exogenous compounds (drugs, toxins).[15,16] Although these effects are not easy to control in most cases, they should be documented so that they can be taken into account when interpreting results from veterinary clinical pathology assays.

Nonbiological preanalytical factors affecting veterinary clinical pathology testing include technical effects owing to techniques associated with sample collection, handling, and storage. For equids, sodium or potassium EDTA is the preferred anticoagulant for use in the blood collection tubes for hematology assays. When collecting blood into EDTA tubes, proper proportions between blood and anticoagulant should be adhered to because an excess of EDTA can result in red blood cell (RBC) shrinkage, which will falsely decrease the mean corpuscular volume (MCV) and increase the mean corpuscular hemoglobin concentration (MCHC).[17] Gentle inversion

Table 1
Comparison of hematologic and serum biochemical values in various donkey populations and horses

	UK Donkeys (Burden et al,[6] 2016)		US Donkeys (Zinkl et al,[27] 1990)		Catalonian Donkeys (Folch et al,[5] 1997; Jordana et al,[42] 1998)		UK Donkeys (French & Patrick,[26] 1995)		Horses (Animal Health Diagnostic Center Reference Ranges[d])	
	SI Units	Conventional Units	SI Units	Conventional Units	SI Units	Conventional Units	SI Units	Conventional Units	SI Units	Conventional Units
PCV										
Mean ± SD	—	—	0.38 ± 0.05 L/L	38 ± 5% (n = 166)	0.36 ± 0.05 L/L	36 ± 5% (n = 98)	—	—	—	—
2.5%–97.5%	0.27–0.42 L/L	27%–42% (n = 137)	—	—	—	—	—	—	—	—
5%–95%	—	—	—	—	—	—	0.25–0.38 L/L	25%–38% (n = 4215)	0.31–0.48 L/L	31%–48%
Hb										
Mean ± SD	—	—	131 ± 17 g/L	13.1 ± 1.7 g/dL (n = 166)	122.8 ± 22.7 g/L	12.3 ± 2.3 g/dL (n = 98)	—	—	—	—
2.5%–97.5%	89–147 g/L	8.9–14.7 g/dL (n = 137)	—	—	—	—	—	—	—	—
5%–95%	—	—	—	—	—	—	90–153 g/L	9–15.3 g/dL (n = 4210)	118–159 g/L	11.8–15.9 g/dL
RBC										
Mean ± SD	—	—	$6.65 ± 1.05 × 10^{12}$/L	$6.65 ± 1.05 × 10^{6}$/μL (n = 166)	$6.87 ± 1.22 × 12^{12}$/L	$6.87 ± 1.22 × 10^{6}$/μL (n = 98)	—	—	—	—
2.5%–97.5%	$4.4\text{–}7.1 × 10^{12}$/L	$4.4\text{–}7.1 × 10^{6}$/μL (n = 137)	—	—	—	—	—	—	—	—
5%–95%	—	—	—	—	—	—	$4\text{–}7.3 × 10^{12}$/L	$4\text{–}7.3 × 10^{6}$/μL (n = 8995)	$6.6\text{–}9.7 × 10^{12}$/L	$6.6\text{–}9.7 × 10^{6}$/μL
MCV										
Mean ± SD	—	—	57.9 ± 5.5 fL	$57.9 ± 5.5 \; \mu m^{3}$ (n = 166)	52.6 ± 7.5 fL	$52.6 ± 7.5 \; \mu m^{3}$ (n = 98)	—	—	—	—

2.5%–97.5%	53–67 fL	53–67 µm³ (n = 137)	—	—	57–79 fL	57–79 µm³ (n = 4235)	43–55 fL	43–55 µm³
5%–95%	—	—	—	—	57–79 fL	57–79 fL	—	43–55 fL
MCH								
Mean ± SD	19.9 ± 1.9 pg	19.9 ± 1.9 pg	19.9 ± 1.9 pg (n = 166)	18.4 ± 2.2 pg	18.4 ± 2.2 pg (n = 98)	—	—	—
2.5%–97.5%	17.6–23.1 pg	17.6–23.1 pg (n = 137)	—	—	—	—	—	—
5%–95%	—	—	—	—	18.9–28.6 pg	18.9–28.6 pg (n = 4238)	15–20 pg	15–20 pg
MCHC								
Mean ± SD	343 ± 11 g/L	343 ± 11 g/L	34.3 ± 1.1 g/dL (n = 166)	347 ± 12.8 g/L	34.7 ± 1.3 g/dL (n = 98)	—	—	—
2.5%–97.5%	310–370 g/L	31–37 g/dL (n = 137)	—	—	—	—	—	—
5%–95%	—	—	—	—	314–391 g/L	31.4–39.1 g/dL (n = 4239)	330–360 g/L	33–36 g/dL
WBC								
Mean ± SD	$10.3 \pm 2.5 \times 10^9/\text{L}$	$10.3 \pm 2.5 \times 10^3/\mu\text{L}$ (n = 165)	$10.7 \pm 2.9 \times 10^9/\text{L}$	$10.7 \pm 2.9 \times 10^3/\mu\text{L}$ (n = 98)	—	—	—	—
2.5%–97.5%	—	—	—	—	—	—	—	—
5%–95%	—	—	—	—	$6.1\text{–}16.1 \times 10^9/\text{L}$	$6.1\text{–}16.1 \times 10^3/\mu\text{L}$ (n = 4239)	$5.2\text{–}10.1 \times 10^9/\text{L}$	$5.2\text{–}10.1 \times 10^3/\mu\text{L}$
Segmented neutrophils								
Mean ± SD	$4.7 \pm 1.7 \times 10^9/\text{L}$	$4.7 \pm 1.7 \times 10^3/\mu\text{L}$ (n = 165)	$4.5 \pm 1.2 \times 10^9/\text{L}$	$4.5 \pm 1.2 \times 10^3/\mu\text{L}$ (n = 98)	—	—	—	—
2.5%–97.5%	$2.4\text{–}6.3 \times 10^9/\text{L}$	$2.4\text{–}6.3 \times 10^3/\mu\text{L}$ (n = 138)	—	—	—	—	—	—
5%–95%	—	—	—	—	$2.2\text{–}13.3 \times 10^9/\text{L}$	$2.2\text{–}13.3 \times 10^3/\mu\text{L}$ (n = 4213)	$2.7\text{–}6.6 \times 10^9/\text{L}$	$2.7\text{–}6.6 \times 10^3/\mu\text{L}$

(continued on next page)

Table 1
(continued)

	UK Donkeys (Burden et al,[6] 2016)		US Donkeys (Zinkl et al,[27] 1990)		Catalonian Donkeys (Folch et al,[5] 1997; Jordana et al,[42] 1998)		UK Donkeys (French & Patrick,[26] 1995)		Horses (Animal Health Diagnostic Center Reference Ranges[d])	
	SI Units	Conventional Units	SI Units	Conventional Units	SI Units	Conventional Units	SI Units	Conventional Units	SI Units	Conventional Units
LYMPH										
Mean ± SD	—	—	4.4 ± 1.7 $\times 10^9/L$	4.4 ± 1.7 $\times 10^3/\mu L$ (n = 165)	5.3 ± 2.4 $\times 10^9/L$	5.3 ± 2.4 $\times 10^3/\mu L$ (n = 98)	—	—	—	—
2.5%–97.5%	2.2–$9.6 \times 10^9/L$	2.2–$9.6 \times 10^3/\mu L$ (n = 138)	—	—	—	—	—	—	—	—
5%–95%	—	—	—	—	—	—	1.8–$7.8 \times 10^9/L$	1.8–$7.8 \times 10^3/\mu L$ (n = 4212)	1.2–$4.9 \times 10^9/L$	1.2–$4.9 \times 10^3/\mu L$
MONO										
Mean ± SD	—	—	0.51 ± 0.29 $\times 10^9/L$	0.51 ± 0.29 $\times 10^3/\mu L$ (n = 165)	0.22 ± 0.19 $\times 10^9/L$	0.22 ± 0.19 $\times 10^3/\mu L$ (n = 98)	—	—	—	—
2.5%–97.5%	0–$0.75 \times 10^9/L$	0–$0.75 \times 10^3/\mu L$ (n = 138)	—	—	—	—	—	—	—	—
5%–95%	—	—	—	—	—	—	0–$0.80 \times 10^9/L$	0–$0.80 \times 10^3/\mu L$ (n = 4167)	0–$0.6 \times 10^9/L$	0–$0.6 \times 10^3/\mu L$
EOS										
Mean ± SD	—	—	0.58 ± 0.53 $\times 10^9/L$	0.58 ± 0.53 $\times 10^3/\mu L$ (n = 165)	0.68 ± 0.54 $\times 10^9/L$	0.68 ± 0.54 $\times 10^3/\mu L$ (n = 98)	—	—	—	—
2.5%–97.5%	0.1–$0.9 \times 10^9/L$	0.1–$0.9 \times 10^3/\mu L$ (n = 138)	—	—	—	—	—	—	—	—
5%–95%	—	—	—	—	—	—	0.09–1.15 $\times 10^9/L$	0.09–1.15 $\times 10^3/\mu L$ (n = 4158)	0–1.2 $\times 10^9/L$	0–1.2 $\times 10^3/\mu L$

BASO

Mean ± SD	—	$0.04 \pm 0.05 \times 10^9$/L	$0.04 \pm 0.05 \times 10^3/\mu$L (n = 165)	$0.02 \pm 0.06 \times 10^9$/L	$0.02 \pm 0.06 \times 10^3/\mu$L (n = 98)	—	—	—	—
2.5%–97.5%	$0\text{–}0.066 \times 10^9$/L	$0\text{–}0.066 \times 10^3/\mu$L (n = 138)	—	—	—	—	—	—	—
5%–95%	—	—	—	—	—	$0\text{–}0.05 \times 10^9/\mu$L	$0\text{–}0.05 \times 10^3/\mu$L (n = 3581)	$0\text{–}0.3 \times 10^9/\mu$L	$0\text{–}0.3 \times 10^3/\mu$L

PLT

Mean ± SD	—	$330 \pm 110 \times 10^9$/L	$330 \pm 110 \times 10^3/\mu$L (n = 89)	$234.1 \pm 82.9 \times 10^9$/L	$234.1 \pm 82.9 \times 10^3/\mu$L (n = 98)	—	—	—	—
2.5%–97.5%	$95\text{–}384 \times 10^9$/L	$95\text{–}384 \times 10^3/\mu$L (n = 137)	—	—	—	—	—	—	—
5%–95%	—	—	—	—	—	—	—	$94\text{–}232 \times 10^9$/L	$94\text{–}232 \times 10^3/\mu$L

Na

Mean ± SD	141 ± 4 mmol/L	141 ± 4 mEq/L (n = 108)	—	—	—	—	—	—	—
2.5%–97.5%	128–138 mmol/L	128–138 mEq/L (n = 137)	—	—	—	—	—	—	—
5%–95%	—	—	—	—	—	—	—	134–142 mmol/L	134–142 mEq/L

K

Mean ± SD	4.2 ± 0.6 mmol/L	4.2 ± 0.6 mEq/L (n = 108)	—	—	—	—	—	—	—
2.5%–97.5%	3.2–5.1 mmol/L	3.2–5.1 mEq/L (n = 137)	—	—	—	—	—	—	—
5%–95%	—	—	—	—	—	—	—	2.4–4.8 mmol/L	2.4–4.8 mEq/L

Cl

Mean ± SD	102 ± 3 mmol/L	102 ± 3 mEq/L (n = 108)	—	—	—	—	—	—	—
2.5%–97.5%	96–106 mmol/L	96–106 mEq/L (n = 136)	—	—	—	—	—	—	—

(continued on next page)

Table 1
(continued)

	UK Donkeys (Burden et al,[6] 2016)		US Donkeys (Zinkl et al,[27] 1990)		Catalonian Donkeys (Folch et al,[5] 1997; Jordana et al,[42] 1998)		UK Donkeys (French & Patrick,[26] 1995)		Horses (Animal Health Diagnostic Center Reference Ranges[d])	
	SI Units	Conventional Units	SI Units	Conventional Units	SI Units	Conventional Units	SI Units	Conventional Units	SI Units	Conventional Units
5%–95%	—	—	—	—	—	—	—	—	95–104 mmol/L	95–104 mEq/L
Urea nitrogen										
Mean ± SD	—	—	3.0 ± 0.8 mmol/L	18 ± 5 mg/dL (n = 215)	6.01 ± 1.3 mmol/L	36.1 ± 7.7 mg/dL (n = 97)	—	—	—	—
2.5%–97.5%	1.5–5.2 mmol/L	9.0–31.2 mg/dL (n = 138)	—	—	—	—	—	—	—	—
5%–95%	—	—	—	—	—	—	1.9–7.6 mmol/L	11.4–46.6 mg/dL (n = 4213)	1.7–3.7 mmol/L	10–22 mg/dL
Creat										
Mean ± SD	—	—	97.24 ± 26.52 µmol/L	1.1 ± 0.3 mg/dL (n = 108)	93.7 ± 19.5 µmol/L	1.06 ± 0.22 mg/dL (n = 97)	—	—	—	—
2.5%–97.5%	53–118 µmol/L	0.60–1.33 mg/dL (n = 138)	—	—	—	—	—	—	—	—
5%–95%	—	—	—	—	—	—	53–141 µmol/L	0.60–1.6 mg/dL (n = 1135)	70.7–132.6 µmol/L	0.8–1.5 mg/dL
Ca										
Mean ± SD	—	—	2.95 ± 0.2 mmol/L	11.8 ± 0.8 mg/dL (n = 215)	—	—	—	—	—	—
2.5%–97.5%	2.2–3.4 mmol/L	8.8–13.6 mg/dL (n = 118)	—	—	—	—	—	—	—	—
5%–95%	—	—	—	—	—	—	—	—	2.7–3.2 mmol/L	10.8–12.9 mg/dL

Total protein										
Mean ± SD	—	—	73 ± 6 g/L[b]	7.3 ± 0.6 g/dL[b] (n = 166); 7.2 ± 0.7 g/dL[a] (n = 215)	66.2 ± 6.8 g/L[b]	6.62 ± 0.7 g/dL[b] (n = 98)	—	—	—	—
2.5%-97.5%	58-76 g/L[a]	5.8-7.6 g/dL[a] (n = 138)	—	—	—	—	—	—	—	—
5%-95%	—	—	—	—	—	—	58-82 g/[c]	5.8-8.2 g/dL[c] (n = 4218)	54-70 g/L[a]	5.4-7.0 g/dL[a]
alb										
Mean ± SD	—	—	33 ± 3 g/L	3.3 ± 0.3 g/dL (n = 215)	26.8 ± 3.6 g/L	2.68 ± 0.36 g/dL (n = 97)	—	—	—	—
2.5%-97.5%	21.5-31.6 g/L	2.15-3.16 g/dL (n = 137)	—	—	—	—	—	—	—	—
5%-95%	—	—	—	—	—	—	20-34 g/L	2-3.4 g/dL (n = 1688)	29-36 g/L	2.9-3.6 g/dL
glob										
Mean ± SD	—	—	39 ± 7 g/L	3.9 ± 0.7 g/dL (n = 215)	—	—	—	—	—	—
2.5%-97.5%	32-48 g/L	3.2-4.8 g/dL (n = 137)	—	—	—	—	—	—	—	—
5%-95%	—	—	—	—	—	—	29-53 g/L	2.9-5.3 g/dL (n = 1682)	23-38 g/L	2.3-3.8 g/dL
AST										
Mean ± SD	—	—	487 ± 119 U/L	487 ± 119 U/L (n = 214)	254 ± 57 U/L	254 ± 57 U/L (n = 97)	—	—	—	—
2.5%-97.5%	238-536 U/L	238-536 U/L (n = 137)	—	—	—	—	—	—	—	—
5%-95%	—	—	—	—	—	—	59-199 U/L	59-199 U/L (n = 4197)	222-489 U/L	222-489 U/L
GLDH										
Mean ± SD	—	—	—	—	—	—	—	—	—	—

(continued on next page)

Table 1
(continued)

	UK Donkeys (Burden et al,[6] 2016)		US Donkeys (Zinkl et al,[27] 1990)		Catalonian Donkeys (Folch et al,[5] 1997; Jordana et al,[42] 1998)		UK Donkeys (French & Patrick,[26] 1995)		Horses (Animal Health Diagnostic Center Reference Ranges[a])	
	SI Units	Conventional Units	SI Units	Conventional Units	SI Units	Conventional Units	SI Units	Conventional Units	SI Units	Conventional Units
2.5%–97.5%	1.2–8.2 U/L	1.2–8.2 U/L (n = 136)	—	—	—	—	—	—	—	—
5%–95%	—	—	—	—	—	—	0.4–8 U/L	0.4–8 U/L (n = 3543)	2–10 U/L	2–10 U/L
ALP										
Mean ± SD	—	—	236 ± 75 U/L	236 ± 75 U/L (n = 215)	—	—	—	—	—	—
2.5%–97.5%	98–252 U/L	98–252 U/L (n = 138)	—	—	—	—	—	—	—	—
5%–95%	—	—	—	—	—	—	150–563 U/L	150–563 U/L (n = 1567)	88–261 U/L	88–261 U/L
GGT										
Mean ± SD	—	—	69 ± 29 U/L	69 ± 29 U/L (n = 108)	48 ± 22 U/L	48 ± 22 U/L (n = 97)	—	—	—	—
2.5%–97.5%	14–69 U/L	14–69 U/L (n = 138)	—	—	—	—	—	—	—	—
5%–95%	—	—	—	—	—	—	8–49 U/L	8–49 U/L (n = 4220)	8–33 U/L	8–33 U/L
Total bilirubin										
Mean ± SD	—	—	1.71 ± 3.42 µmol/L	0.1 ± 0.2 mg/dL (n = 215)	0.86 ± 0.51 µmol/L	0.05 ± 0.03 mg/dL (n = 97)	—	—	—	—
2.5%–97.5%	0.1–3.7 µmol/L	0.006–0.22 mg/dL (n = 138)	—	—	—	—	—	—	—	—
5%–95%	—	—	—	—	—	—	1.4–7.7 µmol/L	0.08–0.45 mg/dL (n = 4212)	8.55–35.9 µmol/L	0.5–2.1 mg/dL

CK

Mean ± SD	—	64 ± 43 U/L (n = 108)	64 ± 43 U/L (n = 108)	195 ± 104 U/L	195 ± 104 U/L (n = 97)	—	—	—	—
2.5%–97.5%	128–525 U/L	128–525 U/L (n = 137)	—	—	—	—	—	—
5%–95%	—	—	—	15–149 U/L	15–149 U/L (n = 4218)	171–567 U/L	171–567 U/L

TG

Mean ± SD	—	—	0.84 ± 0.37 mmol/L	74.8 ± 32.5 mg/dL (n = 97)	—	—
2.5%–97.5%	0.6–2.8 mmol/L	53.1–248 mg/dL (n = 138)	—	—
5%–95%	—	0.2–4.3 mmol/L	17.7–380.9 mg/dL	0.16–0.73 mmol/L	14–65 mg/dL (n = 3176)

Cholesterol

Mean ± SD	—	108 ± 30 mg/dL (n = 215)	2.79 ± 0.76 mmol/L	1.84 ± 0.68 mmol/L	71.1 ± 26.3 mg/dL (n = 97)	—
2.5%–97.5%	1.4–2.9 mmol/L	54.14–112.1 mg/dL (n = 137)	—
5%–95%	—	1.76–3.44 mmol/L	68–133 mg/dL

Reference ranges are given as mean ± SD, 2.5% to 97.5% percentiles, or 5% to 95% percentiles. The analyzed sample size is included in parentheses.

Abbreviations: PCV, packed cell volume; Hb, hemoglobin concentration; RBC, red blood cell count; MCV, mean cell/corpuscular volume; MCH, mean cell hemoglobin concentration; WBC, white blood cell count; LYMPH, lymphocytes; MONO, monocytes; EOS, eosinophils; BASO, basophils; PLT, platelet count; Na, sodium (Na); K, Potassium; Cl, chloride; Creat, creatinine; Ca, calcium; alb, albumin; glob, globulin; AST, aspartate aminotransferase; GLDH, glutamate dehydrogenase; ALP, alkaline phosphatase; GGT, gamma-glutamyl transferase; CK, creatine kinase; TG, triglycerides.

a Serum total protein.
b Plasma total protein.
c Unknown if serum or plasma.
d RIs established at the Animal Health Diagnostic Center of Cornell University (from at least 120 adult healthy horses).
Data from Refs. [5,6,26,27,42]

of the tube several times (not shaking) or rolling the tube between your hands after collection will help to avoid the formation of clots within the sample by assuring that the anticoagulant is properly mixed with the sample. If large clots or even microclots should form, they can cause errors in the hematology cell counts and can clog instrument lines in the automated analyzers.[17] The tubes should then be properly labeled with the patient identification, the owner's name, and the date the sample was collected. Although there are no firmly established guidelines for stability of all hematology analytes at various temperatures and times after collection, it is generally accepted as the best practice to analyze the samples as soon as possible after collection, ideally within 2 hours. When this is not possible, as is the case when samples must be shipped to an external diagnostic laboratory, 2 to 3 air-dried, unstained, blood smears should be prepared from the EDTA whole-blood sample to accompany the remaining blood sample to the laboratory. Examination of these smears is useful because if the blood sample is not analyzed within a few hours, several blood cell changes may occur that can alter the results. For instance, platelets often form clumps when collected in EDTA tubes, falsely decreasing the platelet count (pseudothrombocytopenia), which is well documented in horses.[18] When this is suspected, collecting blood samples in heparin- or citrate-containing tubes is indicated. The effect of EDTA on platelet clumping in donkeys is unknown. White blood cell (WBC) morphology can be altered, and RBCs will swell with time (usually >24 hours) and may lyse.[19] If the samples are to be shipped to a laboratory, the slides should be carefully packaged within a sturdy slide mailer and protected from direct exposure to ice packs, which can result in condensation and cell lysis on the slides. The EDTA whole-blood sample should be kept chilled before analysis, roughly at refrigeration temperatures (4°C). Therefore, if shipment is required, the EDTA whole-blood sample should be sent in an insulated box with a frozen ice pack. On should avoid freezing the sample to avoid subsequent hemolysis and ship the samples via a courier for overnight delivery to the desired diagnostic laboratory.

For routine biochemical analysis, serum or heparin plasma is the sample required. In most cases, these 2 samples can be expected to yield very similar results, although there are some predictable differences between specific analytes. For example, potassium and phosphate concentrations and lactate dehydrogenase activity will be higher in serum than plasma because these analytes leak from the cells during clot formation.[13] Because of the fact that plasma contains fibrinogen and other clotting factors, the protein and globulin values will be higher in plasma than serum. For times when expedited biochemical analysis is required, collection into a heparin tube is advised because there is no need to wait for a clot to form so the sample can be centrifuged and analyzed immediately. When using a heparin tube, keep in mind that underfilling of the tube can cause errors in the results. Also, the tubes must be inverted or gently rolled to mix after collection. If there is going to be a delay of more than 2 hours before analyzing the sample, the sample should be centrifuged, and the serum or plasma should be separated from the cells. The same is also true when serum separator (Corvac) tubes are used. Once the serum or plasma has been separated, it can be refrigerated for up to 48 hours before testing. The final sample should be labeled properly as previously described for hematology testing, including labeling it with the appropriate designation of either "serum" or "plasma" because the appearance of both can be otherwise indistinguishable. If samples must be shipped to a diagnostic laboratory, the separated serum or plasma should be sent in a plain tube with an ice pack, for overnight delivery. If long-term storage of samples is required, they may be frozen at −20°C.

HEMOGRAM

A hemogram or complete blood count (CBC) assesses the numbers, proportions, and morphologic characteristics of the RBCs (erythrogram), WBCs (leukogram), and the platelets (thrombogram). It may also include a measurement of the total solids in the plasma and a description of the visual characteristics of the plasma. Some laboratories will include a crude measure of fibrinogen using a heat precipitation method in a routine CBC for a large animal.

Information regarding specific hematologic and biochemical parameters for donkeys, mules, and hinnies, which have been established with large sample sizes, following ASVCP guidelines, is very scarce or nonexistent. For this reason, the results obtained from hematology and biochemical analytes in donkeys and their hybrids are often compared with reference ranges that have been established for horses, which is problematic given the evidence for the hematologic and biochemical differences that exist between these species.[6,15,20–24] Given the previously mentioned study limitations that have affected much of the donkey-specific clinical pathology values in the literature and the preanalytical factors as well, the following information regarding the hemogram findings should be likewise interpreted with caution. Although subjectively valuable, whenever possible, specific references should be examined in detail before transference of values is assumed.

ERYTHROGRAM

In adult mammals, erythrocytes (RBC) are predominantly produced by the bone marrow.

Many RBC parameters can be measured with automated analyzers, including RBC count, RBC mass (hematocrit, HCT), and hemoglobin concentration (Hb). Packed cell volume (PCV) is an alternative to HCT for quantifying RBC mass. PCV is assessed by determining the percentage of RBCs per volume of blood present in centrifuged microhematocrit tubes. Previous publications have demonstrated RBC counts lower in donkeys compared with horses.[5,6,25,26] Some studies have also shown RBC counts to decrease with increasing age in donkeys.[8,27] Zinkl and colleagues[27] hypothesized this greater RBC count in young donkeys to be associated with smaller RBCs, possibly due to iron deficiency, although iron was not measured in this study, nor is a single measure of iron predictive of deficiency owing to diurnal variation and variations between measurements and actual iron stores in the bone marrow.[25,26] Foals also have smaller and more numerous RBCs than adult horses, and this is considered a physiologic difference.[28] The same decrease in RBC count with increasing age was also found to be true for lactating donkeys and for various breeds and donkeys in specific geographic locations, including Catalonian donkeys, Pêga donkeys, Ragusana donkeys of Sicily, and donkeys in the Czech and Slovak Republics.[5,20,24,29,30] There is also some limited research looking at blood parameters in periparturient versus lactating donkeys. RBC count and HCT were higher during late pregnancy than at the time of foaling and during lactation, possibly due in part to increased water intake and fluid loss, respectively.[31] Some studies also showed sex-related differences in the mean RBC count with male donkeys having slightly higher means.[5] Other studies demonstrated just the opposite, with female donkeys having higher mean RBC counts.[32] Reticulocytes were not observed or not mentioned in the published literature on hematologic values in donkeys, which aligns with the general lack of reticulocytosis in horses.[16,25,32]

In addition to the parameters already discussed, other RBC indices are also commonly assessed as part of a complete erythrogram, including mean RBC size

(MCV), size variation (red blood cell distribution width, RDW), mean Hb content (mean corpuscular hemoglobin, MCH), and mean Hb concentration of the RBCs (MCHC). Because HCT, as reported by most hematology analyzers, is a calculation based on RBC size and count (HCT = (MCV × RBC)/10), discrepancies between HCT and PCV may be due to inaccurate RBC count or MCV as measured by the analyzer or altered packing of RBC in the microhematocrit tube used to measure PCV.[16] Microcytosis, macrocytosis, and normocytosis denote decreased, increased, and normal MCV values, respectively. Because Hb carries oxygen via the RBC, Hb serves as an accurate measure of oxygen-carrying capacity of the RBCs in the absence of hemolysis or Hb dysfunction. MCHC and MCH are both calculated values that depend on the measured Hb concentration (MCH = (Hb × 10)/RBC and MCHC = (Hb/HCT or PCV) × 100).[31] Hypochromic, hyperchromic, and normochromic are the terms used to describe decreased, increased, and normal MCHC (erythrocyte Hb concentration) values, respectively.

Several studies reported higher values for MCV, MCH, and/or MCHC in older donkeys compared with younger donkeys.[20,30] The donkeys in the study by Dezzutto and colleagues[20] were also lactating, and a greater MCH was seen in late-lactation versus early-lactation jennets. Conflicting relationships were reported in regard to RBC indices and gender, with some studies finding increased MCV, MCH, and/or MCHC in female donkeys,[27,30] and others finding increased MCH and MCHC in male donkeys.[33] Others also reported increases in MCH and MCV with increasing age in donkeys, associated with increases in PCV and Hb and decreases in RBC count.[2,5,21] An increase in MCH with increasing age was also documented in hinnies.[2] This same study showed a decrease in RDW associated with increasing age for donkeys, horses, and mules.

Other RBC morphologic features, such as the presence of inclusions, variations in RBC shape, and the pattern of arrangement, are best characterized by blood smear examination prepared from peripheral blood with a hematologic stain applied.

LEUKOGRAM

Peripheral blood leukocytes consist of neutrophils, eosinophils, and basophils (collectively called granulocytes) as well as lymphocytes and monocytes (collectively called mononuclear cells). With the exception of lymphocytes, each of these cells is produced and matures in the bone marrow. Although lymphocytes are produced by the bone marrow, they mature and proliferate in other lymphoid tissue.

Values for the total WBC count and the differential cell counts can be produced from automated analyzers but should always be confirmed with manual examination of at least 100 WBCs on a stained blood smear. The absolute differential cell count is crucial to assess because significant changes in the numbers of multiple cell types can leave the total WBC count within the RI. The blood smear examination is also useful for assessing WBC morphology, such as immature neutrophils, and evidence of accelerated granulopoiesis (band neutrophils and toxic change, respectively), dysplastic changes, reactive lymphocytes, other nuclear or cytoplasmic changes, and infectious agents.[16] Similar to the erythrogram, many leukogram parameters for donkeys appear to differ from those values established for horses.[6]

Total WBC counts tend to decrease with age across several donkey breeds and geographic regions.[23,24,26] Eosinophils showed a positive correlation with age in donkeys in most studies[20,21,24,30] with the exception of 1 study that found the opposite.[5] Likewise, conflicting results regarding the association between age and neutrophil counts also exist with some showing a decrease with age and others an increase with age.[5,30] WBC counts associated with gender also appear conflicting with female donkeys tending to have higher neutrophil values than male donkeys in some studies [15,25] and lower values than male donkeys in others.[24,27,34]

Although limited in number, studies examining the hematologic values of donkey foals have found some significant differences in the WBC values compared with horse foals, necessitating care when interpreting the leukogram in this species.[9,15]

WBC values for late gestation, after foaling, and lactating donkeys have also been examined, and WBC counts appear to be increased at foaling as compared with preparturition and postparturition.[31]

THROMBOGRAM

Platelets function in the initial hemostatic process of hemostatic plug formation in damaged vasculature. As described above with other preanalytical considerations, prompt analysis of samples is necessary for accurate platelet counts. Platelet values appear to fluctuate in the first several weeks of life for donkey foals and differ from values in adult donkeys.[9,15]

A NOTE ABOUT HYBRIDS

Literature regarding clinical pathology of mules and hinnies is extremely rare. One study compared hematological and biochemical values of clinically healthy mules, hinnies, horses, and donkeys and found significant differences between mules and hinnies in regard to RBC, WBC, magnesium, bilirubin, creatinine, and aspartate aminotransferase (AST), although further studies on larger populations are needed.[2] McLean and colleagues[2] used an automated hematology analyzer and found that the RBC and WBC counts were significantly lower, and the eosinophil differential count (EOS) was significantly higher in this group of hinnies compared with the mules. However, the hinnies in this study were also significantly older, and previous studies in donkeys have demonstrated a reduction in RBC and WBC counts and an increase in EOS with increased age as described above. As demonstrated in horses, some cell count results may vary depending on the automated analyzer used as well as between automated analyzers and manual differential cell counts.[19,35]

BLOOD PARASITES

Blood smear examination can also be useful for identification of hemoparasites. *Babesia caballi* and *Theileria equi* are the protozoans responsible for equine piroplasmosis (EP) in all members of the *Equus* genus, including donkeys and their hybrid crosses.[36] Although EP is endemic in many parts of the world, especially in tropical and subtropical climates, it is also reportable to the World Organization for Animal Health. EP is transmitted by several ticks of the genera *Hyalomma*, *Dermacentor*, and *Rhipicephalus*.[37] Contaminated needles and syringes are also capable of transmitting *T equi*. Both *T equi* and *B caballi* are intraerythrocytic parasites that invade and lyse RBCs, resulting in hemolytic anemia. In general, *B caballi* infection tends to result in milder clinical disease than that caused by *T equi*. EP in donkeys rarely causes acute disease characterized by anemia, fever, swollen eyelids, constipation, and/or splenomegaly.[36] These acute cases may be diagnosed via identification of the parasites in a blood smear examination, in which they may appear as dark dots, rings, or pear-shaped marks within RBCs.[36] EP can also result in a more chronic presentation with very nonspecific clinical signs, including weight loss, poor performance, and partial anorexia. In addition, EP in donkeys can also result in an asymptomatic infection, and often with a lower parasitemia than that typically seen in infected horses.[36] For that reason, these chronic carrier cases often require serologic testing for diagnosis. Although donkeys infected with EP may show very nonspecific signs or no clinical signs at all, they frequently have abnormal clinical pathology findings. Decreased RBC count, PCV, Hb, and Platelet Count (PLT) and increased MCH, MCHC, and WBC are common hematologic findings associated with EP in donkeys.[38,39] Currently, there is no safe and effective treatment available to clear the carrier state in donkeys, so serologic assays performed on these animals typically result in positive titers for life.[36,37]

Trypanosomiasis is another disease associated with hemoprotozoan parasites found in many parts of the world. This includes those *Trypanosoma* species that require the tsetse fly (*Glossina* spp) for transmission (*Theileria congolense* and *Theileria brucei*). *T brucei* is especially deadly to horses, but donkeys seem to be more resistant to severe disease, although serious and acute illness can occur, marked by fever, anemia, icterus, enlarged lymph nodes, and petechial hemorrhages of the mucous membranes.[36] *Theileria vivax* (which can be transmitted mechanically) and *T congolense* typically produce slightly milder clinical disease in infected equids, including anorexia, edema, and wasting.[36] *Theileria evansi* is spread mechanically by horse and stable flies. It can result in weight loss, weakness, anemia, hemoglobinuria, fever, edema, and neurologic signs or a chronic, asymptomatic, carrier state, which is more common in donkeys and mules.[34] Interestingly, transplacental transmission of *T evansi* was demonstrated in a jennet to her foal following experimental infection.[40] Dourine, caused by *Theileria equiperdum*, is transmitted mechanically during mating and is the only trypanosome that is not transmitted by an insect vector. It is also primarily a tissue parasite and rarely invades the blood. Blood smear examination or use of the centrifugation method may allow for detection of trypanosomes in acute cases with high levels of parasitemia (with the exception of *T equiperdum*, which is better diagnosed by microscopy of direct smears of fluid from infected genitalia).[36] Polymerase chain reaction (PCR) assays on EDTA whole blood can be used for diagnosis of acute disease if blood smear examinations are unrewarding. For more chronic disease states, diagnosis must rely on serologic testing modalities.

Anaplasma phagocytophilum, the causative agent of anaplasmosis in equids, is transmitted by tick vectors of the *Ixodes* species. It has been diagnosed in North and South America and parts of Europe. In equids, the most common clinical signs include fever, partial anorexia, limb edema, and ataxia. Acute anaplasmosis can often be diagnosed via observation of cytoplasmic inclusions (morulae) within neutrophils on a blood smear examination. The most common CBC change noted in this infection is a moderate thrombocytopenia, which should spur a diligent evaluation of the blood smear for organisms. Alternatively, PCR assays can be used to diagnose this disease in the early stages. With more prolonged exposure, serology tests (such as an indirect fluorescent antibody assay) can be used to look for rising titers.[36]

SERUM BIOCHEMISTRY
Hyperlipidemia and Metabolic Disease

The incidence and high mortality associated with hyperlipidemia in the donkey warrant careful evaluation of the pertinent biochemical findings that are used to support diagnosis of this disease. Opalescent serum facilitates a preliminary diagnosis, which is often confirmed by measuring serum TG concentrations.

Discrepancies across the literature in how TG are to be used to diagnose this condition highlight the fundamental difference between a value lying outside the RI and one that has diagnostic utility: a combination of sensitivity and specificity, for diagnosing a clinical disease. A value may fall well outside a RI before having diagnostic utility. The gold-standard diagnosis of the clinical disease relies on demonstration of fatty infiltrates in the liver, which is not clinically practiced nor is incorporated into most of the studies investigating diagnosis of this disease in donkeys. In the donkey, this is further confounded by the difficulties in generating breed-specific RIs. RIs for TG across breeds and studies vary greatly. A recent comparison of a bench top analyzer and point-of-care meter yielded RI of 0.82 to 3.14 mmol/L (73–278 mg/dL) and 0.87 to 3.02 mmol/L (77–267 mg/dL), respectively, in donkeys. The study included 42 healthy donkeys (breeds were not further specified) for generation of the RI, and 6 with hypertriglyceridemia were included in validation assays.[41] Metabolic parameters are affected more than many other biochemical analytes by environment, nutrition, and management practices. In a study of 45 healthy donkeys (44 mammoth and 1 miniature donkey) residing in Bryan, Texas, TG concentrations for one-third of the donkeys were above the laboratory's published reference ranges for the adult horse (Texas Veterinary Medical Diagnostic Laboratory). The donkeys were on pasture and not fed a grain diet in the study. Cholesterol concentration is not as extensively relied on for the diagnosis of hyperlipidemia, but has similar variability in reported ranges across donkey herds, breeds, and studies.[15,22,30,42]

In a retrospective analysis of 449 clinical cases of hyperlipidemia (defined as serum TG >4.4 mmol/L; 389.7 mg/dL based on the RI generated at the Donkey Sanctuary) and presence of clinical signs (not otherwise specified), 72% of the afflicted animals had another concurrent disease present.[43] In this study, hyperlipidemia was identified in 6% of the control donkeys that were devoid of clinical signs of illness. Of note, the mean serum TG concentration was much higher in nonsurvivors (14.2 mmol/L; 1257.8 mg/dL) compared with survivors (9.3 mmol/L; 823.7 mg/dL). Body condition score was not associated with an increased risk, whereas specific management practices were. One such practice was bedding on chopped cardboard, which has previously been reported to be a risk factor for colic in donkeys in the United Kingdom.[44] Time will tell if other bedding substrates that are enticing to donkeys cause similar issues in North America. Other studies have reported higher thresholds for clinically diagnosing the disease, up to 5.7 mmol/L; 504 mg/dL and associated a poor prognosis with concentrations exceeding 33.9 mmol/L; 3002.6 mg/dL.[45,46]

Another parameter pertinent to the evaluation of metabolic state that is confounded by large discrepancies in published RIs and divergent management practice is glucose. Intervals for glucose range from 96.77 ± 22.10 mg/dL (5.37 ± 1.23 mmol/L) reported in Albino donkeys[47] down to 58.35 ± 10.40 mg/dL (3.24 ± 0.58 mmol/L) in Brazilian donkeys (n = 40),[22] and even lower in Poitou donkeys (49.13 ± 3.17 mg/dL; 2.73 ± 0.18 mmol/L).[1] The procedural details provided in these publications failed to provide a maximum timeframe between blood collection and serum separation; thus, an in vitro consumption of glucose as a preanalytical variable remains a consideration.[22] Differences of this magnitude have the potential to affect clinical decisions. The use of sodium fluoride tubes to prevent enzymatic use of glucose has been used in some studies, but RIs are meant to facilitate interpretation of data generated from samples that match preanalytical procedures that the laboratory anticipates submitting clinicians would use. The authors discourage this approach because these types of tubes are rarely used for routine biochemical testing. In a separate study comparing biochemical parameters in obese and nonobese donkeys, the small differences in glucose reported: 84.2 ± 2.2 mg/dL (4.67 ± 0.12 mmol/L) compared with 74.5 ± 1.4 mg/dL (4.14 ± 0.08 mmol/L) (mean ± standard deviation [SD]), respectively, are likely of limited clinical utility.[48] The difference between these 2 stratified groups of donkeys falls within the 20% total allowable error for glucose provided in current recommendations from the ASVCP.

In addition to discrepancies in TG concentrations, reported levels of regulatory hormones are also divergent in the donkey literature. Plasma insulin and TG concentrations have been reported to positively correlate with naturally occurring disease in 1 study.[49] Unfortunately, as it is in the horse, diagnostic utility of single insulin measurement is limited in both sensitivity and specificity. Studies evaluating dynamic testing in the donkey are lacking. One study reported lower insulin concentrations in the donkey as compared with published RIs for the horse. However, this study failed to provide validation details documenting acceptable performance of the insulin assay for the donkey sample and analyzed predominantly mammoth donkeys.[50] In another study, the donkey (62 healthy animals, predominantly Andalusians) had insulin concentrations within the RI for the adult horse. In that study, dilution of plasma from a healthy donkey with experimentally induced hyperglycemia was used to verify specificity of the insulin assay used.[48] At the authors' institution, assay performance for the donkey has not been explicitly evaluated, but most donkeys analyzed have insulin concentrations that fall within the established RI for horses. However, it is important to note that most of these animals were evaluated because of a clinical suspicion for metabolic disease; thus, the range of insulin in clinically healthy donkeys may be lower than this group reflects (Dr. Barbara Schanbacher, Personal Communication, 2019).

An important note that has been recognized by investigators publishing in this area is that the marked increase in large lipoprotein particles that often occurs in hyperlipidemia can cause a solute exclusion effect and falsely lower electrolyte concentrations if an indirect ion-selective electrode method is used.[51] Indirect methods are used on most bench-top chemistry analyzers in referral laboratories, whereas direct (undiluted) procedures are often used in point-of-care testing. The different methodologies can yield vastly discrepant results (eg, pseudohyponatremia if a lipemic sample is analyzed with an indirect method), and donkey clinicians should be aware of the method used in the reference laboratory.

Enzymology

The clinical interpretation of serum enzyme activities in the donkey has largely been extrapolated from the horse. There are limited reports specifically evaluating diagnostic utility of serum enzyme activities in the donkey. Thus, the authors hypothesize that most clinical decisions are based on extrapolation from the horse or clinical experience. There are a few reports of marked changes in serum enzyme activities in association with particular diseases. For example, acute necrotizing pancreatitis owing to grain overload was reported to manifest with a marked increase in lipase and amylase activities.[52] The diagnostic sensitivity and specificity for these 2 enzymes in tandem for diagnosis of pancreatitis in the donkey are unknown.

Creatine kinase (CK) activity is higher in donkey foals for the first day of life, as has been reported in horses, and this is speculated to result from muscle compression during delivery.[15] Some studies found higher CK activity in specific donkey breeds associated with lean muscle mass, as has been reported in human athletes.[30,53] In greyhounds, an example of a canine athlete, serum creatinine concentrations are higher than reported for other breeds, but CK activity is no different.[54] A mild increase in serum CK activity was reported in a mule with *Neospora hughesi*–mediated equine protozoal myeloencephalitis.[55]

Serum Proteins

Clinical interpretation of protein parameters in donkeys depends on assessment of hydration status, breed, sex, age, lifestyle, and pathologic processes. In a donkey study in the Czech and Slovak Republics (n = 112), total protein concentration was higher in male donkeys, and older donkeys had higher globulin concentrations. The same trend toward higher albumin and total protein concentrations was documented in male Brazilian donkeys.[8] Female lactating donkeys 2 years of age had higher concentrations of alpha-2 globulins, and lower concentrations of albumin and gamma globulins compared with young donkeys between 3 and 10 years, and those older than 10 years of age as semiquantified by cellulose acetate electrophoresis.[20]

BODY CAVITY FLUIDS

No specific literature exists establishing upper limits of protein concentration and nucleated cell count in the normal fluid of body cavities of donkeys. Thus, the current limits used in the horse to distinguish normal cavity fluid (a transudate) from an exudative effusion must be used. Similarly, most of the differential diagnoses for effusions in horses and donkeys share significant overlap. For example, the bicavitary transudative effusions associated with an atypical presentation of *A phagocytophilum* infection have been documented in both the horse and the donkey. Interestingly, the pathophysiologic mechanism proposed for this clinical manifestation is vasculitis, which in the authors' experience tends to cause a higher protein concentration in the effusion than what was documented in the report (protein <2.0 g/dL).[56]

CEREBROSPINAL FLUID ANALYSIS

In the single published report specifically evaluating normal cerebrospinal fluid (CSF) in the donkey, results obtained were similar to what has been reported in the horse. The study evaluated serum and CSF from the lumbosacral space in adult miniature donkeys: 10 female donkeys and 10 male donkeys. Samples were clear and colorless with a specific gravity less than 1.002 and a nucleated cell count of 2 to 4 cells/μL. Only small lymphocytes were seen. The study also measured various biochemical analytes and compared the concentrations to serum; the gradients of the analytes measured are of unknown clinical utility at this time.[57]

EVALUATION OF THE RESPIRATORY SYSTEM

The tracheal wash and bronchoalveolar lavage are 2 common diagnostic tools used to evaluate the upper and lower airways, respectively, in both the horse and the donkey. The authors are not aware of divergent recommendations in the general evaluation of these samples for cytologic evidence of a respiratory disease process. Of specific note, the donkey is a reservoir for *Dictyocaulus arnfieldi* and typically can tolerate a high parasite burden without clinical disease. This can lead to high shedding and exposure to disease-susceptible horses in copasturing scenarios. Infested animals may have increased eosinophil counts in their tracheal and bronchoalveolar fluids. In a recent case report, coinfection with *Streptococcus equi* ssp *zooepidemicus* group C and asinine herpesvirus 5 were hypothesized to have contributed to the clinical disease. Pituitary pars intermedia dysfunction, corticosteroid administration, and overworking of donkeys are also associated with increased incidence of clinical disease.[58] The *D arnfieldi* infection is patent in the donkey, and larvae can be found in the feces via a modified Baermann method, whereas this is not the case in the horse.[59]

COAGULATION TESTING

Published reports to date highlight clinical relevant differences in coagulation testing between donkeys and horses; thus, use of equine RI or control material is not recommended. In a study of 38 healthy Andalusian donkeys and 29 Andalusian horses, both activated partial thromboplastin time (aPTT) and prothrombin time (PT) were significantly shorter in the donkey as compared with the horse. Thus, use of horse RIs may lead to underdiagnoses of hypocoagulable states in donkeys. Fibrin degradation products and D-dimers were higher in donkeys as compared with horses.[60] In a separate study, routine coagulation tests and individual coagulation factors were quantified by mixing the donkey sample with factor-deficient human plasmas over a range of proportions and measuring the recovery of clotting function. The study included 80 healthy Andalusian and crossbred donkeys along with 40 horses. The donkeys again had shorter PTs and aPTTs, although only the former achieved statistical significance. The donkeys also had significantly higher levels of factors VIIa, IX, and XI as well as proteins C and S. By thromboelastography, the activated clot time, time to peak, and clot formation rate were all shorter in the donkey. Importantly for interpretation of these differences, fibrinogen concentration and platelet counts were not different between the donkeys and the horses tested.[61]

SUMMARY

The stoic nature of donkeys and their hybrids is appreciated by those who work closely with them, and it can make diagnosis of disease challenging. Clinical pathology assays can provide a wealth of information necessary to arrive at an accurate diagnosis, but caution should be taken when interpreting results given the considerations described in this article. Further donkey and mule-specific research in the field of clinical pathology is needed to overcome the limitations that have been identified.

REFERENCES

1. Gupta AK, Varshney JP, UP. Comparative studies on biochemical indices in different breeds of equines. Indian Vet J 1994;71:26–30.

2. McLean AK, Wang W, Navas-Gonzalez FJ, et al. Reference intervals for hematological and blood biochemistry reference values in healthy mules and hinnies. Comp Clin Path 2016;25(4):871–8.

3. Friedrichs KR, Harr KE, Freeman KP, et al. ASVCP reference interval guidelines: determination of de novo reference intervals in veterinary species and other related topics. Vet Clin Pathol 2012;41(4):441–53.

4. Gutierrez JP, Marmi J, Goyache F, et al. Pedigree information reveals moderate to high levels of inbreeding and a weak population structure in the endangered Catalonian donkey breed. J Anim Breed Genet 2005;122(6):378–86.

5. Folch P, Jordana J, Cuenca R. Reference ranges and the influence of age and sex on haematological values of the endangered Catalonian donkey. Vet J 1997;154(2):163–8.

6. Burden FA, Hazell-Smith E, Mulugeta G, et al. Reference intervals for biochemical and haematological parameters in mature domestic donkeys (Equus asinus) in the UK. Equine Vet Educ 2016;28(3):134–9.

7. Morrow LD, Smith KC, Piercy RJ, et al. Retrospective analysis of post-mortem findings in 1,444 aged donkeys. J Comp Pathol 2011;144(2–3):145–56.

8. Zakari FO, Ayo JO, Rekwot PI, et al. Effects of age and season on haematological parameters of donkeys during the rainy and cold–dry seasons. Int J Biometeorol 2015;59(12):1813–24.

9. Veronesi MC, Gloria A, Panzani S, et al. Blood analysis in newborn donkeys: hematology, biochemistry, and blood gases analysis. Theriogenology 2014;82(2): 294–303.

10. Gloria A, Veronesi MC, Carluccio R, et al. Biochemical blood analysis along pregnancy in Martina Franca jennies. Theriogenology 2018;115:84–9.

11. Bain MS. Determination of albumin in caprine serum. Res Vet Sci 1986; 41(1):82–4.

12. Bush V, Reed RG. Bromocresol purple dye-binding methods underestimate albumin that is carrying covalently bound bilirubin. Clin Chem 1987;33(6):821–3.

13. Garcia Moreira V, Beridze Vaktangova N, Martinez Gago MD, et al. Overestimation of albumin measured by bromocresol green vs bromocresol purple method: influence of acute-phase globulins. Lab Med 2018;49(4):355–61.

14. Ueno T, Hirayama S, Sugihara M, et al. The bromocresol green assay, but not the modified bromocresol purple assay, overestimates the serum albumin concentration in nephrotic syndrome through reaction with alpha2-macroglobulin. Ann Clin Biochem 2016;53(Pt 1):97–105.

15. Sgorbini M, Bonelli F, Rota A, et al. Hematology and clinical chemistry in Amiata donkey foals from birth to 2 months of age. J Equine Vet Sci 2013;33(1):35–9.

16. Walton RM. Equine clinical pathology. Chichester (Unite Kingdom): John Wiley & Sons, Inc.; 2013. p. 15–35.

17. Braun J-P, Bourges-Abella N, Geffre A, et al. The preanalytic phase in veterinary clinical pathology. Vet Clin Pathol 2015;44(1):8–25.

18. Hinchcliff KW, Kociba GJ, Mitten LA. Diagnosis of EDTA dependent pseudo-thrombocytopenia in a horse. J Am Vet Med Assoc 1993;203(12):1715–6.

19. Bauer N, Nakagawa J, Dunker C, et al. Evaluation of the automated hematology analyzer Sysmex XT-2000iV compared to the ADVIA (R) 2120 for its use in dogs, cats, and horses. Part II: accuracy of leukocyte differential and reticulocyte count, impact of anticoagulant and sample aging. J Vet Diagn Invest 2012;24(1):74–89.

20. Dezzutto D, Barbero R, Valle E, et al. Observations of the hematological, hematochemical, and electrophoretic parameters in lactating donkeys (Equus asinus). J Equine Vet Sci 2018;65:1–5.

21. Laus F, Spaterna A, Faillace V, et al. Reference values for hematological and biochemical parameters of mixed breed donkeys (Equus asinus). Wulfenia J 2015;22(1):294–304.

22. Mori E, Fernandes WR, Mirandola RMS, et al. Reference values on serum biochemical parameters of Brazilian donkey (Equus asinus) breed. J Equine Vet Sci 2003;23(8):358–64.

23. Folch P, States WU. Reference ranges and the influence of age and sex on donkey 1997;154(2):163–8.

24. Girardi AM, Marques LC, de Toledo CZP, et al. Hematological variables of the Pêga donkey (Equus asinus) breed: influence of age and sex. Comp Clin Path 2015;24(2):335–42.

25. Gupta A, Varshney J, Ghei J, et al. Some haemato-biochemical studies in Indian donkeys (Equus asinus). Indian Vet J 1992;69:21–4.

26. French J, Patrick V. Reference values for physiological, haematological and biochemical parameters in domestic donkeys (Equus asinus)itle. Equine Vet Educ 1995;7(1):33–5.

27. Zinkl JG, Mae D, Guzman Merida P, et al. Reference ranges and the influence of age and sex on hematologic and serum biochemical values in donkeys (Equus asinus). Am J Vet Res 1990;51(3):408–13.

28. Harvey JW, Asquith RL, McNulty PK, et al. Haematology of foals up to one year old. Equine Vet J 1984;16(4):347–53.

29. Caldin M, Furlanello T, Solano-Gallego L, et al. Reference ranges for haematology, biochemical profile and electrophoresis in a single herd of Ragusana donkeys from Sicily (Italy). Comp Clin Path 2005;14(1):5–12.

30. Sedlinská M, Horáčková E, Vyvial M, et al. Biochemical and haematological profile of donkeys in the Czech and Slovak republics: influence of age and sex. Acta Vet Brno 2017;86(2):151–7.

31. Bonelli F, Rota A, Corazza M, et al. Hematological and biochemical findings in pregnant, postfoaling, and lactating jennies. Theriogenology 2016;1:1–6.

32. Nayeri G. Blood characteristics of the adult donkey. Zentralbl Veterinarmed A 1978;25:541–7.

33. Babeker EA, Abdalbagi Y. Hematological profile of donkey (Equus asinus) breed in White Nile State, Sudan. Sci Rep 2014;10:218–28.

34. Mori E, Mirandola RMS, Ferreira RR, et al. Reference values on hematologic parameters of the Brazilian donkey (Equus asinus) breed. J Equine Vet Sci 2004; 24(7):271–6.

35. Tvedten HW, Korcal D. Automated differential leukocyte count in horses, cattle, and cats using the Technicon H-1E hematology system. Vet Clin Pathol 1996; 25(1):14–22.

36. Brooke. The working equid veterinary manual. 8th edition. Essex (United Kingdom): Whittet Books Limited; 2013. p. 469–500.

37. Kumar S, Kumar R, Sugimoto C. A perspective on Theileria equi infections in donkeys. Jpn J Vet Res 2009;56(4):171–80.

38. Davitkov D, Davitkov D, Vucicevic M, et al. A molecular and haematological study of *Theileria equi* in Balkan donkeys. Acta Vet Hung 2017;65(2):234–41.

39. Laus F, Spaterna A, Faillace V, et al. Clinical investigation on Theileria equi and Babesia caballi infections in Italian donkeys. BMC Vet Res 2015;11:100.

40. Kumar R, Kumar S, Virmani N, et al. Journal of equine veterinary science transplacental transmission of Trypanosoma evansi from experimentally infected donkey mare to neonatal foal. J Equine Vet Sci 2015;35(4):337–41.

41. Pongratz MC, Junge HK, Riond B, et al. Validation of the Accutrend Plus point-of-care triglyceride analyzer in horses, ponies, and donkeys. J Vet Emerg Crit Care (San Antonio) 2016;26(5):682–90.

42. Jordana J, Folch P, Cuenca R. Clinical biochemical parameters of the endangered Catalonian donkey breed: normal values and the influence of sex, age, and management practices effect. Res Vet Sci 1998;64(1):7–10.

43. Burden FA, Du Toit N, Hazell-Smith E, et al. Hyperlipemia in a population of aged donkeys: description, prevalence, and potential risk factors. J Vet Intern Med 2011;25(6):1420–5.

44. Cox R, Burden F, Gosden L, et al. Case control study to investigate risk factors for impaction colic in donkeys in the UK. Prev Vet Med 2009;92(3):179–87.

45. Tarrant JM, Campbell TM, Parry BW. Hyperlipaemia in a donkey. Aust Vet J 1998; 76(7):466–9.

46. Naylor JM, Kronfeld DS, Acland H. Hyperlipemia in horses: effects of undernutrition and disease. Am J Vet Res 1980;41(6):899–905.

47. Cubeddu GM, Bini PP, Floris B, et al. Costanti ematiche dell'asinello bianco dell'asinara. Boll Soc Ital Biol Sper 1991;67:577–84.

48. Mendoza FJ, Estepa JC, Gonzalez-De Cara CA, et al. Energy-related parameters and their association with age, gender, and morphometric measurements in healthy donkeys. Vet J 2015;204(2):201–7.
49. Forhead AJ, Dobson H. Plasma glucose and cortisol responses to exogenous insulin in fasted donkeys. Res Vet Sci 1997;62(3):265–9.
50. Dugat SL, Taylor TS, Matthews NS, et al. Values for triglycerides, insulin, cortisol, and ACTH in a herd of normal donkeys. J Equine Vet Sci 2010;30(3):141–4.
51. Burtis C, Ashwood E, Bruns D. Tietz fundamentals of clinical chemistry. In: Sawyer B, editor. Scool of allied health sciences TTUHSC. 8th edition. Saunders; 2008. p. 434–5. St Louis (MO).
52. Kiuchi MG, Souto HB, Kiuchi T, et al. Case report. Medicine 2015;94(46):e2094.
53. Brancaccio P, Maffulli N, Limongelli FM. Creatine kinase monitoring in sport medicine. Br Med Bull 2007;81-82(1):209–30.
54. Zaldívar-López S, Marín LM, Iazbik MC, et al. Clinical pathology of Greyhounds and other sighthounds. Vet Clin Pathol 2011;40(4):414–25.
55. Finno CJ, Eaton JS, Aleman M, et al. Equine protozoal myeloencephalitis due to Neospora hughesi and equine motor neuron disease in a mule. Vet Ophthalmol 2010;13(4):259–65.
56. Restifo MM, Bedenice D, Thane KE, et al. Cavitary effusion associated with Anaplasma phagocytophilum infection in 2 equids. J Vet Intern Med 2015;29(2): 732–5.
57. Mozaffari AA, Samadieh H. Analysis of serum and cerebrospinal fluid in clinically normal adult miniature donkeys. N Z Vet J 2013;61(5):297–9.
58. The Donkey Sanctuary. The Clinical Companion of the Donkey. 1st Edition. Leicestershire (UK): Matador; 2017. p. 153-4.
59. Grimes C, Culang D. What is your diagnosis? Transtracheal wash from a donkey. Vet Clin Pathol 2018;47(1):162–3.
60. Mendoza FJ, Perez-Ecija RA, Monreal L, et al. Coagulation profiles of healthy andalusian donkeys are different than those of healthy horses. J Vet Intern Med 2011;25(4):967–70.
61. Perez-Ecija A, Mendoza FJ. Characterisation of clotting factors, anticoagulant protein activities and viscoelastic analysis in healthy donkeys. Equine Vet J 2017;49(6):734–8.

Genetics, Evolution, and Physiology of Donkeys and Mules

Margaret M. Brosnahan, DVM, PhD

KEYWORDS

- Equine • Cytogenetics • Evolution • Genomics • Hybrid • Mule • Hinny • Donkey

KEY POINTS

- The species that make up the genus *Equus* are closely related in geologic time, but are karyotypically diverse, with chromosome numbers ranging from 2n = 32 to 2n = 66.
- Despite karyotype variability, interspecies breeding between all members of the genus can produce offspring that are healthy and viable, yet most often sterile.
- Cytogenetic studies and recent advances in genome sequencing and applied genomics have improved our understanding of the evolutionary relationships between equine species.
- Veterinarians focusing their clinical practice on the domestic horse are likely to encounter donkeys and the horse–donkey hybrids, the mule and the hinny.
- Characteristics unique to donkeys and hybrids may be clinically important, and should be considered in the diagnosis and treatment of disease in these animals.

INTRODUCTION

Donkeys, horses, and zebras make up the sole genus *Equus* in the family Equidae. The domestic donkey, *Equus africanus asinus*, is a subspecies of the African wild ass, along with the Nubian and Somali wild asses. The remaining living members of the genus include 2 species of Asian wild ass, 3 species of zebra, the domestic horse, and Przewalski's horse.[1] Although the number of chromosomes in these species ranges from 2n = 32 in Hartmann's zebra to 2n = 66 in Przewalski's horse,[2,3] interspecies breeding can produce healthy, but most often sterile, hybrid offspring. The most commonly encountered of these is the mule, produced by the mating of a mare and a jack donkey. The reciprocal cross, a stallion and a jenny donkey, produces the hinny.

Domestication of the donkey occurred an estimated 5000 years ago. Domestic populations originated from 2 discrete wild ass populations, most probably in Northeast

Disclosure Statement: The author has nothing to disclose.
College of Veterinary Medicine, Midwestern University, 19555 North 59th Avenue, Cactus Wren Hall 336-P, Glendale, AZ 85308, USA
E-mail address: mbrosn@midwestern.edu

Africa.[4] Domesticated donkeys were brought to South America in the fifteenth century from both Spanish and Northern African sources, and eventually to the West Indies. Catalan and other European breeds of donkey were imported to North America in the eighteenth and nineteenth centuries.[5,6] The existence of the horse–donkey hybrids is documented back to at least 3000 years ago. Mules were prized for many tasks from farming to harness racing in ancient Greece, and were bred as draft animals throughout Europe for centuries, most notably in France and Italy. In North America, mules were favored for military and agricultural purposes beginning in the 1700s.[7] In the present day, the donkey population is estimated to be at least 40 million animals worldwide.[8] Donkeys and their hybrids are used throughout the world as work or pack animals, for pleasure and competitive equestrian activities, and as companions. In some regions where there is increasing interest in donkey milk as a food staple because of its favorable nutrient profile, the donkey can be considered a production animal.[9]

Veterinarians who focus their clinical practice on the domestic horse may be asked to work on other equids, or may seek out such opportunities through equitarian initiatives. Donkeys and horse–donkey hybrids are the most likely to be encountered, but on occasion zebras and the less common zebroid hybrids may be presented by zoos or private owners.[10] A basic understanding of the evolutionary relationship between these species and the chromosomal makeup of their hybrids may be helpful to practitioners in several ways. First, it reinforces the important concept that each is in fact a distinct species and that "donkeys are not just little horses." Each species first evolved for adaptation to a different climate, horses on the cooler Eurasian grasslands, and donkeys in the hotter, drier African deserts.[8] Some then were domesticated and selectively bred for specific purposes. Subsequently, interspecies breeding was undertaken, creating hybrid offspring with unique chromosomal, physical, and physiologic characteristics. This process has resulted in differences in anatomy and physiology between domestic horses and other equids that are relevant to clinical practice. Second, it may help the practitioner to adapt their knowledge of the domestic horse in the safest and most effective way in situations where research on other equids is lacking. Third, it will improve the practitioner's general understanding of cytogenetics and when this may be a valuable clinical tool to investigate breeding, fertility problems, or developmental anomalies. Fourth, it will foster an appreciation for the natural and cultural histories of living equids and the humans that share their habitats.[11–13] Competent veterinary care is important for the welfare of working equids in developing countries, and for the conservation of those that are rare or endangered such as Grevy's zebra[14] and many Italian donkey breeds.[15] Finally, it will create an awareness of current genomics technologies, and the many ways in which the equid genomes have contributed to scientific research and continue to do so in the postgenomic era.[16]

CYTOGENETICS
Evolution of Equine Karyotypes

Today's equid species evolved from a common ancestor that lived approximately 4 million years ago. It was at about this time that the domestic horse became the first to diverge from the common lineage. The African asses, of which the domestic donkey is a member, were the next to diverge, approximately 2.1 million years ago, with the final split between Asiatic asses and zebras occurring about 1.9 million years ago.[2]

Although these timeframes are considered to be quite recent in geological time, subsequent chromosomal evolution occurred comparatively rapidly.[2] The defining karyotypes of each surviving species therefore show wide variation in number and structure, reflective of the cumulative effects of chromosomal rearrangements, including centromere repositioning, translocations, and inversions.[1,17,18] Centromere repositioning is a process by which a new centromere forms and the original one ceases to function but the rest of the chromosome retains its integrity. This process has occurred many times in the evolution of the genus *Equus* and the formation of the equid species.[19] Centric fusion or Robertsonian translocation is thought to be the most common type of translocation in equid evolution,[2] and it is a single such event involving chromosome 5 from the domestic horse and chromosomes 23 and 24 from Przewalski's horse that distinguishes the karyotypes of these 2 species.[3,20]

Historically, the scientific investigation of equine karyotypes arose from a desire to understand the problem of infertility, particularly in the equine hybrids.[21] More recently, and with the advent of increasingly sophisticated genomics techniques, equine karyotypes and genomes have become important tools for the study of speciation, domestication,[22] and epigenomics. The ability to identify the parent of origin of the chromosomes of hybrids makes them particularly useful as model organisms for the study of parental imprinting and chromosome organization within the nucleus.[23,24] Equid chromosomes also have unique structural characteristics, such as satellite free centromeres, that facilitate investigation of the basic biological principles of chromosome structure.[25]

Although early reports of chromosome numbers in the domestic horse varied, it was determined definitively in 1959 that the domestic horse had a diploid chromosome number of 64. Since that time, the standard karyotype of the domestic horse has undergone periodic revision for the clarification and improvement of uniform reporting in the face of new banding and mapping technologies.[26–28] Shortly thereafter, the diploid chromosome number in the domestic donkey was identified correctly as 62, with 1 notable gross difference from the horse being the presence of more metacentric chromosomes.[29] As with the horse, subsequent work has refined the standard presentation of the donkey karyotype,[26,30] characterized evolutionarily significant structural components such as the evolutionary new centromere on donkey chromosome (EAS) 13,[2] and identified horse and human homologues.[21,31–33]

Equine hybrids typically have a diploid chromosome number that is the sum of the haploid chromosome number of each parent. The horse–donkey hybrids each have a diploid number of 63, reflecting 32 from the horse parent and 31 from the donkey parent.[26,29] Similar findings have been made in the investigation of donkey–zebra and horse–zebra hybrids. The offspring of a domestic donkey sire and a Grevy zebra dam possessed 48 chromosomes, with 31 from the donkey and 17 presumed from the zebra,[34] whereas a diploid number of 53 was found in a domestic donkey—Burchell's zebra hybrid, including 22 from the zebra sire and 31 from the donkey dam.[35] The presentation of hybrid karyotypes understandably lacks the paired chromosome layout characteristic of the karyotypes of distinct species, and instead they often are ordered by centromere position.[26] Although conventional karyotyping methods historically resulted in hybrid karyotypes in which the parent of origin of some chromosomes was uncertain,[26] newer chromosome painting technologies have resulted in complete and accurate karyotypes for even the less common equine hybrids.[35]

Effect of Karyotypes on Fertility

The outcome of these highly variable but evolutionarily proximate karyotypes is that although equids of different species may interbreed and produce viable offspring, those offspring, such as mules, hinnies, and zebroid hybrids, are most commonly infertile. In male hybrids, meiosis fails in primary spermatocytes because of an inability of chromosomes to pair properly at the synaptic stage, although rarely normal gametes may form. Hybrid females are born with few oocytes.[36] *Prdm9*, a gene encoding a methyltransferase specific to meiosis and known to be associated with sterility in hybrid mice, does not seem to play a role in equine hybrid sterility.[37] Cytogenetic studies have demonstrated the theoretic potential for the formation of multivalents during meiotic chromosome pairing to result in viable, genetically complete gametes with a haploid number of 28 to 35. Successful breeding with a donkey or horse of the opposite sex could then occur, producing offspring with a diploid chromosome number anywhere from 59 to 67.[38]

The notable exception to hybrid infertility is the domestic horse–Przewalski's horse hybrid, which is consistently fertile. The effect of the Robertsonian translocation is the formation of a trivalent during meiosis. Offspring of the hybrids and a domestic horse may have diploid chromosome numbers of 64 or 65 and resemble a domestic horse or Przewalski's horse, respectively.[39,40]

Clinical Cytogenetics

Cytogenetics techniques have proven to be useful tools in the assessment of clinical problems of the horse, including sex reversal syndromes, and developmental anomalies attributed to aberrant autosomes.[27,41] These techniques can be equally useful for those working on donkeys and hybrids, particularly with respect to conservation efforts, for example, with rare or endangered donkey breeds when assessing infertility is of paramount importance. Specifically with respect to hybrids, cytogenetic analysis has been used to confirm[42] or refute[43] the occasional claims of hybrid fertility. More recently, a multiplex polymerase chain reaction test using mitochondrial DNA has been developed to allow identification of hinnies and mules via molecular rather than cytogenetic means when their breeding is unknown.[44]

GENOME SEQUENCING

Technology enabling whole genome sequencing has been of significant benefit to our understanding of the evolution of equine species as well as for the investigation of clinical diseases at the molecular level. The genome sequence of the domestic horse was published in 2009.[45] The first assembly of the donkey genome was produced in 2013,[46] and additional assemblies of the donkey genome have been generated since that time.[1,47–49] Most recently, the genomes of all remaining living equids were sequenced, along with that of the extinct quagga. A comparison of all equine genomes suggests that gene flow has occurred between equine species, supporting the possibility of fertile hybrids rather than complete reproductive isolation in the evolution of these species.[17]

GENETIC DIVERSITY

Genetic diversity has been investigated extensively in individual donkey breeds and in geographically defined populations. In the former case, this represents conservation efforts aimed at preserving breeds of historical and cultural importance. Diminished use of donkeys in agriculture resulted in near extinction of breeds such as the Martina Franca donkey of Italy, long prized for mule breeding because of its tall stature.[50] Similar efforts have been undertaken for breeds in Spain,[51] Portugal,[52] and Brazil.[53] This contrasts with observations in North America, where no similar studies are reported. Despite their role in the history of the American West, donkeys are considered exotic species and have more frequently been the target of extermination rather than conservation.[11]

In the second instance, genetic diversity is investigated as a mean to refine the identification of the centers of donkey origin and domestication to areas of Africa,[54] Serbia,[55] and Central and South America.[5] Studies of genetic diversity have been supported by techniques such as microsatellite typing,[15,56] computer modeling and pedigree analysis,[50,53] and mitochondrial DNA analysis.[57,58] Pathogen-driven selection has been assessed using variation in major histocompatibility genes as well as microsatellites.[59]

PHENOTYPIC DIVERSITY

Genetics necessarily influence the phenotypic diversity observed in living donkey breeds, with the physical characteristics of hybrids a function of the species, breed, and gender of each parent. Of equal importance for veterinarians accustomed to practicing on the domestic horse is an appreciation for the differences that exist between the domestic horse and other equids and hybrids. The implication of genetic variation across the equine species and hybrids as described elsewhere in this article is that the data generated specifically for the horse, such as laboratory reference ranges, drug doses, husbandry practices, and procedural techniques, may not be directly applicable to non-caballine equids. In some instances, these differences have already been identified at a molecular level, whereas for others our knowledge is based purely on phenotype. Representative differences that are or may be of clinical significance are described briefly here.

Hair Coat and Coat Color

Donkey hair is lighter and shorter than horse hair, and unlike horses, donkeys do not grow winter coats. The length and thickness of the coat, and therefore its role in thermoregulation, do not vary significantly with season. This is likely a result of donkeys evolving in warmer and drier climates than horses, and is an important consideration in husbandry practices. The mule hair coat is overall more similar to the horse, although intermediate between the horse and donkey in some respects. Mules do seem to grow winter coats.[60] The rare Poitou donkey of France is well-known for its long haircoat, unique among equids and caused by recessive mutations in the fibroblast growth factor 5 (FGF5) gene.[61]

Coat color associations with genetic disease in the donkey are not identified in the literature as for the domestic horse.[62–65] Known genetic mutations affecting coat color in donkeys include a recessive mutation in the melanocortin 1 receptor (MC1R) gene producing a red coat,[66] and a mutation in the agouti signaling protein (ASIP) gene resulting in the absence of light points.[67] White spotting is caused by a mutation in the KIT gene.[68] Albinism caused by a recessive mutation in the tyrosinase (TYR) gene has been identified in a population of feral donkeys in Italy.[69] These donkeys have adapted to sun exposure via increased serum retinol.[70]

Serology and Hematology

Differences are evident between the serum proteomes of the donkey and horse, with the mule being more similar to the donkey.[71] The hemoglobin structure of the donkey and horse differ from each other, with mule hemoglobin having characteristics of both.[72] Coagulation profiles differ between donkeys and horses.[73,74] Differences in red blood cell antigens between the donkey and the horse are well-known to result in a high incidence of neonatal isoerythrolysis in mule foals.[75,76]

Metabolic Parameters

Evidence exists for differences in both glucose and lipid metabolism between donkeys and horses.[77–79] This may be a function of the different environments in which they evolved. Donkeys show a more rapid decrease in glucose and lower levels of lactate than horses during low and high intensity exercise, respectively.[80] Thyroid hormone and melatonin concentrations are higher in the serum of donkeys than of horses.[81,82]

Musculoskeletal Anatomy

Radiographic parameters of the normal donkey foot differ from those of the horse, and may affect the evaluation of the laminitic foot.[83] Physes of the distal limb in the donkey close later than in the horse.[84] Variations exist in the vertebral formulas of the donkey and horse.[85]

Respiratory Tract

The donkey has a deep pharyngeal recess and narrower nasal ventral meatus, which can create difficulty in the passage of a nasogastric tube.[86]

Ocular System

Ultrasonographically obtained biometric measurements made of donkey eyes suggest that they are considerably smaller than horse eyes.[87]

Behavior, Social Structure, and Intelligence

Social behaviors including dominance and preference to associate with the same species have been observed in ponies, donkeys, and mules living in herd setting, and have been attributed to a genetic basis.[88] Intelligence in mules that surpasses that of the horse or the donkey is attributed to hybrid vigor.[89]

Infectious and Parasitic Diseases

Donkeys seem to be less susceptible to infection with equine infectious anemia virus,[90] and mules may be less likely to develop EHV-1 myeloencephalopathy after infection.[91] In these cases, infected animals may act as silent carriers of disease. Donkeys are known to be the natural hosts of the lungworm *Dictyocaulus arnfieldi*, maintaining patent but clinically inapparent infections. Horses, by contrast, develop clinical signs following infection, typically from cohabitation with donkeys.[92] The epidemiology of lungworm in horse–donkey hybrids has not been studied in depth.

SUMMARY

An understanding of the evolution and genetics of the genus *Equus* and its extant species is of benefit to veterinarians working in equine practice as well as those interested in conservation. When working with non-caballine equids, veterinarians should always consider that direct application of data relevant to the horse may be suboptimal in their diagnosis and treatment.

REFERENCES

1. Renaud G, Petersen B, Seguin-Orlando A, et al. Improved de novo genomic assembly for the domestic donkey. Sci Adv 2018;4(4):eaaq0392.
2. Musilova P, Kubickova S, Vahala J, et al. Subchromosomal karyotype evolution in Equidae. Chromosome Res 2013;21(2):175–87.

3. Ahrens E, Stranzinger G. Comparative chromosomal studies of E. caballus (ECA) and E. przewalskii (EPR) in a female F1 hybrid. J Anim Breed Genet 2005; 122(Suppl 1):97–102.

4. Beja-Pereira A, England PR, Ferrand N, et al. African origins of the domestic donkey. Science 2004;304(5678):1781.

5. Jordana J, Ferrando A, Miro J, et al. Genetic relationships among American donkey populations: insights into the process of colonization. J Anim Breed Genet 2016;133(2):155–64.

6. Katic U. The transportation of mules from South America to the West Indies in the 1860s. Hist Med Vet 1998;23(1):3–23.

7. Savory TH. The mule. Sci Am 1970;223(6):102–9.

8. Senior JM. Not small horses: improving treatments for donkeys. Vet Rec 2013; 173(12):292–3.

9. Ali M, Baber M, Hussain T, et al. The contribution of donkeys to human health. Equine Vet J 2014;46(6):766–7.

10. Wiedner EB, Lindsay WA, Isaza R. Management of zebras and zebra hybrids (zebroids). Compend Contin Educ Vet 2012;34(9):E4.

11. Wills J. Brighty, donkeys and conservation in the Grand Canyon. Endeavour 2006;30(3):113–7.

12. Berger TE, Peters J, Grupe G. Life history of a mule (c. 160 AD) from the Roman Fort Biriciana/WeiBenburg (Upper Bavaria) as revealed by serial stable isotope analysis of dental tissues. Int J Osteoarchaeol 2010;20:158–71.

13. Devriese L. From mules, horses and livestock to companion animals: a linguistic-etymological approach to veterinary history, mirroring animal and (mainly) human welfare. Vlaams Diergeneeskd Tijdschr 2012;81:237–46.

14. Rubenstein D, Low Mackey B, Davidson Z, et al. Equus grevi. The IUCN Red List of Threatened Species. 2016: e.T7950A89624491.

15. Colli L, Perrotta G, Negrini R, et al. Detecting population structure and recent demographic history in endangered livestock breeds: the case of the Italian autochthonous donkeys. Anim Genet 2013;44(1):69–78.

16. Short RV. The contribution of the mule to scientific thought. J Reprod Fertil Suppl 1975;(23):359–64.

17. Jonsson H, Schubert M, Seguin-Orlando A, et al. Speciation with gene flow in equids despite extensive chromosomal plasticity. Proc Natl Acad Sci U S A 2014;111(52):18655–60.

18. Trifonov VA, Musilova P, Kulemsina AI. Chromosome evolution in perissodactyla. Cytogenet Genome Res 2012;137(2–4):208–17.

19. Carbone L, Nergadze SG, Magnani E, et al. Evolutionary movement of centromeres in horse, donkey, and zebra. Genomics 2006;87(6):777–82.

20. Myka JL, Lear TL, Houck ML, et al. FISH analysis comparing genome organization in the domestic horse (Equus caballus) to that of the Mongolian wild horse (E. przewalskii). Cytogenet Genome Res 2003;102(1–4):222–5.

21. Raudsepp T, Christensen K, Chowdhar BP. Cytogenetics of donkey chromosomes: nomenclature proposal based on GTG-banded chromosomes and depiction of NORs and telomeric sites. Chromosome Res 2000;8(8):659–70.

22. Kimura B, Marshall FB, Chen S, et al. Ancient DNA from Nubian and Somali wild ass provides insights into donkey ancestry and domestication. Proc Biol Sci 2011;278(1702):50–7.

23. Hepperger C, Mayer A, Merz J, et al. Parental genomes mix in mule and human cell nuclei. Chromosoma 2009;118(3):335–47.

24. Wang X, Miller DC, Harman R, et al. Paternally expressed genes predominate in the placenta. Proc Natl Acad Sci U S A 2013;110(26):10705–10.

25. Giulotto E, Raimondi E, Sullivan KF. The unique DNA sequences underlying equine centromeres. Prog Mol Subcell Biol 2017;56:337–54.

26. Eldridge F, Blazak WF. Horse, ass, and mule chromosomes. J Hered 1976;67(6): 361–7.

27. Lear TL, Bailey E. Equine clinical cytogenetics: the past and future. Cytogenet Genome Res 2008;120(1–2):42–9.

28. Richer CL, Power MM, Klunder LR, et al. Standard karyotype of the domestic horse (Equus caballus). Committee for standardized karyotype of Equus caballus. The Second International Conference for Standardization of Domestic Animal Karyotypes, INRA, Jouy-en Josas, France, 22nd-26th May 1989. Hereditas 1990; 112(3):289–93.

29. Benirschke K, Brownhill LE, Beath MM. Somatic chromosomes of the horse, the donkey and their hybrids, the mule and the hinny. J Reprod Fertil 1962;4:319–26.

30. Di Meo GP, Perucatti A, Peretti V, et al. The 450-band resolution G- and R-banded standard karyotype of the donkey (Equus asinus, 2n = 62). Cytogenet Genome Res 2009;125(4):266–71.

31. Raudsepp T, Chowdhary BP. Construction of chromosome-specific paints for meta- and submetacentric autosomes and the sex chromosomes in the horse and their use to detect homologous chromosomal segments in the donkey. Chromosome Res 1999;7(2):103–14.

32. Raudsepp T, Kijas J, Godard S, et al. Comparison of horse chromosome 3 with donkey and human chromosomes by cross-species painting and heterologous FISH mapping. Mamm Genome 1999;10(3):277–82.

33. Raudsepp T, Otte K, Rozell B, et al. FISH mapping of the IGF2 gene in horse and donkey-detection of homoeology with HSA11. Mamm Genome 1997;8(8):569–72.

34. Benirschke K, Low RJ, Brownhill LE, et al. Chromosome studies of a donkey-grevy zebra hybrid. Chromosoma 1964;15:1–13.

35. Iannuzzi A, Pereira J, Iannuzzi C, et al. Pooling strategy and chromosome painting characterize a living zebroid for the first time. PLoS One 2017;12(7): e0180158.

36. Chandley AC, Jones RC, Dott HM, et al. Meiosis in interspecific equine hybrids. I. The male mule (Equus asinus X E. caballus) and hinny (E. caballus X E. asinus). Cytogenet Cell Genet 1974;13(4):330–41.

37. Steiner CC, Ryder OA. Characterization of Prdm9 in equids and sterility in mules. PLoS One 2013;8(4):e61746.

38. Yang F, Fu B, O'Brien PC, et al. Refined genome-wide comparative map of the domestic horse, donkey and human based on cross-species chromosome painting: insight into the occasional fertility of mules. Chromosome Res 2004;12(1): 65–76.

39. Chandley AC, Short RV, Allen WR. Cytogenetic studies of three equine hybrids. J Reprod Fertil Suppl 1975;(23):356–70.

40. Short RV, Chandley AC, Jones RC, et al. Meiosis in interspecific equine hybrids. II. The przewalski horse/domestic horse hybrid. Cytogenet Cell Genet 1974; 13(5):465–78.

41. Halnan CR. Equine cytogenetics: role in equine veterinary practice. Equine Vet J 1985;17(3):173–7.

42. Ryder OA, Chemnick LG, Bowling AT, et al. Male mule foal qualifies as the offspring of a female mule and jack donkey. J Hered 1985;76(5):379–81.

43. Trommershausen-Bowling A, Millon L. Centric fission in the karyotype of a mother-daughter pair of donkeys (Equus asinus). Cytogenet Cell Genet 1988;47(3): 152–4.

44. Franco MM, Santos JB, Mendonca AS, et al. Short Communication Quick method for identifying horse (Equus caballus) and donkey (Equus asinus) hybrids. Genet Mol Res 2016;15(3).

45. Wade CM, Giulotto E, Sigurdsson S, et al. Genome sequence, comparative analysis, and population genetics of the domestic horse. Science 2009;326(5954): 865–7.

46. Orlando L, Ginolhac A, Zhang G, et al. Recalibrating Equus evolution using the genome sequence of an early Middle Pleistocene horse. Nature 2013; 499(7456):74–8.

47. Bertolini F, Scimone C, Geraci C, et al. Next generation semiconductor based sequencing of the donkey (Equus asinus) genome provided comparative sequence data against the horse genome and a few millions of single nucleotide polymorphisms. PLoS One 2015;10(7):e0131925.

48. Huang J, Zhao Y, Bai D, et al. Corrigendum: donkey genome and insight into the imprinting of fast karyotype evolution. Sci Rep 2015;5:17124.

49. Huang J, Zhao Y, Bai D, et al. Donkey genome and insight into the imprinting of fast karyotype evolution. Sci Rep 2015;5:14106.

50. Rizzi R, Tullo E, Cito AM, et al. Monitoring of genetic diversity in the endangered Martina Franca donkey population. J Anim Sci 2011;89(5):1304–11.

51. Navas FJ, Jordana J, Leon JM, et al. A model to infer the demographic structure evolution of endangered donkey populations. Animal 2017;11(12):2129–38.

52. Quaresma M, Martins AM, Rodrigues JB, et al. Pedigree and herd characterization of a donkey breed vulnerable to extinction. Animal 2014;8(3):354–9.

53. Santana ML Jr, Bignardi AB. Status of the genetic diversity and population structure of the Pega donkey. Trop Anim Health Prod 2015;47(8):1573–80.

54. Rosenbom S, Costa V, Al-Araimi N, et al. Genetic diversity of donkey populations from the putative centers of domestication. Anim Genet 2015;46(1):30–6.

55. Stanisic LJ, Aleksic JM, Dimitrijevic V, et al. New insights into the origin and the genetic status of the Balkan donkey from Serbia. Anim Genet 2017;48(5):580–90.

56. Bordonaro S, Guastella AM, Criscione A, et al. Genetic diversity and variability in endangered Pantesco and two other Sicilian donkey breeds assessed by microsatellite markers. ScientificWorldJournal 2012;2012:648427.

57. Cozzi MC, Valiati P, Cherchi R, et al. Mitochondrial DNA genetic diversity in six Italian donkey breeds (Equus asinus). Mitochondrial DNA A DNA Mapp Seq Anal 2018;29(3):409–18.

58. Vilstrup JT, Seguin-Orlando A, Stiller M, et al. Mitochondrial phylogenomics of modern and ancient equids. PLoS One 2013;8(2):e55950.

59. Vranova M, Alloggio I, Qablan M, et al. Genetic diversity of the class II major histocompatibility DRA locus in European, Asiatic and African domestic donkeys. Infect Genet Evol 2011;11(5):1136–41.

60. Osthaus B, Proops L, Long S, et al. Hair coat properties of donkeys, mules and horses in a temperate climate. Equine Vet J 2018;50(3):339–42.

61. Legrand R, Tiret L, Abitbol M. Two recessive mutations in FGF5 are associated with the long-hair phenotype in donkeys. Genet Sel Evol 2014;46:65.

62. Bellone RR, Holl H, Setaluri V, et al. Evidence for a retroviral insertion in TRPM1 as the cause of congenital stationary night blindness and leopard complex spotting in the horse. PLoS One 2013;8(10):e78280.

63. Sandmeyer LS, Bellone RR, Archer S, et al. Congenital stationary night blindness is associated with the leopard complex in the Miniature Horse. Vet Ophthalmol 2012;15(1):18–22.

64. Brooks SA, Gabreski N, Miller D, et al. Whole-genome SNP association in the horse: identification of a deletion in myosin Va responsible for Lavender Foal syndrome. PLoS Genet 2010;6(4):e1000909.

65. Metallinos DL, Bowling AT, Rine J. A missense mutation in the endothelin-B receptor gene is associated with Lethal White Foal Syndrome: an equine version of Hirschsprung disease. Mamm Genome 1998;9(6):426–31.

66. Abitbol M, Legrand R, Tiret L. A missense mutation in melanocortin 1 receptor is associated with the red coat colour in donkeys. Anim Genet 2014;45(6):878–80.

67. Abitbol M, Legrand R, Tiret L. A missense mutation in the agouti signaling protein gene (ASIP) is associated with the no light points coat phenotype in donkeys. Genet Sel Evol 2015;47:28.

68. Fenn DJ, Raudsepp T, Cothran EG, et al. Validation of a candidate causative mutation for white spotting in donkeys. Anim Genet 2017;48(1):124–5.

69. Utzeri VJ, Bertolini F, Ribani A, et al. The albinism of the feral Asinara white donkeys (Equus asinus) is determined by a missense mutation in a highly conserved position of the tyrosinase (TYR) gene deduced protein. Anim Genet 2016;47(1): 120–4.

70. Cappai MG, Lunesu MG, Accioni F, et al. Blood serum retinol levels in Asinara white donkeys reflect albinism-induced metabolic adaptation to photoperiod at Mediterranean latitudes. Ecol Evol 2017;7(1):390–8.

71. Henze A, Aumer F, Grabner A, et al. Genetic differences in the serum proteome of horses, donkeys and mules are detectable by protein profiling. Br J Nutr 2011; 106(Suppl 1):S170–3.

72. Isaacs WA. Gene expression in an interspecific hybrid: analysis of hemoglobins in donkey, horse, and mule by peptide mapping. Biochem Genet 1970;4(1): 73–85.

73. Mendoza FJ, Perez-Ecija RA, Monreal L, et al. Coagulation profiles of healthy Andalusian donkeys are different than those of healthy horses. J Vet Intern Med 2011;25(4):967–70.

74. Perez-Ecija A, Mendoza FJ. Characterisation of clotting factors, anticoagulant protein activities and viscoelastic analysis in healthy donkeys. Equine Vet J 2017;49(6):734–8.

75. McClure JJ, Koch C, Traub-Dargatz J. Characterization of a red blood cell antigen in donkeys and mules associated with neonatal isoerythrolysis. Anim Genet 1994;25(2):119–20.

76. Traub-Dargatz JL, McClure JJ, Koch C, et al. Neonatal isoerythrolysis in mule foals. J Am Vet Med Assoc 1995;206(1):67–70.

77. Mendoza FJ, Aguilera-Aguilera R, Gonzalez-De Cara CA, et al. Characterization of the intravenous glucose tolerance test and the combined glucose-insulin test in donkeys. Vet J 2015;206(3):371–6.

78. Mendoza FJ, Estepa JC, Gonzalez-De Cara CA, et al. Energy-related parameters and their association with age, gender, and morphometric measurements in healthy donkeys. Vet J 2015;204(2):201–7.

79. Mendoza FJ, Gonzalez-Cara CA, Aguilera-Aguilera R, et al. Effect of intravenous glucose and combined glucose-insulin challenges on energy-regulating hormones concentrations in donkeys. Vet J 2018;240:40–6.

80. Mueller PJ, Jones MT, Rawson RE, et al. Effect of increasing work rate on metabolic responses of the donkey (Equus asinus). J Appl Physiol (1985) 1994;77(3): 1431–8.
81. Mendoza FJ, Perez-Ecija RA, Toribio RE, et al. Thyroid hormone concentrations differ between donkeys and horses. Equine Vet J 2013;45(2):214–8.
82. Guillaume D, Zarazaga LA, Malpaux B, et al. Variability of plasma melatonin level in pony mares (Equus caballus), comparison with the hybrid: mules and with jennies (Equus asinus). Reprod Nutr Dev 2006;46(6):633–9.
83. Collins SN, Dyson SJ, Murray RC, et al. Radiological anatomy of the donkey's foot: objective characterisation of the normal and laminitic donkey foot. Equine Vet J 2011;43(4):478–86.
84. Van Thielen B, Willekens I, Van der Schicht A, et al. Radiography of the distal extremity of the manus in the donkey foal: normal images and quantitative characterization from birth to 2 years of age: a pilot study. Anat Histol Embryol 2018; 47(1):71–83.
85. Jamdar MN, Ema AN. A note on the vertebral formula of the donkey. Br Vet J 1982;138(3):209–11.
86. Lindsay FE, Clayton HM. An anatomical and endoscopic study of the nasopharynx and larynx of the donkey (Equus asinus). J Anat 1986;144:123–32.
87. Laus F, Paggi E, Marchegiani A, et al. Ultrasonographic biometry of the eyes of healthy adult donkeys. Vet Rec 2014;174(13):326.
88. Proops L, Burden F, Osthaus B. Social relations in a mixed group of mules, ponies and donkeys reflect differences in equid type. Behav Processes 2012;90(3): 337–42.
89. Proops L, Burden F, Osthaus B. Mule cognition: a case of hybrid vigour? Anim Cogn 2009;12(1):75–84.
90. Cook SJ, Cook RF, Montelaro RC, et al. Differential responses of Equus caballus and Equus asinus to infection with two pathogenic strains of equine infectious anemia virus. Vet Microbiol 2001;79(2):93–109.
91. Pusterla N, Mapes S, Wademan C, et al. Investigation of the role of mules as silent shedders of EHV-1 during an outbreak of EHV-1 myeloencephalopathy in California. Vet Rec 2012;170(18):465.
92. Soulsby L, Trawford AF, Matthews JB, et al. Donkey: hero or villain of the parasite world? Past, present and future. Vet Parasitol 2004;125(1–2):43–58.

Donkey Nutrition and Malnutrition

Faith A. Burden, BSc, PhD[a],*, Nicola Bell, BSc, MSc[a]

KEYWORDS

- Donkey • Mule • Ass • Nutrition • Feeding

KEY POINTS

- Donkeys are more efficient at digesting low nutritional quality fibers than horses or ponies and have a lower maintenance energy requirement.
- A diet based on fibrous forages and limited grazing is usually sufficient for the majority of donkeys kept as companion animals.
- Working or production donkeys should be provided with a diet based on fiber; they often need supplementation with high-energy feeds.
- The dull donkey with a poor appetite is a clinical emergency, because they are highly prone to developing hyperlipemia, which may be life threatening.
- Body condition scoring and weight estimation for donkeys should use available species-specific systems; those designed for horses are not appropriate.

INTRODUCTION

The domestic donkey is a unique equid species whose ancestor the African Wild Ass (*Equus africanus*) evolved to survive in semi-arid, mountainous environments with sparse food sources and intermittent access to water.[1] Domesticated only for approximately 6000 years, the donkey has been vital to many communities throughout the world as a draught animal.[2] There are currently approximately 46 million donkeys and 10 million donkey hybrids globally[3] with the vast majority of these living and working in low- and middle-income countries. A recent resurgence of interest in products such as donkey meat, milk,[4] and products made from their skins, particularly within China,[5] is also meaning this species is increasingly being farmed on an intensive scale for production purposes. In recent times, the donkey has found a role as a pet and companion with a growing interest in the use of donkeys for therapeutic purposes for vulnerable children and adults.

Disclosure Statement: None.
a Research Department, The Donkey Sanctuary, Slade House Farm, Sidmouth, Devon EX10 0NU, UK
* Corresponding author.
E-mail address: faith.burden@thedonkeysanctuary.org.uk

Although there is significant shared heritage between the donkey and horse, they are remarkably different in their physical traits, behavior and nutritional requirements. Treatment of the donkey as a "small horse with big ears," particularly when formulating diets, frequently leads to compromised health and welfare because the innate needs of this unique species are not met. This review aims to provide the reader with an overview of the specific needs of the donkey and practical advice for the management of common nutritional challenges.

THE ORIGINS OF THE DONKEY

Today's domestic donkey and the world's feral and semi-feral donkeys are descendants of the African wild ass (*E africanus*).[1,6] A separate branch of wild asses evolved in Asia, including the onager (*Equus hemionus*) and kiang (*Equus kiang*), no species of which has been domesticated but whom share many characteristics with African wild asses. African wild asses evolved to live in semi-arid, often mountainous, environments with sparse, highly fibrous food sources, dispersed water access, and wildly fluctuating temperatures. Steep terrain with narrow, rocky mountain paths contrasts with the ancestral home of the donkeys' cousin, the horse, that would inhabit open grassy plains. Although certain characteristics, such as size, type, color, and temperament have changed since the donkey was domesticated in North Africa, the donkey has retained much of its ancestor's behavior, for example, social and feeding behaviors.

FEEDING BEHAVIOR

Under natural conditions, donkeys spend most of the day foraging.[7,8] The ancestors of the domestic donkey survived on lignin-rich, low-energy, fibrous plants that they would have to range over long distances (20–30 km/d) for most of the day (14–18 hours).[9] To increase their potential source of food in their natural environment, donkeys have evolved to be browsers as well as grazers,[10] with woody shrubs and trees being potential food sources when grasses and other low vegetation are not abundant. Donkeys are highly effective at selecting the most nutrient-dense plants available and evidence shows that they take longer to chew their feedstuffs than do horses fed the same diet.[11] Donkeys kept in domestic environments rarely have the opportunity to exhibit this combination of natural behaviors without significant effort being made to enrich the natural environment and provide appropriate exercise. The donkey is a hindgut fermenter and has evolved as a trickle feeder; this more or less continuous feeding suits the digestive system of the donkey, which has a relatively small stomach but voluminous large colon and caecum.[12] In the colon and cecum, there is a microbial breakdown of feed, especially fibrous materials, that was not digested in the small intestine.

FEEDING THE HEALTHY DONKEY

When compared with horses, donkeys are very efficient at digesting poor nutritional quality fiber, in particular highly fibrous roughage such as straw.[11,13,14] These adaptations may be beneficial for working donkeys and allow them to thrive on feed sources that would be inadequate for horses and ponies managed under similar conditions. The donkey's superior digestive efficiency is linked to a longer mean retention time of feed in the gastrointestinal tract. One study showed an mean retention time of 39 hours for donkeys compared with 30 hours for ponies fed the same rations.[13] Maintenance energy requirements for donkeys are lower than horses, with stated levels varying between 50% and 75% of what would be required by a similar size horse, depending on activity level and season.[11,15] The daily maintenance intake for donkeys has been estimated at 1.3% to 1.8% of bodyweight in dry matter.[11,15] The donkeys' adaptation to thrive on poor nutritional quality feed can easily lead to obesity, in particular companion donkeys when fed the same way as horses and ponies.[12,16] Obesity is also a risk when donkeys are kept with horses or ponies and are not fed and managed differently. Many donkey health problems may result from the provision of high-energy diets, including obesity, which may influence metabolic and hormonal imbalances,[16] hyperlipemia,[17] and laminitis.[18] In these conditions, excess energy storage as metabolically active adipose tissue can lead to the inappropriate mobilization of lipids, insulin resistance, and enzyme dysregulation.

Practical Feeding

Donkeys should be fed a diet of sufficient quantity to maintain them in good condition (normal weight and a body condition score of 2.5–3.0 of 5 measured using a donkey-specific body condition scoring system),[19] to avoid them becoming underweight or overweight and to allow them to express their natural behaviors. A diet which is high in fiber and low in energy and nonstructural carbohydrates (NSC; starches and sugars) is ideal.[12] These diets are best supplied using straws (barley or wheat straw, checked to have few seed heads) or stover (the leaves and stalks of field crops such as corn, maize, or sorghum), which may be supplemented with a variable proportion of coarse, low-energy hay, haylage, and/or grazing depending on what is available locally,[12,20] the donkey's body condition, the time of year, and the prevailing weather conditions. Safe logs and branches should also be provided to satisfy the donkey's natural browsing behaviors.

Donkeys should be fed rations in a trickle feeding manner over a 24-hour period to ensure sufficient chewing time, because their digestive system is adapted to a continuous intake of food with a high fiber content. Chewing promotes production of saliva, which acts as a lubricant and neutralizes the continuous gastric acid secretion. Regular dental examinations should ascertain that the donkey is able to cope with fibrous diets and any transition to this type of diet should be made gradually to decrease the risk of gastrointestinal impaction.[21] Where possible and when dental health is good, straw should be provided ad libitum, should help reduce boredom and unwanted behaviors such as the chewing of fences and other wooden structures.

SUPPLEMENTARY FEEDING

Although many donkeys can live on a diet of straw supplemented appropriately with grass and/or hay or haylage with supplemented vitamins and minerals as necessary, certain individuals, such as pregnant and lactating jennies, young growing donkeys, working donkeys, or stallions kept for breeding purposes, have higher energy needs owing to their level of exercise or basic needs.[20,22] Therefore, they may need to be supplemented with higher energy, fiber- or oil-based feeds such as alfalfa, unmolassed beet pulp, or rice bran. Such higher energy feeds should be given in small rations mixed with appropriate roughage such as an unmolassed short chopped fiber that is divided throughout the day (≥2–3 meals per day depending on the amount of feed with each meal being no more than 1 kg and ideally <500 g for a 200-kg donkey). The amount should be adjusted to the current level of energy expenditure for the donkey. The use of cereal grain-based feeds is discouraged in donkeys because their use increases the risk of donkeys developing gastric ulcers,[23] laminitis, and colic.[21] Where cereal grains or molasses are included to increase the palatability or energy density of feeds, it is advised that combined starch and sugar levels (NSCs) do not exceed 15% and ideally should be less than 10%.

VITAMINS, MINERALS, AND PROTEIN

Little research has been carried out to establish the protein, vitamin, and mineral requirements of donkeys.[12] Protein metabolism and utilization in the donkey seems to be complex, and experience would indicate that donkeys can survive on low-quality protein containing diets better than can horses as evidenced by their ability to survive, breed, work, and grow on forages containing low-quality protein. Vitamin and mineral levels advised for horses seem to provide optimal levels for donkeys and can be safely extrapolated.[24]

PROVISION OF WATER

Donkeys are well-known for their thirst tolerance, which should not be confused with their water requirements. Water requirements for donkeys are similar to that of horses and vary considerably depending on workload, ambient temperature, and water content of feed, as well as during pregnancy and lactation. Donkeys will typically drink 5% to 10% of their body weight daily,[20] and lactating jennies and donkeys with a high level of activity such as working donkeys may need more. In the donkey's natural habitats, water is normally in short supply and widely dispersed. This condition has led to donkeys being more thirst tolerant than horses and to them being able to rehydrate rapidly (20–30 L within a few minutes) without adverse effects.[25] It is common also for donkeys to maintain a normal appetite even when dehydrated,[26] a trait that may lead to late diagnosis of dehydration and concurrent issues such as impaction colic.

Donkeys may be very exacting about drinking from unfamiliar or contaminated water sources, leading them to tolerate excessive dehydration meanwhile maintaining a seemingly normal appetite. To prevent impaction colic, care must therefore be taken to provide clean, palatable water from suitable containers. In addition, many donkeys seem to dislike very cold water and geriatric or vulnerable animals may benefit from warmed water in the winter months to maintain appropriate levels of hydration.[19] During periods of cold weather, water sources such as troughs and buckets should be inspected several times a day to ensure that they are free from ice and are providing fresh water. In routinely cold climates, the provision of heated troughs is appreciated by donkeys.

BODY CONDITION SCORING

Weighing or weight estimation and body condition scoring are extremely useful tools to assess the general condition and health status of donkeys when carried out on at least a monthly basis. Often the first obvious sign of deteriorating health is a gradual loss of weight. Weight gain is easier to deal with if noticed early. Weight can be obtained using electronic scales; however, most owners do not have access to this type of equipment. In such cases, the use of a weight estimation calculator and a body condition scoring system specifically designed for donkeys are encouraged. Further details about weight estimation and condition scoring can be found at the Donkey Sanctuary website (www.thedonkeysanctuary.org.uk; **Fig. 1**).[19] The Henneke body scoring system for horses[27] is not useful for donkeys owing to species-specific differences in body shape, conformation, muscle mass, and

DONKEY BODY CONDITION SCORE CHART

Accurate Body condition scoring is a hands-on process for feeling the amount of muscle and fat that are covering the donkey's bones. Using this chart as a guide, feel the coverage over the bones in five specific areas listed below. Fat deposits may be unevenly distributed especially over the neck and hindquarters. Some resistant fat deposits may be retained in the event of weight loss or may calcify (harden). Careful assessment of all areas should be made and combined, to give an overall score. When deciding on the correct course of action following condition scoring, you might have to take into consideration the age of the donkey and any veterinary conditions they have. Aged donkeys can be hard to condition score due to lack of muscle bulk and tone giving thin appearance dorsally with dropped belly ventrally, while overall condition may be reasonable. If in doubt, get advice from your vet.

Condition score	Neck and shoulders	Withers	Ribs and belly	Back and loins	Hindquarters
1. Poor (very thin)	Neck thin, all bones easily felt. Neck meets shoulder abruptly, shoulder bones felt easily, angular.	Dorsal spine and withers prominent and easily felt.	Ribs can be seen from a distance and felt with ease. Belly tucked up.	Backbone prominent, can feel dorsal and transverse processes easily.	Hip bones visible and felt easily (dock and pin bones). Little muscle cover. May be cavity under tail.
2. Moderate (underweight)	Some muscle development overlying bones. Slight step where neck meets shoulders.	Some cover over dorsal withers, spinous processes felt but not prominent.	Ribs not visible but can be felt with ease.	Dorsal and transverse processes felt with light pressure. Poor muscle development either side of midline.	Poor muscle cover on hindquarters, hip bones felt with ease.
3. Ideal	Good muscle development, bones felt under light cover of muscle/fat. Neck flows smoothly into shoulder, which is rounded.	Good cover of muscle/ fat over dorsal spinous processes, withers flow smoothly into back.	Ribs just covered by light layer of fat/muscle, ribs can be felt with light pressure. Belly firm with good muscle tone and flattish outline.	Can feel individual spinous or transverse processes with pressure. Muscle development either side of midline is good.	Good muscle cover over hindquarters, hip bones rounded in appearance, can be felt with light pressure.
4. Overweight (fat)	Neck thick, crest hard, shoulder covered in even fat layer.	Withers broad, bones felt with pressure.	Ribs dorsally only felt with firm pressure, ventral ribs may be felt more easily. Belly over developed.	Can only feel dorsal and transverse processes with firm pressure. May have slight crease along midline.	Hindquarters rounded, bones felt only with pressure. Fat deposits evenly placed.
5. Obese (very fat)	Neck thick, crest bulging with fat and may fall to one side. Shoulder rounded and bulging with fat.	Withers broad, bones felt with firm pressure.	Large, often uneven fat deposits covering dorsal and possibly ventral aspect of ribs. Ribs not palpable dorsally. Belly pendulous in depth and width.	Back broad, difficult to feel individual spinous or transverse processes. More prominent crease along mid line fat pads on either side. Crease along midline bulging fat either side.	Cannot feel hip bones, fat may overhang either side of tail head, fat often uneven and bulging.

Fig. 1. Donkey body condition score chart. (*Courtesy of* The Donkey Sanctuary, Devon, UK.)

adipose tissue distribution.[28,29] The donkey has an angular frame and often a pendulous abdomen. The abdominal shape may be in part owing to the relatively high large colon capacity to accommodate fiber,[13] abdominal fat, and a slackness of abdominal muscles, which is more evident in sedentary and geriatric animals. Regardless of the body condition, as a part of the assessment it is important to palpate the animal. Donkeys can have coarse, thick coats, especially in winter or when suffering from pituitary pars intermedia dysfunction, and appearances are often deceptive.[19] Donkeys frequently develop a fatty crest,[28,29] which may fall over to one side of the neck. Once in situ, these deposits rarely disappear, even with dieting, and may remain in a donkey that is in otherwise good condition. Fat pads are common on the buttocks and the dorsal and lateral thorax, and donkeys often carry significant abdominal fat (often up to 8 cm, but increasing up to 14 cm in the obese donkey). When such fat pads are longstanding, they may become calcified and therefore, extremely hard, such pads will never be lost through dieting and should be ignored when condition scoring.

FEEDING FOR COMMON CONDITIONS

The majority of donkeys manage very well on basic rations. However, there are cases that require special feeding.

Underweight Donkeys

Before dietary changes can be made, a thorough clinical assessment should be carried out, including observation of feeding behavior and assessment of feeding and management practices (such as hobbling/tethering), a thorough dental examination, blood sampling to assess overall health (with particular attention to liver and kidney function, pituitary pars intermedia dysfunction, and equine metabolic syndrome) and assessment of the parasitic burden.[28] In working donkeys, assessment of workload and availability of feedstuffs during working hours is useful, because not having access to adequate feedstuffs when energy demands are high will lead to a poor body condition score with negative health consequences.

Working and companion donkeys with low body condition scores may have concurrent dental disease,[30,31] liver disease, other health issues, or problems with companion animals such as bullying or separation grief.[19] A holistic approach to resolving all underlying causes is essential. When managing animals that require an improvement in body condition, it is important to encourage energy intake throughout the day by providing, for example, higher quantities of hay, soaked unmolassed beet pulp, or a short-chopped fiber product.[19,28]

OBESITY

As in all species, obesity is a major welfare issue for donkeys that predisposes to a number of diseases. Recent studies have shown that obese donkeys have higher insulin concentrations,[32] which are associated with a history of laminitis (endocrinopathic laminitis) and may worsen with grazing. Dietary management of obese donkeys is challenging and requires ongoing veterinary input. An inappropriate diet is often compounded by lack of exercise, issues with other donkeys, separation grief, and equine metabolic syndrome. Although obesity is uncommon in working donkeys, those that are worked infrequently or are kept for production purposes may also be at risk of obesity and related issues.

Before embarking on a management plan for an obese donkey, a dental check to ensure the animal can be given a diet based on long-stem straw or stover should be done along with an assessment of the donkey's ability to exercise. Where appropriate, evaluation of hematologic and biochemical parameters is indicated to assess underlying diseases, but also to determine triglyceride values before dietary changes to prevent hyperlipemia. Donkeys with elevated triglycerides (>2.8 mmol/L)[33] should have an exercise program initiated before dietary changes are made. Once levels decrease to within the normal range,[33] dietary changes may be introduced.

Dietary management for obese or laminitic animals or those with equine metabolic syndrome that have healthy teeth should focus on straw with very limited grazing in warm climates, and straw with limited hay when weather is cold (<10°C). If there are concerns about nutritional deficiency, vitamin, mineral, and protein supplements designed for equids may be provided in appropriate quantities. Pasture management should be part of the plan, with intake being restricted by the use of temporary electric fencing. A guide of less than 0.2 acre (less than 0.08 ha) per donkey of short cropped pasture is reasonable, and benefits from rotation.[28] Evidence suggests that fructan levels in grass are rarely sufficient to trigger ration-induced laminitis owing to disrupted fermentation in the hindgut. It is likely that high NSC (simple sugars, starches, fructans) levels in grasses promote excessive insulin secretion and the development of endocrinopathic laminitis.[34] It is therefore extremely important to maintain a healthy grass sward, because NSC levels can be high in lush pastures but also in frosty grass and grass stressed by drought or overgrazing.

Although seemingly an easy option, the management of obesity in donkeys by decreasing the time grazing has limited effect on total dietary intake because they may spend more time at pasture eating rather than exercising and carrying out social behaviors.[11] This may then be followed by long periods of confinement, which only exacerbates the issue. To encourage donkeys to lose weight, they should be appropriately exercised. As mentioned, donkeys should have their body condition scored and weight estimated monthly. Progress when dieting donkeys may be slow, and perseverance is essential. Rapid weight loss should be avoided owing to metabolic complications. It often takes weeks for weight loss to be noticed; however, once the process begins, weight loss should be gradual. The aim should be to lose 2% to 3% of body weight monthly.

HYPERLIPEMIA AND THE INAPPETENT DONKEY

Donkeys are prone to developing hyperlipemia,[17] a complex metabolic disturbance that is associated with almost any disease and stressing factor of donkeys.[17] Avoiding hyperlipemia is imperative in dull and inappetent donkeys, which should be viewed as a clinical emergency. Hyperlipemia secondary to other clinical conditions is common (72% of hyperlipemia cases in 1 study), and the mortality rate may be as high as 49%.[17] Prevention through reduction of stress and maintenance of appetite is important; dealing with pain associated with any primary disease process is critical. Many sick donkeys will maintain an appetite and should be given a diet similar to that normally provided.[35] Offering small tasty meals and forages along with the opportunity to browse and graze is also helpful. Hospitalized donkeys may be provided with straw if this is what they are accustomed to. When nonsteroidal anti-inflammatory drugs are prescribed, caution must be exercised and frequent evaluation and recording of fecal output and gut sounds should be undertaken.[35] Nutritional management of sick donkeys often focuses on the need to stimulate the donkey's appetite, although molasses and cereal grains can be used successfully in the short term, they can be detrimental in the long term. Alternatively, donkeys should be tempted to eat with the addition of safe fruit and vegetables, dried mint and fenugreek, unmolassed beet pulp, fruit juices, or yeast extracts to a base fiber feed.[19] Donkeys bond extremely strongly[36] and to prevent further decline it is essential to ensure the sick donkey's companion is close by, even within a hospital setting.

Where appetite is significantly decreased or absent, consideration may be given to nasogastric tubing, intravenous fluids, or parenteral nutrition to maintain a positive energy balance until voluntary feeding is reestablished.[35,37] When administering frequent treatments by nasogastric tube or oral drenching, the potential for exacerbating or predisposing to hyperlipemia from stress must be balanced with the clinical needs. Some animals may benefit from a small bore feeding tube rather than frequent tubing, which can also be used to administer fluids and electrolytes. In anorectic animals for more than 2 days, oral fluids should be supplemented with potassium because hypokalemia can alter energy homeostasis and may lead to ileus. Inclusion of 1 g of potassium chloride per liter of oral fluids should be sufficient, alongside normal tubing preparations. Patients should be fed fiber-rich products, such as a rolled or ground instant oat cereal produced for humans. Prebiotics and probiotics are administered by some clinicians when managing hyperlipemia donkeys. Consideration should be given to gastric protectants.[19]

DENTAL DISEASE

Dental disease is common in donkeys, particularly geriatrics,[30,31,38] and this often leads to an inability to chew long fiber forages, causing gradual weight loss with associated depression and lethargy. In serious cases, dental pain can lead to a donkey becoming inappetent and predisposed to hyperlipemia.[17] For these animals, it is essential to replace long fiber forages with alternative fiber sources that can be easily chewed and digested. Short-chopped products designed for laminitic equines are suitable, and many of the low-energy products can be used to replace all fiber sources. Chopped fiber forages should be provided frequently throughout the day and be fed to dry matter intake requirements. Although the feeding of such products ad libitum may lead to gorging in the short term, intake may self-regulate after a few weeks, and care should be taken to monitor weight throughout this period with restrictions put in place if unwanted weight is gained.

Donkeys that do not require such drastic changes in diet can be given small, frequent feeds of high fiber concentrates and unmolassed sugar beet pulp, alongside forage.

LAMINITIS

In the acute stages of laminitis, it is essential to remove any contributory dietary factors. The donkey should be removed from pasture and given a high-fiber, low NSC diet.[19] Maintaining fiber intake is essential because a negative energy balance will likely lead to hyperlipemia. Straw may be fed to laminitic donkeys but with decreased mobility frequent checks must be carried out on gut motility and fecal output. A short-chopped forage with an NSC content of less than 10% is ideal to maintain the animal in the short term and decrease the risk of impaction. Hay may be fed, but it is important to be aware that NSC levels in most hay is high and may be inappropriate. Where available, haylage may be suitable, a high-fiber product with declared NSC content should be used. Sloppy feeds of unmolassed beet are useful to encourage water intake and assist with the administration of drugs. Long-term management of the chronic laminitic is the same as that already described for obese animals.

LIVER AND KIDNEY DISEASE

Dietary management is a key component of a treatment plan for donkeys suffering from liver or kidney disease. The donkey with liver disease needs a low protein diet to decrease intestinal ammonia production. Such a diet, with less than 8% protein, can be met by grass, hay, straw, and pasture. In addition, it is important to avoid alfalfa or cereal-based feeds and levels of fat within the diet should be controlled with supplementary oil being discouraged.

Animals with kidney disease should have a diet low in calcium and protein (<8%) and, where possible, should be maintained on hay and pasture. Legumes such as alfalfa and clover contain high levels of protein and calcium, and should be avoided. Where extra energy is required it can be supplied in the form of high oil supplements.

FEEDING IN PREGNANCY

Nutrient requirements for pregnancy and lactation in the donkey have yet to be established.[20] Guidelines for donkeys are extrapolated from horse and pony data and make use of practical experience.[19,28] In the final trimester, the female donkey will have a greater energy requirement, and it is important to supply high-quality protein, vitamins, and minerals as the fetus develops.[20] To supply these nutrients, the energy density and quality of forages must be increased. The hay, haylage, or grazing portion of the diet should be gradually increased until it constitutes the majority of the diet and a supplement containing vitamins, minerals, and protein, with low NSC levels as designed for small ponies should be provided. If good quality hay, haylage, or grazing is not available, supplementation with alfalfa or unmolassed beet pulp is useful. During pregnancy, the digestive tract capacity decreases, which may lead to the female donkey being unable to satisfy the energy requirements of herself and the foal. This is a major predisposing factor for hyperlipemia and care should be taken to ensure energy requirements are met.[35]

During lactation, the female donkey should receive adequate, good quality pasture and hay. Supplementation with vitamin and mineral products, chopped alfalfa, or high-fiber concentrates may also be indicated. Hyperlipemia remains a concern in the lactating donkey and owners should monitor appetite and provide adequate feed. The foal should be allowed to pick at the dam's feed in preparation for weaning. Foals should grow steadily and it is best practice to monitor the weight and condition of the foal every 2 weeks, growth curves are not yet available for donkey foals.[20] If the rate of growth is too rapid, any supplementary nutritional intake should be restricted, but with appropriate vitamin and mineral supplementation. If the foal is stunted, appropriate supplementary feeding may be advised.

SUMMARY

The donkey is supremely adapted to survive on food that would be inadequate for most other equines. The donkey's ability to digest highly fibrous forages, its thirst tolerance and ability to maintain appetite even when dehydrated has led to an animal able to survive in some of the world's most inhospitable places. Although still commonly found working across the globe, the donkey also faces new challenges as a production and companion animal where environmental conditions and feed provision is very different to that found in the species' natural environment. The donkey should be fed a diet high in fiber and low in energy and NSC, which is best supplied using straws and moderate quality hay and grazing. Such a diet should be complemented with an enriched natural environment allowing opportunities to browse and exercise and carry out other natural behaviors. Dietary management of the donkey is essential to avoid health issues and ensure well-being and should be seen as the foundation of a healthy animal experiencing a high welfare state. Further information relating to donkey and mule nutrition is available from The Donkey Sanctuary.

REFERENCES

1. Rossel S, Marshall F, Peters J, et al. Domestication of the donkey: timing, processes, and indicators. Proc Natl Acad Sci U S A 2008;105:3715–20.
2. Ali M, Baber M, Hussain T, et al. The contribution of donkeys to human health. Equine Vet J 2014;46:766–7.
3. FAOSTAT. Live animals (data). Available at: http://www.fao.org/faostat/en/#data/QA. Accessed January 21, 2019.
4. Souroullas K, Aspri M, Papademas P. Donkey milk as a supplement in infant formula: benefits and technological challenges. Food Res Int 2018;109:416–25.
5. Zhu M, Weng Q. China: will the donkey become the next pangolin? Equine Vet J 2018;50(2):276.
6. Beja-Pereira A. African origins of the domestic donkey. Science 2004;304(5678):1781.
7. Moehlman PD. Behavioral patterns and communication in feral asses (Equus africanus). Appl Anim Behav Sci 1998;60:125–69.
8. Klingel H. Observations on social organization and behaviour of African and Asiatic wild asses (Equus africanus and E. hemionus). Z Tierpsychol 1977;44:323–31.
9. Smith DG, Pearson RA. A review of the factors affecting the survival of donkeys in semi-arid regions of sub-Saharan Africa. Trop Anim Health Prod 2005;37:1–19.

10. Aganga AA, Tsopito CM. A note on the feeding behaviour of domestic donkeys: a Botswana case study. Appl Anim Behav Sci 1998;60:235–9.

11. Wood SJ. Some factors affecting the digestible energy requirements and dry matter intake of mature donkeys. Edinburgh (UK): PhD Thesis: University of Edinburgh; 2010.

12. Smith DG, Burden FA. Practical donkey and mule nutrition. In: Geor R, Coenen M, Harris P, editors. Equine applied and clinical nutrition. Philadelphia: Saunders; 2013. p. 304–16.

13. Pearson RA, Archibald RF, Muirhead RH. The effect of forage quality and level of feeding on digestibility and gastrointestinal transit time of oat straw and alfalfa given to ponies and donkeys. Br J Nutr 2001;85:599–606.

14. Faith Burden FA, Thiemann A. Donkeys are different. J Equine Vet Sci 2015;35: 376–82.

15. Carretero-Roque L, Colunga B, Smith DG. Digestible energy requirements of Mexican donkeys fed oat straw and maize stover. Trop Anim Health Prod 2005; 37:123–42.

16. Mendoza FJ, Estepa JC, Gonzalez-De Cara CA, et al. Energy-related parameters and their association with age, gender, and morphometric measurements in healthy donkeys. Vet J 2015;204:201–7.

17. Burden FA, Du Toit N, Hazell-Smith E, et al. Hyperlipemia in a population of aged donkeys: description, prevalence, and potential risk factors. J Vet Intern Med 2011;25:1420–5.

18. Morrow LD, Smith KC, Piercy RJ, et al. Retrospective analysis of post-mortem findings in 1,444 aged donkeys. J Comp Pathol 2011;144:145–56.

19. Evans L, Crane M, editors. The clinical companion of the donkey. London: Matador Publishing; 2018.

20. Martin-Rosset W. Donkey nutrition and feeding: nutrient requirements and recommended allowances—a review and prospect. J Equine Vet Sci 2018;65:75–85.

21. Cox R, Burden F, Gosden L, et al. Case control study to investigate risk factors for impaction colic in donkeys in the UK. Prev Vet Med 2009;92(3):179–87.

22. Pearson RA, editor. Donkey, mules and horses in tropical agricultural development. Edinburgh, United Kingdom: University of Edinburgh Press; 1991. p. 86–95.

23. Burden FA, Gallagher J, Thiemann AK, et al. Necropsy survey of gastric ulcers in a population of aged donkeys: prevalence, lesion description and risk factors. Animal 2009;3:287–93.

24. National Research Council (U.S.), Committee on Nutrient Requirements of Horses. Donkeys and other equids. In: Nutrient requirements of horses. 6th rev. edition. Washington, DC: National Academies Press; 2007. p. 268–79.

25. Schmidt-Nielsen K. Desert animals. Physiological problems of heat and water. Oxford, United Kingdom: Oxford University Press; 1964.

26. Dill DB, Youssef MK, Cox CR, et al. Hunger vs. thirst in the burro (Equus asinus). Physiol Behav 1980;24:975–8.

27. Henneke DR, Potter GD, Kreider JL, et al. Relationship between condition score, physical measurements and body fat percentage in mares. Equine Vet J 1983; 15(4):371–2.

28. Burden F. Practical feeding and condition scoring for donkeys and mules. Equine Vet Educ 2012;24:589–96.

29. Valle E, Raspa F, Giribaldi M, et al. A functional approach to the body condition assessment of lactating donkeys as a tool for welfare evaluation. PeerJ 2017;5: e3001.

30. du Toit N, Burden FA, Dixon PM. Clinical dental examinations of 357 donkeys in the UK. Part 1: prevalence of dental disorders. Equine Vet J 2009;41:390–4.
31. du Toit N, Gallagher J, Burden FA, et al. Post mortem survey of dental disorders in 349 donkeys from an aged population (2005-2006). Part 1: prevalence of specific dental disorders. Equine Vet J 2008;40:204–8.
32. McLean A, Nielsen B, Yokoyama M, et al. Insulin resistance in standard donkeys (Equus asinus) of three body conditions-thin, moderate, and obese. J Equine Vet Sci 2009;29(5):406–7.
33. Burden FA, Hazell-Smith E, Mulugeta G, et al. Reference intervals for biochemical and haematological parameters in mature domestic donkeys (Equus asinus) in the UK. Equine Vet Educ 2016;28(3):134–9.
34. Katz LM, Bailey SR. The pathogenesis of equine acute laminitis. Equine Vet J 2016;44:752–61.
35. Durham AE, Thiemann AK. Nutritional management of hyperlipaemia. Equine Vet Educ 2015;27(9):482–8.
36. Murray L, Byrne K, D'Eath RB. Pair-bonding and companion recognition in domestic donkeys, Equus asinus. Appl Anim Behav Sci 2013;143:67–74.
37. Thiemann AK. Clinical approach to the dull donkey. Practice 2013;35:470–6.
38. Rodrigues JB, Dixon PM, Bastos E, et al. A clinical survey on the prevalence and types of cheek teeth disorders present in 400 Zamorano-Leonés and 400 Mirandês donkeys (Equus asinus). Vet Rec 2013;173:581.

30. du Toit N, Burden FA, Dixon PM. Clinical dental examinations of 357 donkeys in the UK. Part 1: prevalence of dental disorders. Equine Vet J. 2009;41:390–4.

31. du Toit N, Gallagher J, Burden FA, et al. Post mortem survey of dental disorders in 349 donkeys from an aged population (2005–2006). Part 1: prevalence of specific dental disorders. Equine Vet J. 2008;40:204–8.

32. McLean AK, Nielsen B, Yokoyama M, et al. Insulin resistance in standard donkeys (Equus asinus) of three body conditions: thin, moderate, and obese. J Equine Vet Sci. 2009;29(5):405–7.

33. Dosi MC, Hazell-Smith E, Mahibata G, et al. Reference intervals for biochemical and haematological parameters in mature domestic donkeys (Equus asinus) in the UK. Equine Vet Educ. 2018;30(10):516–21.

34. Katz LM, Bailey SR. The pathogenesis of equine acute laminitis. Equine Vet J. 2012;44(6):752–61.

35. Durham AE, Thiemann AK. Nutritional management of hyperlipaemia. Equine Vet Educ. 2015;27(9):482–8.

36. McLean AK, Byrne J, Delrate FS. Pasture grass and companion's opinion in the domestic donkey stimulus. Appl Anim Behav Sci. 2013;143:87–94.

37. Thiemann AK. Clinical approach to the dull donkey. In Pract. 2013;35:470–6.

38. Rodrigues JB, Dixon PM, Bastos E, et al. A clinical survey on the prevalence and types of cheek teeth disorders present in 400 Zamorano–Leones and 400 Mirandes donkeys (Equus asinus). Vet Rec. 2013;173:581.

Donkey and Mule Welfare

Eric Davis, DVM, MS

KEYWORDS

- Welfare • Donkey • Burro • Feral • Herbivore • Wildlife • Ejiao • Working equine

KEY POINTS

- Donkeys and mules have supported man for millennia and are currently critical to the lives of the poorest rural and urban humans.
- Working donkeys and mules suffer from poor harness, lack of veterinary care, improper nutrition, and a low status and value, despite their usefulness.
- In the wealthier societies, donkeys especially are seen as pets, and often suffer significant health problems owing to physiologic differences from *Equus caballus*.
- There are large feral populations of donkeys in parts of the world that are seen as invasive pests, an economic resource, or a natural progression of megafauna in the Anthropocene.
- Recent market developments in Traditional Chinese Medicine have led to major shifts in donkey populations, degraded welfare, and a push to intensively farm these animals.

INTRODUCTION

The donkey has been a partner of man for millennia, carrying the earliest pastoralists and traders, pulling chariots of pharaohs and kings, and bringing the prophets to the holy cities.[1] Early on the cross between *Equus caballus* and *Equus asinus* proved to be an especially useful animal for travel and agriculture. Even today, these stoic and hardy animals have often made the lives of women, children, and old men of the world's poorest rural communities easier. Despite noble and tireless service, the reputation of the donkey has been one of denigration, its contributions forgotten or belittled, and its loads often increased to inhumane levels.[2] In the twenty-first century world donkey, populations can be divided into 4 groups, based on geography and the socioeconomic standing of the human societies in which they exist: (1) working rural and urban donkey of the poorer countries of the world, (2) the donkeys in companion animal populations primarily in the richer parts of the planet, such as North America and Western Europe, (3) the feral herds of *E asinus*, and wild members of the species *Equus africanus*, in the western hemisphere, Australia, and east Africa, and (4) the new paradigm in which millions of donkeys

Disclosure Statement: The author has no relationships with a commercial company that has a direct financial interest in subject matter or materials discussed in this article.
Veterinary Medicine & Epidemiology, UC Davis-International Animal Welfare Training Institute, School of Veterinary Medicine, 2108 Tupper Hall, One Shields Avenue, Davis, CA 95616, USA
E-mail address: ewdavis@ucdavis.edu

Vet Clin Equine 35 (2019) 481–491
https://doi.org/10.1016/j.cveq.2019.08.005
0749-0739/19/Crown Copyright © 2019 Published by Elsevier Inc. All rights reserved.

are intensively farmed in China and elsewhere dedicated to the production of *ejiao* and other industrial products.[3] All of these populations have significant welfare problems, which have the potential to get much worse as human population increases and the climate of the planet continues to warm, with attendant changes in agriculture, land use, and water availability.

WORKING DONKEY AND MULE POPULATIONS

From the very earliest human civilizations, the progenitors of the modern donkey served as an essential beast of burden, assisting man with nomadic pastoralism and trade, first in East and North Africa, and later in the Middle East and Asia. The hardy *E asinus*, descended from the wild *E africanus*, stoic and easily trainable, offered advantages as a method of transport over the previously domesticated large herbivores, the ox and the sheep.[4] Besides being able to carry more load than sheep or goats, and walking faster than oxen, the equine digestive system requires less water for proper functioning.[4,5] As a result, in Saharan and sub-Saharan Africa, the donkey likely made improvements in trade and nomadic pastoralism possible. As societies became more sophisticated, donkeys were used to pull chariots of leaders and warriors, based on predynastic gravesites at places like Abydos, in upper Egypt.[1]

Well-established in the Middle East and North Africa as an essential part of trade and travel from the most ancient of times, donkeys were distributed throughout Europe by the Roman Empire, which used them for transport and farming, as well as the production of mules.[6] As part of this dispersion, donkeys came to the British Isles in 43 AD with the Roman subjugation of the Iron Age tribes that lived there. Similarly, trade along the Silk Road brought the donkey and mule to Central Asia and the Far East.[6,7]

The same advantages of donkeys that made them essential to the ancient civilizations of the Old World made them useful as Europeans moved to explore and conquer the Western Hemisphere and Australia. The donkey's stoicism, desert adaptation, and strength, as well as their importance in the breeding of mules, made them one of the first domestic creatures to be carried to these new lands. Even before the conquest of Mexico and the continents of North and South America, donkeys were a part of the second voyage of Christopher Columbus, to the island of Hispaniola in 1495. The Spanish highly valued mules for both riding and draught and were quick to begin breeding programs to produce them after their destruction of the Aztec empire in 1519.[8] These mules served not only for further expeditions seeking gold and fame in the arid Sonoran life zone, but also for the growing mining and cattle ranching operations that spread from Texas, across Mexico and Central America, and into South America as far as Tierra del Fuego. Over the next 500 years donkeys remained a part of industry and agriculture in the Western Hemisphere, with actual increases in numbers with human population and booms in gold and silver mining in the nineteenth century.[6,8]

As with the Americas, donkeys were first imported into Australia, because of their durability and minimal water needs. Sir Thomas Elder, a Scottish businessman and stockman with several large land holdings, imported numbers of donkeys to Western Australia in 1866. Along with camels, which Elder also introduced to the continent, they were used as pack animals in the vast stretches of dry grassland and scrub that made up the Australian Outback. The environments in both in Australian and south western North America are highly suited to the donkey's biology, which, although it made them useful into the 1920s, also resulted in their being seen as pests and an invasive species, as discussed elsewhere in this article.[9,10]

There remain large numbers of working draught donkeys in use in the twenty-first century, which serve the poorest of populations in all the areas where they are used. Although the exact population size is difficult to verify, their numbers have been estimated to be around 39 million as of 2010.[1,2] Cultural prejudice against donkeys has resulted in a situation where they are not only undervalued, but often completely forgotten by aid agencies and nongovernmental organizations (NGOs). This situation is truly disheartening considering the degree to which they carry the loads of most under-resourced classes, and particularly women and children.[11,12]

In the face of all this, working donkey populations have actually expanded in areas such as East Africa and South Asia, where hard manual labor and transport is often done by those that are the least powerful in societies (women and children). Working donkeys represent an improvement in their standard of living.[4] At the same time, the very people who benefit from the donkey often lack experience with their care and behavior, resulting in misreading of the animal's motivations and abilities. Such inexperience is expressed as poorly handled and overworked animals, in which the signs of pain are ignored and husbandry needs are not met.[12]

Of course, the reasons for this mistreatment vary from individual to individual, and society to society. Although it would be very difficult to identify the relative frequency of injury caused by ignorance versus cruelty, there is no doubt that humans may neglect the welfare of their working donkeys when they themselves are on the brink of starvation and exhaustion. Further, as people around the world are increasingly more able to access media that gives them a view of cars, trucks, and other conveyances from the wealthy Western world, the donkey's low esteem and value seem to be magnified. Experience shows that young people who are often the ones doing the menial jobs associated with donkey power, take out their frustrations on the very animals that serve them by overworking and beating.[13,14]

Excessive loading and long work hours are often listed as one of the main welfare problems for the working donkey and mule. Although this can occur in rural, as well as urbanized settings, as a rule, the more industrial the tasks given to donkeys, the more severe the physical requirements. Particularly notorious in this area are the manufacturing of bricks, which use donkeys or mules to transport both wet molded bricks and the dried product in North Africa, the Middle East, and the Indian subcontinent.[15,16] Similarly, donkeys working in coal mines in Pakistan and India are loaded very heavily and carry the coal up steep grades to exit the mines (M. Tariq, personal communication, 2018).

The harness used on donkeys and mules varies widely and, if improperly constructed, can have a very detrimental effect on the animal's welfare. Although we have found the construction and padding of pack saddles in certain areas, like the Sierra Gorda of Mexico, to be well-made and appropriate for donkeys, those who use the animals in places like this have a tradition of relying on their burros, going back generations. The proper design and construction of packing equipment requires skill and a time commitment, and access to natural fibers, which are less abrasive than the hard polypropylene twine that has taken over much of the world, owing to its durability, strength, and low cost. Particularly where donkeys have been introduced as pack animals to human populations in which they replace women or children as beasts of burden, harnesses tend to be made out of whatever can be found cheaply and easily. This is the case in much of East Africa, where donkeys are harnessed with nothing more than a strap around their neck, without attention to padding, angle of draught, or the differences in anatomy between donkeys and oxen.[4,13]

The wounds that result from inappropriately hard and abrasive tying materials or simply throwing bags, made of synthetic fibers, across the animal's back, cause pressure points on the withers and over the lumbar spine. These points then develop severe abrasions, which become infected, and do not heal. Because animals must remain in work, because their owners cannot or will not rest them, the lesions spread, with a large degree of separation between the wound edges and the underlying fasciae and periosteum. The cavity then fills with exudate, making granulation and healing impossible until the animal is either rested for a prolonged period of time or the damaged tissue is surgically removed and stabilized with sutures, release incisions, and a stent bandage. Of course, the equipment and skill required to achieve this requisite therapy is generally lacking. Eventually the lesions involve the underlying bone, resulting in a downward spiral of pain and loss of usefulness, until the donkey is abandoned or killed, with the carcass rendered or used to feed zoo animals.[17]

Other factors make the situation worse in urban settings. With limited resources and knowledge, owners use the same undesirable harness making materials and designs, but in addition, poorly constructed and chronically overloaded carts, usually constructed from the undercarriage of cars or small trucks, compound the problem. These vehicles are heavy, have increased ground friction because of the wide tires used when conveyances are motorized, and lack brakes. Further, the low axel placement, relative to the point at which the animal is attached to the cart, causes much of the weight to come down on the animal's back, especially when decelerating or going downhill. Such design results in fatigue and skin lesions, as the poorly padded harness cuts into the animal's withers and top line.[17,18] Even in huge megalopolis cities, like Cairo, one can see donkeys or mules pulling these carts through dense traffic. The animals are forced to work harder to keep up with the moving cars and trucks, and breath extremely polluted air in the process. In addition, urban cart donkeys have to work on hard, often hot, pavement without proper hoof protection or traction.[17]

Another impediment to the welfare of donkeys working in industrial and urban settings is the lack of proper nutrition. Although donkeys can survive on coarse feedstuffs owing to digestive adaptations that evolved in very marginal environments, finding adequate and safe food sources, where no access to pasture is possible, is a serious challenge. Donkeys are either fed the least expensive of feedstuffs, such as chaff or, even, garbage, or are left to simply fend for themselves. With the amount of completely indigestible materials, such as wrapping plastics, in urban waste dumps and alongside road ways, donkeys often ingest this refuse of modern civilization, resulting in intestinal impactions that can often be fatal. Again, veterinary care is generally not available to the owners of working donkeys at an affordable price, making affected animals suffer severely. The same is true of lacking dental care and vaccination for such common and easily preventable diseases as tetanus.[19] The owners of the working donkey, no matter how much they rely on their animals, can rarely afford medical care of any kind, even if it were available. Although a number of international NGOs provide intermittent clinics at low or no cost, regular care by skilled veterinarians or paraprofessionals is lacking in the vast majority of locations, rural or urban. The donkey that gets its teeth examined, is deparasitized, or receives a routine surgery with anesthesia and asepsis, is a lucky animal who happened to be in the right place at the right time.[20]

Although there have been some attempts to raise the status of donkeys by a few equine- and donkey-oriented groups, mostly based in the United Kingdom, international animal protection NGOs have concentrated far more on companion animal welfare. Volunteer veterinary groups tend to concentrate on dogs, cats, and horses, and generally do not address the root problems of poor care and working conditions in donkeys or mules in an organized fashion. Similarly, global development agencies tasked with improving food production and local industries do not value donkeys, making them nearly invisible. Rather than recognizing the contribution of donkeys in transport of products, water, and fuel, they are seen as an anachronism or ignored all together.

Perhaps one of the most egregious threats to donkeys stems from the political and military situation in the Middle East, South Asia, and parts of Africa. The mixture of young armed men, used to killing and torture, and the presence of an undervalued and ridiculed animal make for some truly awful outcomes for donkeys in these regions. These range from sadistically using donkeys as targets for bullets, bayonets, and knives to the weaponization of pack animals with improvised explosive devices. Because donkeys are common in places like Afghanistan and Syria, and are easily trained to travel on roads unguided, they are ideal vectors for the delivery of deadly explosives in the asymmetrical wars of the twenty-first century.[12,13]

COMPANION ANIMAL DONKEYS IN NORTH AMERICA, WESTERN EUROPE, AND AUSTRALIA

Paradoxically, donkeys in the wealthier countries can suffer from different problems than their toiling brethren in the developing world. Donkeys and mules once had an economic function in places like the rural parts of Europe, Ireland, and North America; however, today they are kept primarily as pets. A limited number of enthusiasts take their donkeys and mules quite seriously in sports such as packing, pack racing, and driving, the majority of donkeys in the First World are seen as amusing novelties, whose main function is to eat pasture.

The same adaptations that have made donkeys so valuable to the poor result in a number of health problems when donkeys find themselves in an environment with plentiful food and water, and where they are not required to work. Owners of donkeys in the West tend to see them as "horses with long ears," and often remain ignorant of their particular metabolism, digestion, and anatomy. Certainly the most common health problems in donkeys in the United States and the UK are related to obesity.[21] Their very efficient digestive system and insulin resistance (relative to horses) puts them at risk of condition such as endocrinopathic laminitis, where climate makes pasture growth nearly continuous throughout the year or high digestible energy feedstuffs, such as alfalfa, are the norm for equine diets. Further, in moist environments such as the British Isles and the Eastern United States, donkey's hooves, adapted to the driest of deserts, absorb excessive moisture, delaminate, and develop abscesses (J. Rodriguez, personal communication, 2015.).[22] Most veterinary professionals in equine practice lack training and experience in donkey management and health care, because the schools from which they graduated lack faculty with interest in donkeys and mules. Of course it would be unreasonable to expect novice owners to have any better idea of how to care for their donkeys, a problem that is compounded by the tendency for people to use nonauthoritative, on-line sources, such as social media, to investigate animal care issues or symptoms.

Because animals used for competitions tend to have a higher value, the donkey (rarely involved in shows or other events in the UK or the United States), tend to be owned by individuals with more limited resources and less equine experience. Often these donkeys lack environmental enrichment, being kept in small suburban paddocks, where their only stimulation is daily feeding. The long-lived donkey is also ill-suited to the rapid changes in life situations found in relatively wealthy communities. When donkeys are not something that families rely on for sustenance, it is easy to see them as disposable. This view results in donkeys being relinquished to overcrowded shelters, sold at auction, or simply set free to survive on their own in more rural areas.[5,9] The more valuable mule actually has improved welfare over both donkeys and horses in the wealthier world.[8]

FERAL AND WILD DONKEY POPULATIONS

In several areas in which donkeys were once critical to the economy, there are large feral populations. These include developed countries such as the United States and Australia, but also developing countries like Mexico, Brazil, and some Caribbean islands. As described elsewhere in this article, in the early part of the twentieth century, motorized vehicles and tractors rapidly replaced donkeys. Because these animals were seen to have no economic or food value, many donkeys were simply turned lose on marginal lands. The hardy animals were much better adapted to these environments than cattle or other livestock, and began to thrive with significant increases in population. Presently, there are approximately 15,000 feral donkeys on federal lands in the United States.[23] Estimates of the feral populations of Australia and Brazil are 5 million and 1 to 2 million, respectively.[2,9,24] Similar figures for Mexico are not available. In all of these locations, feral donkeys are seen as pests or invasive species because they compete for scarce resources with sheep and cattle, or, as is the case in the United States, "native" wild species such as the Big Horn Sheep. Depending on the culture and politics of the country involved, attempts to control the feral populations range from hunting to live capture programs, where donkeys are rounded up and either warehoused in long-term holding facilities, put up for adoption, or sold for slaughter.

Animal protection organizations advocate for nonlethal means of population control, and have met with some success in certain situations. Particularly on islands where corralling of feral animals is fairly easy, projects that sterilize male donkeys by castration have been used. However, as a polygamous species, control of female fertility is a more efficient method of limiting population growth. The 2 main methods of decreasing fertility, the porcine zona pellucida vaccine and the anti-GnRH (GonaCon, USDA National Wildlife Research Center) vaccines have been tried as immunocontraceptives in donkeys, although there is little information on efficacy, especially in larger populations that live on extensive tracts of desert in North America and Australia.[25] The problems with the more commonly used contraceptive, the porcine zona pellucida vaccine, are the expense, the need to deliver the agent by injection, and the need to provide booster doses to maintain fertility control. Delivery requires that jennets be gathered and processed in a chute or that they be darted with the vaccine. The former technique involves considerable stress and some danger to the animals. Remote injection by darts, on the other hand, requires that skilled marksmen hunt the animals in very rugged geographic areas or concentrate them by either helicopter herding or feed or water trapping. Immunized jennets must be identified to ensure that their immunity is boosted every year or two. This further compromises the usefulness of immunocontraception. Finally, contraception that does not interfere with the estrus cycle, such as the porcine zona pellucida vaccine, have been criticized by some humane organizations because the females are subjected to repeated breeding and the natural social structure of the wild population is artificially disrupted.[25,26]

Australia has some of the largest nonnative herbivore populations in the world. Camels, water buffalo, cattle, horses, and donkeys were imported to the continent in the nineteenth century. A combination of stray animals and those that were turned out to fend for themselves with the mechanization of agriculture in the twentieth century have thrived in this sparsely populated country. The Australian government has taken a pragmatic approach to these animals, using hunting and slaughter to decrease what many consider a serious environmental problem.[9,10] More recently with the growth of the *ejiao* (donkey hide gelatin) trade, fueled by the increases in disposable wealth in China, the Australian government is considering building slaughter plants to process feral donkeys for their hides. Because donkeys have evolved to live solitary or in small herds, the idea of concentrating animals to provide the volume required to invest in industrial abattoir facilities has been criticized as being inherently inhumane, even if the actual slaughter process adheres to accepted slaughter protocols.[3,27] In contrast, proponents of using feral donkeys from Australia in the *ejiao* trade point out that controlled slaughter for industrial hide harvesting cause less pain and stress to the donkeys involved than hunting by helicopter, not to mention the increase in income to remote rural areas with limited resources.

There are still truly wild donkey populations in the Horn of Africa. The remaining populations of the Nubian (*Equus africanus africanus*) and Somali Wild Ass (*Equus africanus somaliensis*) are listed as critically endangered owing to hunting and habitat loss. The ancient Atlas Wild Ass, which lived in North Africa and is pictured in cave paintings in the Atlas mountains of Morocco, has gone extinct. Although wild asses have been reported as far north and west as northern Chad, the former ranges extended all the way to Syria. As desertification becomes more intense in Africa, with the changing climate, and armed conflicts continue in Sudan, Somalia, and Ethiopia, it seems likely that donkeys, in the range where they originally evolved, will cease to exist in the coming century.[24,28]

As control of feral donkey populations use removal, sterilization, or slaughter, and the original wild donkeys of Africa continue to decrease in numbers, the loss of genetic variability in the species has been identified as a looming problem.[29] There is evidence that isolated feral populations in the southwestern United States have an increased incidence of congenital defects in foals as a result of a shrinking gene pool. The stakeholders in the controversial management of free-living donkey populations must add genetics to the mix of economics, ecological damage, and humane concerns it their discussions on how such donkeys are to be managed.[29]

Although for many years it has been assumed that feral animals such as donkeys are inherently damaging to the natural environment, recent research in the Sonoran life zone has demonstrated that certain donkey behaviors may actually improve the ability of other wildlife to find water and forage in marginal desert environments. This notion has led to an ongoing debate over where feral donkeys fit in to a world of disappearing large herbivore populations.[30]

INDUSTRIAL DONKEY PRODUCTION

In recent decades, the increases in wealth and living standards in China have led to a surge in the market demand for donkey products. Donkeys have existed in China since the caravans of the Silk Road, serving the same purpose in transport and draught that they have in the rest of the world. However, centuries ago, Chinese medicine practitioners began using the gelatinous extract from boiled donkey hides as an elixir. Traditionally this material, called *ejiao*, is thought to have the ability to improve vitality, treat anemia, and even reverse some psychological problems, such as insomnia.[3,27] Because the requirements for high-quality *ejiao* dictated to be produced in Shandong province from the hides of certain black colored donkeys, and because donkeys were valued as draught animals, the supply of this supplement or pharmaceutical was limited. In fact, only the aristocrats and members of the royal family were able to afford *ejiao*. The increase in wealth for the average Chinese citizen began in the late twentieth century, boosting the demand for *ejiao* to astronomical levels. This has been further fueled by new entrepreneurial methods of packaging and marketing the product. Syrups, candy bars, skin ointments, and other forms, decorated with cute cartoons of donkeys, are consumed or given as valued gifts for personal or national occasions.[27,31]

The initial demand for donkey products in China was addressed by slaughtering large numbers of donkeys in the country. By some estimates, the donkey population in China decreased from more than 9 million to less than 3 million by 2017.[27] This massive donkey depopulation increased their value, or at least that of their hides, in other parts of the world. Most notably, in sub-Saharan Africa, large numbers of retired or working donkeys have been diverted into the slaughter chain, for the production of hides, which are then exported to China for *ejiao* processing. The impoverished farmers and teamsters of countries such as Mali and Tanzania face a choice between taking relatively large amounts of money for their draught animals or keeping the donkeys that they and their families rely on to transport water, fuel, and produce. Many, tempted by amounts of cash that they cannot hope to earn any other way, have chosen to sell their donkeys. As has historically been the case with any kind of boom economy, unscrupulous poachers also steal and kill donkeys in these countries, leaving the skinned carcasses to rot.[3,27] The criminality brought on by the hide market is amplified by the egregiously inhumane care of these animals when they are transported and killed. Among other cruelties, it has been reported that many are intentionally starved to death, because it makes them easier to skin. In response, several countries, including Uganda, Tanzania, Botswana, Niger, Burkina Faso, Mali, Senegal, and Nigeria, have banned the export of donkeys for slaughter and the harvesting of donkey hides. However, it is likely that many of these laws are not well-enforced.[2,3]

Countries such as South Africa, Australia, Pakistan, Kenya, and Brazil have taken a different approach and embraced the *ejiao* boom as an agricultural opportunity. This takes the form of using feral donkeys as a natural resource to be managed in a controlled fashion, processed in modern slaughter facilities (often built with Chinese investment), and the products exported to China as part of international trade.[27] In northeastern Brazil, a feedlot operation has been designed to hold 80,000 donkeys gathered from the Nordestino feral donkey herd. In Kenya, a Chinese-funded slaughterhouse kills and processes 450 donkeys every day.[27] Similar operations, using intensive livestock management techniques to raise donkeys, have also been reported from Inner Mongolia, Mexico, and Australia. The largest producer of *ejiao*, the Dong-e E-Jiao Group, based in Shandong, has a large slaughter facility and product manufacturing plant, associated with its feedlot. The complex is 2000 square meters and produces 40 different *ejiao* products from beverages to candy bars to cereals. This corporation also has a donkey museum and hosts an international meeting on donkey health and production every year.[32] The topics of this gathering and the research that the Dong-e Group funds demonstrate the challenges faced by intensive donkey production: contagious disease, nutritional deficiencies, crowding stress, and reproductive failure. Similar problems are encountered when species such as cattle, swine, and chickens have been brought into the realm of industrial agriculture, with attendant welfare concerns. However, the shift from a life in small groups to huge intensive concentration farms is happening much more rapidly with donkeys. For instance, factory farming of swine has been developing since the early twentieth century, giving farmers time to work out the management problems associated with raising large numbers of animals in confinement and for selective breeding to develop livestock that can survive the conditions dictated by economics. Donkeys, in contrast, are forced to make this transition in a decade. It seems quite unlikely that this transition can be made without considerable suffering. Although it is difficult to see how a gelatin product can have medicinal effects beyond increasing protein intake, there have been numerous publications in Chinese journals describing the success of *ejiao* for treating a number of ailments and proposing mechanisms for its efficacy.[33,34]

In Europe, donkey milk production has become a lucrative business. Although not entirely new, promotion of the health benefits of donkey milk and recognition by the medical profession of its benefits to premature infants has led to an increase in small farm milk production in Italy, Spain, and France.[35,36] The supporters of the growth in donkey dairy point out that the value of the product will make it possible for small farmers to keep their donkeys and prevent the extinction of some unique European donkey breeds. Others are concerned about the welfare implications of breeding more donkeys to maintain milk production in a world where donkeys are often abandoned. Will these foals go into the hide production chain or be slaughtered for food in a continent that maintains a market for horsemeat?

SUMMARY AND SEARCHING FOR SOLUTIONS

Perhaps the real issue of donkey welfare is establishing where donkeys will fit in to a mechanized and urbanized world. Do donkeys have a future as draught animals, and, if so, will economic development agencies recognize their contribution to the poorest members of this planet's human population? There is great room for improvement here, something that could benefit both the animals and those who depend on them. It is encouraging that some international equine NGOs are promoting improved care and husbandry of working donkeys and mules, although governmental agencies are slow to follow.[37]

Are donkeys pests in the areas in which they exist in a wild state, or are they a well-adapted large herbivore, and as such, should they be viewed as a resource to biodiversity on a planet that may be seeing the last of such creatures in the coming century?[30,38] Are donkeys livestock, like cattle or swine, which have value for the products of their slaughter? In this context, although they should be treated humanely, should their management be primarily driven by economics? Is the future of donkeys to be pets, like dogs, cats, and horses in the wealthy Western world sustainable? As populations in North America, Europe, and, increasingly Asia, move away from agriculture and rural lives, and have less contact with domestic animals, the basic knowledge of husbandry and an appreciation for the needs of donkeys and mules fades. Is the morbidly obese pet donkey, kept in a small pen without companionship or interesting things to do, not suffering, although in a different way, than its overworked brother in the tropics? The answers to these questions may come partially from science and veterinary medicine, but just as much they are issues of philosophy and values that have implications for all creatures on a shrinking, warming planet. Solutions will take debate, education, and an open-minded commitment by the veterinary and scientific professions, and will have to be global in nature.

REFERENCES

1. Kimura B, Marshal F, Beja-Pereira A, et al. Donkey domestication. Afr Archaeol Rev 2013;30:83–95.
2. McLean A, Navas Gonzales FJ. Can scientists influence donkey welfare? Historical perspective and contemporary view. J Equine Vet Sci 2018;65:25–32.
3. Köhle N. Feasting on donkey skin. In: Golley J, Jaivin L, editors. Prosperity. Canberra (Australia): ANU Press; 2018. p. 176–82.

4. Blench R. The history and spread of donkeys in Africa. In: Starkey P, Fielding D, editors. Donkeys, people and development. A resource book of the An1imal Traction Network for Eastern and Southern Africa (ATNSA). Wageningen (The Netherlands): ACP-EU Technical Centre for Agriculture and Rural Cooperation (CTA); 2000. p. 22–30.

5. Matthews NS, Taylor TS. Veterinary care of donkeys. Ithaca (NY): International Veterinary Information Service; 2004. p. 904–9.

6. Swift A. A brief history of the domestic donkey. In: Donkey time 2017. Available at: https://donkeytime.org/2017/10/10/a-brief-history-of-the-domestic-donkey/. Accessed November 10, 2018.

7. The Donkey Sanctuary. About donkeys - breeds and cross-breeds. In: Knowledge and advice 2017. Available at: https://www.thedonkeysanctuary.org.uk/what-we-do/knowledge-and-advice/about-donkeys. Accessed November 10, 2018.

8. Bough J. Donkeys and mules colonize North America, Australia, and South Africa. In: Bough J, editor. Donkey. London: Reaktion Books Ltd; 2011. p. 22–35.

9. Bough J. From value to vermin: a history of the donkey in Australia. Aust Zoologist 2006;33:388–97.

10. Bayliss P, Yoemans K. Distribution and abundance of feral livestock in the 'Top End' of the northern territory (1985-86), and their relation to population control. Aust Wildl Res 1989;16:651–76.

11. FAOSTAT. Food and agricultural organization of the United Nations. In: FAO statistical database website. Available at: http://faostat.fao.org/site/409/default.aspx. Accessed November 10, 2018.

12. Duggal G. Caught in the middle. In: The donkey sanctuary 2015. Available at: http://www.animalslebanon.org/images/stories/9690-144742750139.pdf. Accessed November 10, 2018.

13. Blakeway S. The multi-dimensional donkey in landscapes of donkey-human interaction. Rel Beyond Anthropocentrism 2014;2:59–77. Available at: http://www.ledonline.it/index.php/Relations/issue/view/54.

14. Itepu F. Donkeys as an alternative draft power source for women in Okavango, Namibia. In: Starkey P, Fielding D, editors. Donkeys, people, and development, a resource book for Animal Traction Network for Eastern and Southern Africa (ATNESA). Wageningen (The Netherlands): ACP-EU Technical Centre for Agricultural and Rural Cooperation (CTA); 2007. p. 244.

15. Burn C, Dennison T, Whay HR. Environmental and demographic risk factors for poor welfare in working horses, donkeys and mules in developing countries. Vet J 2010;186:385–92.

16. Burn C, Dennison D, Whay HR. Relationships between behaviour and health in working horses, donkeys, and mules in developing countries. Appl Anim Behav Sci 2010;126:109–18.

17. Wilson RT. Specific welfare problems associated with working horses. In: Waran N, editor. The welfare of horses. Animal welfare. Dordrecht (The Netherlands): Springer; 2007. p. 203–18.

18. Burn C, Pritchard J, Farajat M, et al. Risk factors for strap-related lesions in working donkeys at the World Heritage Site of Petra in Jordan. Vet J 2008;178:261–9.

19. Pritchard J, Lindberg A, Main DC, et al. Assessment of the welfare of working horses, mules and donkeys, using health and behaviour parameters. Prev Vet Med 2005;69:265–83.

20. Upjohn M, Pfeifer D, Verheyen K. Helping working Equidae and their owners in developing countries: monitoring and evaluation of evidence-based interventions. Vet J 2014;199:210–6.
21. Burden F, Du Toit N, Hazel-Smith E, et al. Hyperlipemia in a population of donkeys: description, prevalence, potential risk factors. J Vet Intern Med 2011;25:1420–5.
22. Crane M. Hoof disorders of the donkey. In: Chuit PA, Montavon S, editors. 10th Congress on equine medicine and surgery. Geneva (Switzerland): International Veterinary Information Service; 2007. p. 154–6.
23. US Department of the Interior Bureau of Land Management. Program data, wild horse and burro program. Available at: https://www.blm.gov/programs/wild-horse-and-burro/about-the-program/program-data. Accessed November 10, 2018.
24. Starkley P, Starkley M. World trends in donkey populations. In: Starkley P, Fielding D, editors. Donkeys people and development, a resource book for the animal traction network of eastern and southern Africa. Waganingen (the Netherlands): FAO; 2000. p. 10–21.
25. Liu I. The zona pellucida vaccine: immunocontraception in wild equines. In The Donkey Welfare Symposium. 2016. Available at: https://vimeo.com/ondemand/donkeywelfare/215191015. Accessed November 10, 2018.
26. Rocha JM, Ferreira-Silva JC, Humberto Fernandes Veloso Neto HF, et al. Immunocastration in donkeys: clinical and physiological aspects. Pferdeheilkunde – Equine Medicine 2018;34:1–5.
27. Mayers A. Under the skin. Sidmouth (United Kingdom): The Donkey Sanctuary; 2017. p. 1–17.
28. Moehlman PD, Kebebe F, Yohannes H. The African wild ass *Equus africanus*: conservation status in the horn of Africa. Appl Anim Behav Sci 1998;60:115–24.
29. NRC (National Research Council). Genetic diversity in free ranging horse and burro populations. In: Palmer GH, editor. Using science to improve the BLM wild horse and burro program: a way forward. Washington, DC: National Academy of Sciences; 2013. p. 143–70.
30. Lundgren E, Ramp D, Ripple W, et al. Introduced megafauna are rewilding the Anthropocene. Ecography (Cop.) 2018;41:857–66.
31. Kriel G. Donkey production: great economic opportunity or potential mine field? Farmer's Weekly 2017;6:36–40.
32. Knowles G. Chinese health fad that is decimating donkey populations worldwide. Post Magazine 2016. Available at: https://www.scmp.com/magazines/post-magazine/long-reads/article/2050424/chinese-health-fad-thats-decimating-donkey. Accessed November 2, 2018.
33. Jianjun G. Treatment of Fufang ejiao syrup for 37 cases of anemia. World Chin Med 2012;4:36–42.
34. Fan H, Liu Yuxi, Kequin X, et al. Characterization and quantification of dermatan sulfate from donkey skin. China Journal of Chinese Materia Medica 1994;4:124–32.
35. Salimei E, Fantuz F, Coppola R, et al. Composition and characteristics of ass's milk. Anim Res 2004;53:67–78.
36. Dezzutto D, Barbero R, Valle E, et al. Observations of the haematological, haematochemical and electrophoretic parameters in lactating donkeys (Equus asinus). J Equine Vet Sci 2018;65:1–5.
37. Varnum A. Working equid use for sustainable livelihoods. Capstone thesis master of public health and international development studies interdisciplinary graduate program. Fort Collins, Colorado: Colorado Stat University; 2017. p. 1–49.
38. Wallach A, Lundgren E, Ripple W, et al. Invisible megafauna. Conserv Biol 2018; 32(4):962–5.

Skin Disorders of the Donkey and Mule

Derek C. Knottenbelt, BVM&S, DVM&S, MRCVS[a],*

KEYWORDS

- Donkey • Mule • Dermatology • Diagnosis • Cutaneous therapy

KEY POINTS

- The donkey's skin is well-adapted to the rigors of a very hot and dry climate, but copes less well with persistent wetting and cold.
- The donkey suffers from infectious and noninfectious dermatologic disorders that can resemble the equivalent states in horses, but often have subtle and sometimes more significant differences.
- Skin disease in donkeys and mules is often presented late in the course of disease so signs are often chronic by the time treatment is sought.
- Since most donkeys are working animals in less developed countries and communities, mistreatment is common and iatrogenic damage and traumatic skin injuries are frequent.
- Mistreatment of minor skin conditions may result in severe complications; the clinician must determine the primary cause to ensure the condition is correctly identified and managed appropriately.

The donkey has for centuries been regarded as a robust and willing servant of mankind and most veterinarians accept that, as a species, it suffers rather fewer skin diseases than most other domestic animals. However, this may be more in the perception than the actuality, because the donkey tends to show few signs of cutaneous discomfort and apart from "pet" circumstances, the donkey has very little advanced veterinary support across the world. The general perception is that the donkey does not feel pain and therefore has no painful conditions—however, this is very far from the truth.

The skin of the donkey is well-adapted to the rigors of direct sunlight and extremes of heat. The donkey has a specific adaptive ability to cope with desert and other high temperature conditions. They preserve water by sweating against the skin and limit the loss of water by allowing the body core temperature to increase significantly before

Disclosure: The author has nothing to disclose.
[a] Equine Medical Solutions, Kildean Industrial & Enterprise Hub, Office 1, Step Building, 146 Drip Road, Stirling FK8 1RW, Scotland
* Equine Medical Solutions, Kildean Industrial & Enterprise Hub, Office 1, Step Building, 146 Drip Road, Stirling FK8 1RW, Scotland.
E-mail address: knotty@equinesarcoid.co.uk

Vet Clin Equine 35 (2019) 493–514
https://doi.org/10.1016/j.cveq.2019.08.006
0749-0739/19/© 2019 Elsevier Inc. All rights reserved.

vetequine.theclinics.com

using body water for cooling. The latter adaptation allows the donkey to restrict the need for heat loss by evaporation and the cooling under the hair coat maximizes the cooling efficiency of sweating. These properties may give the impression that the donkeys' skin is hardy and able to take almost any insult, but quite the reverse is true. The skin of the donkey has much less waterproof protection than the horse and can easily become saturated with rain; therefore, the skin is easily macerated. Nevertheless, the skin of the donkey is possibly liable to fewer of the infectious diseases than other equidae.

The mule also suffers from significant skin disorders, but even less is known about them. Historically, descriptions of skin conditions in mules has relied on army herds of working mules. There are few if any updated texts or evidence-based publications concerning the skin of mules and our current knowledge relies largely on anecdote and personal experiences. In the author's experience, the mule does have skin conditions and physiologic features that are rather more variable than donkeys or horses. This is probably not a surprise but again, this is simply anecdote, and "two anecdotes do not make data."

Despite the vital role played by the donkey and mule in many countries, several of the diseases of the donkey and mule have not been well-characterized and so led to the possibly erroneous concept that the conditions are the same and that the treatments will therefore be the same. The disorders are often given the names of the similar disorders in humans and other animals. This is probably not true, but at least it does provide a framework for clinicians who deal with fewer donkeys than horses.

There is also a dearth of pathologic information about the skin of the donkey that reflects the shameful lack of interest in the species over countless years. The donkeys long-suffering and tolerant nature simply makes the diseases less important in the eyes of the owners or carers. It is certainly true, however, that working donkeys in poorer parts of the world often have a short life span because of the rigors of their lives and their skin afflictions may be a major cause of debility and failure to maintain a healthy and effective working life. Some of the skin disorders that afflict donkeys in tropical climates are very serious both to the donkey itself and to its owners.[1] Zoonotic implications should be considered where dermatophytes, cryptococcus, and histoplasma organisms are endemic.

The major syndromes of donkey dermatology that might be encountered in practice include:

1. Pruritus
2. Nodular skin disease
3. Alopecia
4. Moist/exudative dermatoses
5. Dry dermatosis (flaking and scaling)
6. Pigmentary changes

These syndromes are usually the basis of the owner's complaint and although they are important, it is vital that the clinical examination and further tests are used to refine and improve the diagnostic process. Within each of the 6 syndromes listed, the diagnostic approach needs to consider a further panel of differential diagnoses. This can be summarized broadly into infectious disorders involving viral, bacterial, and fungal disease or noninfectious conditions, which can have multiple origins as outlined in **Table 1**. The diagnostic process is fundamental to the accurate definition of disease and therefore the selection of appropriate therapeutic measures and so there is no circumstance where a clinical examination is not indicated. The clinician

Table 1
Major divisions of skin disease and examples

Classification	Disease Type	Examples in the Donkey
Infection	Virus	Papilloma
	Bacteria	Dermatophilosis
	Fungus	Dermatophytosis/pythiosis/cryptococcosis/histoplasmosis
	Protozoa	Besnoitiosis
	Parasite	Pediculosis/mites/habronemiasis
Noninfectious	Genetic/developmental	Epidermolysis bullosa
	Immunologic/allergic	Pemphigus/Insect bite hypersensitivity/sarcoidosis
	Nutritional	Debility
	Neurologic	Rabies (pruritus)
	Endocrinologic	Pituitary pars intermedia dysfunction
	Trauma	Various/sunburn/photosensitization
	Iatrogenic	Inappropriate chemical applications and medication
	Chemical/toxic	Selenosis/photosensitization
	Neoplastic	Sarcoid/carcinoma/melanoma/histiocytoma

needs to carefully establish whether a clinical sign is a primary or secondary event. The target for the clinician should of course be to establish the primary cause of disease and therefore establishing the primary lesion is critical to the management process overall.

The investigation of dermatologic disorders follows the standard approach, but is often influenced in donkeys by a lack of background information. A logical and comprehensive clinical approach is essential under the circumstances so that as much information can be gleaned as possible in respect of both the animal itself (in case of primary or secondary systemic involvement) or the presenting sign in terms of onset, progression, and prior treatment attempts. Inevitably, because almost every skin disease is directly visible and easily sampled, almost every case can reach a definitive diagnosis. In donkeys and mules, however, there are frequently constraints on economic aspects and on a general lack of evidence-based information. Compromised clinical examination processes lead to mistakes of commission and errors of omission. Clinical satisfaction derives from a logical and comprehensive clinical investigation. Treatment can only be focused when a diagnosis is made. There is no need to guess or to use symptomatic treatment as diagnostic aids in dermatology. The reader is referred to the dermatology texts by Knottenbelt[2] and Scott and Miller[3] for further details of the approach to a dermatology case and the diagnostic tests available for diagnostic confirmation.

INFECTIOUS SKIN DISEASE

Skin infections are relatively common in donkeys and the species is liable to the full range of microorganisms and ectoparasites.

Viral Skin Disease

For the purposes of this article, viral skin disease will not include the asinine sarcoid, which is considered in neoplastic conditions.

The donkey seems less affected by juvenile or adult papilloma than horses. A few cases have been encountered where typical warts are identified.

The donkey is susceptible to equine herpesvirus 3 infection (coital exanthema) and this is usually regarded as a transient venereal infection. It can affect the penis of the stallion and the perineal skin and vulva of the jenny. An acute, florid, inflammatory response with transient vesicles and secondary infection some days after coitus is the classical symptom. Treatment is simply with soothing antibacterial creams and, if the area is significantly painful, human hemorrhoid creams are useful because they contain an antibiotic and local anesthetics. Sexual rest is important because it can spread rapidly and a rest for up to 3 weeks usually allows the stallion to recover and become noninfectious. There does seem to be a carrier status in the males in which immunity is solid for some years. Carrier females are thought to be responsible for the spread and recurrence in a breeding herd, but there may be other mechanisms for it. Many herpesvirus infections have a latent capacity and so recrudescence is likely.

Bacterial Skin Disease

The common bacterial skin diseases of donkeys include:

1. Dermatophilosis
2. Staphylococcal infections, streptococcal furunculosis, and folliculitis
3. Fusobacterial dermatitis and coronitis (*Fusobacterium necrophorum*)

Mixed infections are common in donkeys and the limbs are probably more often affected than the body, but generalized dermatophilosis (*Dermatophilus congolensis*) does occur and can be very difficult to treat.

The immune status of a donkey with extensive skin infections should be established in all cases where the infections are not explicable.

Clinically it is sometimes possible to make an informed guess as to the bacteria involved. A very painful lesion will usually involve Staphylococci and a moderately painful lesion with closely adherent scabs will be streptococcal. Staphylococcal skin infection usually has less exudate, whereas dermatophilus may have more exudate. Dermatophilosis produces focal lesions with a loose scab that leaves a florid red base after removal. The lesion is more irritational than painful. Other bacteria also cause various forms of dermatitis, folliculitis, or furunculosis and it is always important to identify the species involved if possible.

The main differential diagnoses for bacterial skin disease include fungal skin diseases, neoplastic disorders and traumatic injuries. The latter are commonly affected by secondary bacterial infections and even *Habronema* infestation.

A specific diagnosis is important and this should be obtained by culture and, if necessary, biopsy (with or without deep biopsy culture). Once the full spectrum of bacterial involvement is known and the sensitivity profiles established, then rational treatment can be given. For the most part, however, bacterial infections clear spontaneously with good hygiene. It is an important principle of treatment to render the skin inhospitable to bacterial growth. A close clip out and a single antibacterial wash is helpful. Warm water should always be used for therapeutic washes—washing in cold water seldom helps and may prove counterproductive. Blankets, rugs, and bandages should be removed—these items simply increase the local exudation and macerate the skin still further. Furthermore, it is very easy to restrict capillary blood flow and so create a marginal superficial (and occasionally deeper) necrosis of the skin. Ensuring that the skin remains dry and that the donkey is given a healthy diet are important aspects of management. Because the disease is highly contagious under defined environmental and climatic conditions, affected animals should be isolated until they have been treated effectively (**Fig. 1**).

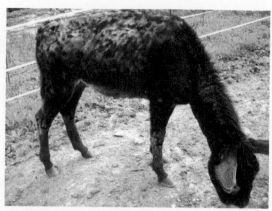

Fig. 1. A typical case of dermatophilosis (rain scald) in a donkey; note the dorsal location of the infection and the pattern of rain run-off. Note also that the animal is in poor body condition, which can make the individual animal more susceptible to the disease. The skin of the donkey has less waterproof properties than that of the horse, so this type of condition can occur in poor climatic conditions where the weather is warm and wet. The organism can be identified in exudate and in skin biopsies.

Fungal Skin Disease

Donkeys are liable to dermatophyte (ringworm) infestation and the clinical features are often less obvious than in horses. Ringworm owing to *Trichophyton* spp. and *Microsporum* spp. dermatophytes are common and present in the usual manner with centrifugally expanding circular patches of alopecia, scaling, and mild exudation (**Fig. 2**). There is seldom any significant pruritus, but the donkey may respond to gentle rubbing of the lesion. More extensive and less well-defined areas may develop in cases affected with certain of the *Trichophyton* spp.

Diagnosis is typically achieved initially by direct microscopy and then culture of hair pluckings from the active outer margin of the lesion, and/or appropriately stained biopsies.[2] Where available, rapid polymerase chain reaction identification obviates the need for prolonged culture. It is important to establish the species involved because control may be affected by the species and its original source.

Treatment involves topical antifungal washes such as enilconazole or natamycin. Oral griseofulvin is commonly prescribed, but there is no real evidence that it is effective at all. Oral konazoles such as fluconazole can be very effective, but they are expensive and little is established on their use in donkeys or mules. The large majority of dermatophytosis cases eventually resolve spontaneously (as in horses), but there may be a significant delay if the donkey is immunocompromised or malnourished. Immunity is reasonably effective and repeat infection with the same organism should not occur for more than 2 years. Vaccine technology has not yet reached the donkey! Spread to other donkeys must be prevented by effective treatment, good hygiene, and isolation of affected animals.

Histoplasmosis

Cutaneous and nasolacrimal histoplasmosis is caused by skin infection with *Histoplasma farciminosum* in donkeys. In both locations, there is ulceration and granulation tissue proliferation (**Fig. 3**). The infection spreads directly from animal to animal and by

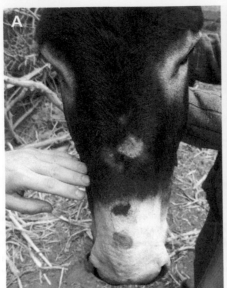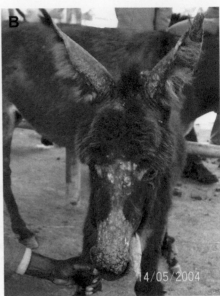

Fig. 2. Typical cases of dermatophytosis. A typical ringworm lesion showing circular alopecic lesions and scaling (*A*). Dermatophyte infections require skin trauma to develop unless the animal is immunocompromised. A more widespread case of dermatophytosis affecting the face and ears (*B*); the species of dermatophyte was not established but both *Microsporum* and *Trichophyton* species affect donkeys from time to time. It is a feature of ringworm in donkeys that some degree of pruritus is relatively common so it is often highly contagious and can become generalized.

vector contact. For the most part, the condition is highly (if slowly) progressive with involvement in particular of traumatized skin (such as the region of the hocks and hind legs). The resulting response causes local exudation and thickening with secondary changes, such as the obstruction (or even destruction) of the nasolacrimal duct. Secondary bacterial infection and even *Habronema* infestation can occur. Probably the commonest sites for this condition in the donkey are within the conjunctiva and nasolacrimal duct (see **Fig. 3** and **Fig. 11**).

Cryptococcosis

Although there remains much uncertainty over the diagnosis of this condition, which can be mistaken for a wide range of similar skin infections, donkeys seem very liable to the disease in tropical climates. Until further evidence is established, the panel of fungal infections that cause the same broad signs can be treated as 1 condition. The epidemiology, clinical features, pathology, and management are all very similar. *Cryptococcus neoformans* is a soil-derived saprophytic opportunistic pathogen that is thought to be transferred into the skin by fly vectors. The commonest site for the infection is the ears. Diagnosis is made from biopsy specimens and the histologic appearance is very typical of the group of pathogens.

Cords, chains, and isolated ulcerating nodules with a characteristic honey like exudate are typically found on the pinnae of affected donkeys (**Fig. 4**). Extensive areas of exudative dermatitis can be found in others areas also, especially in areas where skin trauma and fly attack are combined. The disease causes severe chronic

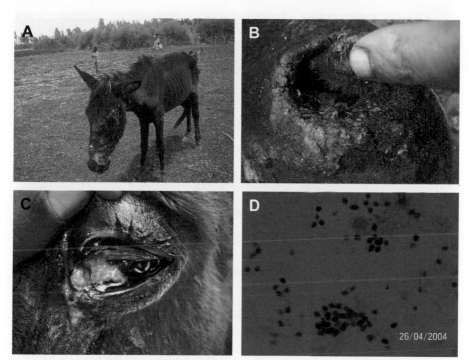

Fig. 3. A mule affected by *Histoplasma farciminosum* (epizootic lymphangitis). The donkey and mule are probably less prone to this infection than horses, but it is nevertheless a devastating and debilitating disease characterized by focal chains and cords of ulcerating nodules (*A*). Nasal and ocular (conjunctival) infections can be life threatening in themselves (*B, C*). The organism can be readily identified in smears and biopsy and it can be cultured readily (*D*). Treatment in largely unrewarding and prevention is the mainstay of management. The disease is widely feared worldwide and is transmitted by biting flies.

debilitating skin inflammation and a cure is hard to achieve. Some affected animals develop a central nervous form of the disease and then usually die.

Treatment is extremely difficult. Prolonged courses of oral potassium iodide and local and systemic konazole medications can help some cases, but the outlook for affected animals is bleak. Systemic fluconazole or itraconazole or even amphotericin B, which is regarded as the drug of choice, can be attempted if the economic situation allows. Interestingly, horses are seemingly much less affected—if at all.

Advanced diagnostic methods such as polymerase chain reaction can be used to reach a more definite diagnosis, but for the most part the management is the same and the prognostic implications are common to all the infections.

Protozoal Skin Disease

Besnoitiosis

In relevant geographic areas, a diffuse scaling dermatitis may be caused by *Besnoitia* spp. protozoa.[4] The changes are typically nonspecific but are often found on the neck region in particular (**Fig. 5**A). The histopathology is said to be distinctive (see **Fig. 5**B). The skin of affected donkeys is often hyperkeratotic and scale and crust arising from self-inflicted trauma as a result of pruritus are common.

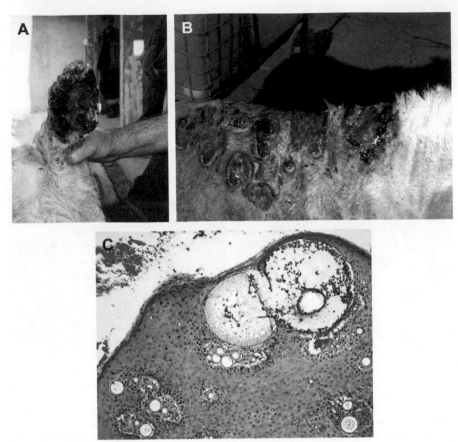

Fig. 4. Typical cases of *Cryptococcus neoformans* infection in donkeys. The lesions are difficult to differentiate from a number of other skin infections including histoplasmosis and glanders (*Burkholderia mallei*) infection (*A, B*). The pleomorphic yeast cells stain a pale blue to pink with H&E and range from 2 to 20 μm in diameter (*C*). There remains controversy over the species involved in this condition and current research is trying to establish the true nature of this infection in donkeys.

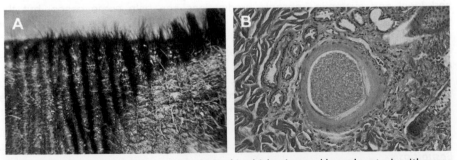

Fig. 5. Typically, *Besnoitia* infection results in skin thickening and hyperkeratosis with prominent scaling and flaking (*A*). The skin can be severely damaged with rugae and lichenification, as demonstrated in this case. The protozoal infection can be identified in biopsy sections, although multiple biopsy samples are often required to confirm the infection. (*B*). Biopsy is the definitive differentiating diagnostic test (**Fig. 5**B). An effective treatment is not reported, although trimethoprim-sulfamethoxazole and ponazuril have been used.

The disease can be moderately or severely pruritic and can therefore be easily mistaken for insect bite hypersensitivity—the latter is rare in donkeys but in any case is commoner than besnoitiosis. The scaling can also be similar to other immune-mediated skin diseases such as pemphigus, cutaneous lupus or sarcoidosis.

Parasitic Skin Disease

A variety of ectoparasites occur in donkeys with the common presenting signs of pruritus and self-inflicted trauma or dermatitis (**Figs. 6–8**). It is important to separate genuine pruritus from insect worry—the latter is usually easily controlled by preventing contact and is usually from flies. Identification of the parasites gives useful information on the likely source of the problem and allows more sensible treatment and prevention strategies. Treatment options are limited in most countries because strong controls on the use of effective insecticidal compounds are enforced. Avermectins given orally or pyrethroids administered topically as washes and powders are anecdotally reported to be marginally effective, but a healthy skin and clean management can be really effective in controlling outbreaks and curing individual cases.

Chorioptic and other mange mite infestations

Chorioptes spp. commonly infest donkeys over the winter months in particular and, although distal limb pruritus is a prominent sign, it can be almost insignificant. In heavy infestations, there may be severe self-trauma and in some cases a hypersensitivity response develops in which the extent of cutaneous inflammation is far worse than the condition warrants (see **Fig. 6**). This is a true hypersensitivity, but it is unclear to what the skin is reacting.

Incidental cases of poultry mite infestation (see **Fig. 7**) and *Psoroptes* spp. infestation (see **Fig. 8**) do occur under defined conditions. Most ectoparasites are opportunistic and prefer other hosts if available, but they can cause severe clinical signs and consequent debility.

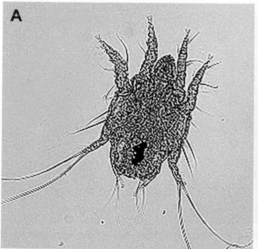
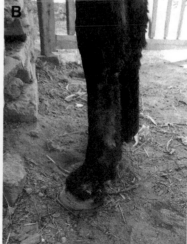

Fig. 6. *Chorioptes equi* affects donkeys occasionally (*A*). The infestation is usually transient, but can cause moderate to severe pruritus (*B*).

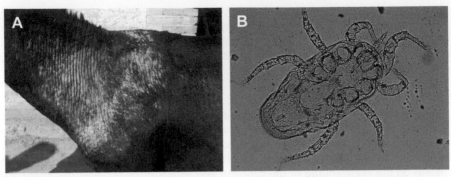

Fig. 7. Severe pruritus arises from highly active mites deriving from poultry contact in particular (*A*). The mites are easily identified in brushings taken from actively pruritic areas (*B*). Usually *Dermanyssus gallinae* is involved.

Pediculosis

Lice are common in donkeys in the UK, but are actually rare in more extensive management systems unless the donkeys are malnourished or otherwise immuno-compromised. Both blood-sucking lice (*Haematopinus* spp.) (**Fig. 9**) and surface- or scale-feeding biting lice (*Werneckiella/Damalinia* spp.) (**Fig. 10**) occur frequently in debilitated and congregated donkeys and mules. Debilitated animals are much more liable to be affected and *Haematopinus asini*, being a blood feeder, adds to the debility with some affected animals being patently anemic.

Lice tend to be moderately species specific and it is not clear if these are the same species that affect horses. In both infestations, pruritus may be seen and although it may be mild the donkey may develop a moth-eaten appearance without marked pruritus. Where pruritus is present, it is usually worse in warm weather and because lice infestations are most prevalent in late winter and early spring the coat alterations are usually obvious. Secondary infections are common in the traumatized skin, but will usually involve opportunistic pathogens rather than severe skin pathogens. The diagnosis is usually not difficult but treatment and control challenges are significant.

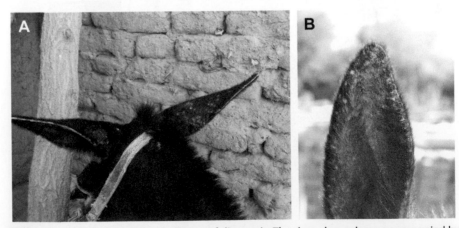

Fig. 8. This case illustrates the challenge of diagnosis. The signs shown here accompanied by pruritus was identified as Psoroptic mange owing to *Psoroptes ovis* (*A*). Almost identical signs arise from fly bite worry, which is usually associated with *Simulium* spp. flies, although these are not usually pruritic (*B*).

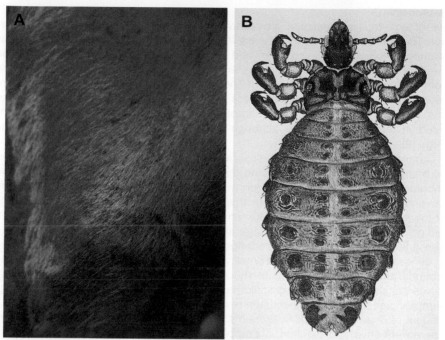

Fig. 9. *Haematopinus asini* affects donkeys more than horses. This is a very prolific parasite, especially when the donkey is debilitated or nutritionally or immunologically compromised. Pruritus is not usually a prominent feature and the parasites are often hard to see because of their dark brown color (*A*). A hand held illuminated magnifying glass usually reveals the parasites. The parasite is a blood feeder and cause severe blood loss in heavy infestations. It is easily recognized microscopically (*B*).

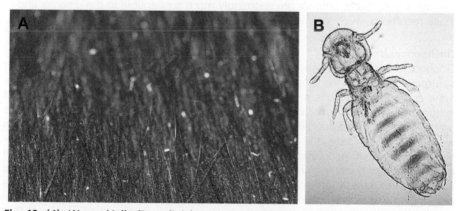

Fig. 10. (*A*). *Werneckiella (Damalinia) equi* are easily seen on the surface of the skin. (*B*). They are large, pale and mobile. Magnification is not usually required to see these parasites.

The parasites are highly contagious so isolation of affected animals and persistent treatment are essential. Oral avermectins and pyrethroid washes and powders can be effective, but do need to be repeated. Overall health and avoiding crowded situations are always helpful.

Habronemiasis

Habronema musca infestation is a relatively common seasonally related skin disorder. The common forms of the disease include a facial form that shows very typical (pathognomonic) facial excoriation and lack of healing that usually starts at the medial canthus of the eye and runs down the face (**Fig. 11**A). Bilateral cases are common (see **Fig. 11**B). It is a common cause of incipient wound healing failure as well (see **Fig. 11**C). It is more or less geographically limited, but climate change has also had an influence on its geographic range. It is still, however, rarely encountered in temperate climates, although it does occur under defined conditions (**Fig. 12**).

Cutaneous habronemiasis was described in 5 donkeys.[5,6] The lesions appeared on many parts of the body, including the medial canthal skin and conjunctiva, the shoulders, the pectoral area, the carpus, and the abdominal wall and prepuce. Several affected animals had more than 1 affected site. The clinical appearance of the lesions associated with habronemiasis were ulcerative areas filled with light red granulation tissue. After curettage, the lower layers revealed, in some cases, a dense fibrous tissue with yellow to beige calcified foci (termed *kunkers*) composed of dense fibrous tissue contained small, caseous, necrotic foci. These also occur in wounds affected by the parasite the case of muscular lesions, but the lower layers consisted of a dense granuloma, without trace of cicatrization. Curettage samples digested with soda solution revealed fragments of nematode larvae reminiscent of *Draschia* spp. or *Habronema* spp. Curettage and excision of the lesion proved effective and resulted in complete healing of the wound by scar tissue formation.

A diagnosis can often be assumed from the characteristic appearance of facial or conjunctival habronemiasis but a biopsy or simply saline brushings as shown in **Fig. 12** can be helpful also.

Treatment with topical ivermectin and steroid is good but more severe cases may require repeated debridement. Oral avermectins have a variable benefit.

The important thing about this condition is the recurrence year on year in susceptible individuals. Some animals are seemingly more susceptible to the disease and in these recurrence every year is to be expected.

Onchocercosis

Onchocercosis is an unusual parasite that afflicts donkeys in some tropical and subtropical regions. The cutaneous clinical signs include ulcerating nodules in the neck and withers regions and sometimes in the digital flexor tendons. The main syndrome that could occur in temperate climates is a focal necrotizing dermatosis on the face or neck predominately that follow from administration of an avermectin wormer. In these cases, the lesions the lesion possibly arises from an immune reaction to the dead microfilaria in the skin capillaries (**Fig. 13**). The withers region and the withers bursa in particular are a focus of serious pathology; the parasites can be found directly in the bursa when a discharging sinus tract develops in this region (**Fig. 14**). The ligamentum nuchae and the digital flexor tendons are natural predilection sites for the adult parasite in donkeys (and horses) and animals that have pain and possibly palpable localized nodules in these areas may be considered to be affected. Ultrasound scanning will help the diagnostic process. The management of onchocercosis is problematic because ideally the parasites need to be removed. The very low incidence of the disease in circumstances where regular avermectin anthelmintic treatment is given suggests that prevention is effective and in any case is far better than a cure.

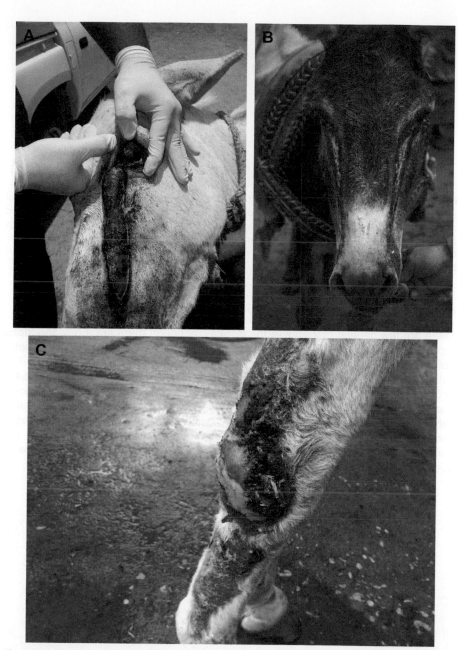

Fig. 11. Primary cutaneous habronemiasis causes marked facial ulceration and often also affects the conjunctivae. The condition can be unilateral (*A*) or bilateral (*B*) and varies in extent and severity between individuals. The common facial form of the disease usually resolves spontaneously in autumn and winter but once an individual has been affected it is very likely to suffer annual deteriorating relapses. Preemptive measures for both prevention or early recognition and treatment are therefore easy to institute. *Habronema musca* also infests wound sites (*C*) and is a common cause of incipient wound healing failure in endemic circumstances.

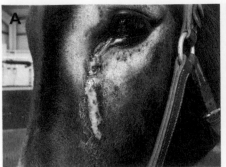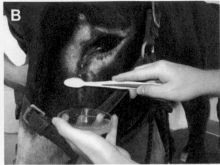

Fig. 12. Cutaneous Habronemiasis in a British Poiteau donkey. The clinical features of facial and ocular habronemiasis are easily recognized at appropriate seasonal times (*A*). This donkey was one of several affected. Diagnosis was confirmed by taking wet brushings from the surface of the open lesion (*B*) and examining for the characteristic larvae under the microscope. Treatment with an ivermectin paste and a steroid cream was simple and curative.

GENETIC AND DEVELOPMENTAL SKIN DISORDERS

There are few genetic diseases of the donkey, although there are a few anecdotal reports of epitheliogenesis imperfecta with large areas of skin missing from birth. Epidermolysis bullosa is also encountered but is exceedingly rare (**Fig. 15**). The author has encountered 1 case of a skin fragility condition that resembled the cutaneous asthenia (Ehlers-Danlos syndrome) that is encountered in other species (including the horse). In this case, the skin was easily traumatized and healed very slowly with large scar formation. The healed skin remained even more fragile and the repeated damage that resulted simply from normal handling was not considered to be acceptable and the donkey was humanely killed at 7 months of age.

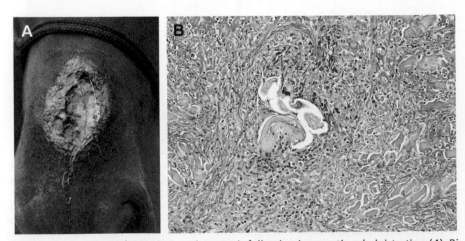

Fig. 13. Cutaneous onchocerciasis with necrosis following ivermectin administration (*A*). Biopsy revealed the remnants of the parasites (*B*). These can be positively identified by polymerase chain reaction methods.

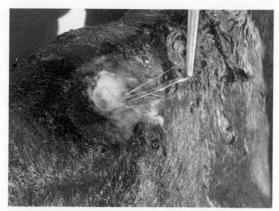

Fig. 14. *Onchocerca cervicalis* adult worms being removed from a withers bursa in a working donkey in Mali. This is a common problem in some parts of the world and a cause of significant morbidity and even mortality.

The donkey is occasionally also liable to dermoid cyst formation and these nodules are typically found in low numbers along the dorsal midline in young donkeys. They contain hair and adnexal structures in a chaotic arrangement. Surgical excision is curative and they do not seem to recur. Little or nothing is known

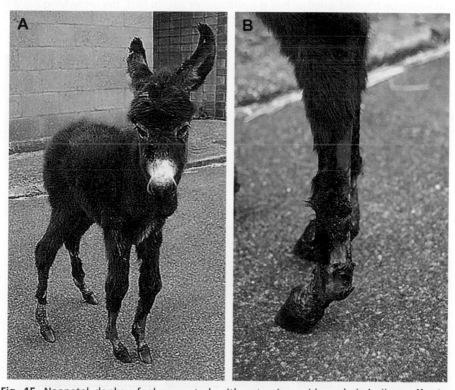

Fig. 15. Neonatal donkey foal presented with extensive epidermolysis bullosa affecting mainly the limb skin (*A, B*). The condition is incurable. (*Courtesy* of Marianne Sloet, DVM, PhD, Dipl. ECEIM, Spec. KNMvD Equine Internal Medicine, Utrecht, Netherlands.)

about the specific genetic or hereditary nature of most of these conditions in donkeys.

IMMUNOLOGIC SKIN DISEASE

The donkey is remarkably free of immune-mediated or autoimmune skin disease with very few reports of cases. The author has, however, encountered several cases of a condition that is indistinguishable both clinically and histologically from pemphigus foliaceus in horses. These cases have been presented with extensive areas of exfoliative hyperkeratotic skin and alopecia with easily epilated hair (**Fig. 16**). Some systemic signs including intermittent fever and distal limb edema were common features. In 1 case, the lesions were sparser and more focal and, in this individual, no systemic signs were present. In the former group, progression was rapid and they failed to respond in the long term to immunosuppressive doses of prednisolone or dexamethasone. In the latter individual case, however, intermittent prednisolone was enough to result in reasonable periods of remission. Keratin and mucocutaneous junctions were affected most obviously. The condition can become generalized and hair loss with circular exudative patches may be encountered. The condition is usually nonpruritic and can be diagnosed from biopsy.

Typical of most autoimmune conditions in most species, the cause of the autoantibody production is hard to establish. Trigger factors, including virus or bacterial infection, drug administration, vaccination, and other systemic and metabolic conditions can easily be blamed whether this is justifiable or not. In fact, the underlying case is seldom identified. A few cases might be due to paraneoplastic pemphigus.

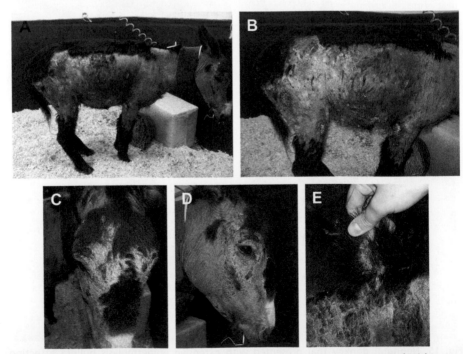

Fig. 16. Pemphigus foliaceus in a donkey. This 9-year-old donkey was presented with extensive hair loss, scaling, and poor body condition (*A–D*). The hair was easily epilated (*E*).

Diagnosis is relatively easily achieved by biopsy but it is very important to avoid any washing, wiping or other interference before biopsy. Multiple biopsies are usually required. It is important to remember that the diagnostic acanthocytes are easily found in the crusts and scales so collection of this into formalin solution can help the diagnostic process.

Although there is no significant published evidence regarding treatment of pemphigus in donkeys, treatment is largely unrewarding and the prognosis is probably very poor. However, high (immunosuppressive) doses of corticosteroids can be attempted; probably the best of these is oral prednisolone (2–4 mg/kg) for the first 7 days and then tapering the dose progressively down to a minimum effective alternate daily dose. There are no data concerning the value of other immunosuppressive drugs such as azathioprine, pentoxifylline aurothioglucose, or methotrexate in donkeys. The risks of laminitis after steroid use in donkeys has not been defined to the author's knowledge and certainly there does not seem to be a higher risk than in horses (in which the risk is probably heavily overstated anyway).

ALLERGIC SKIN DISEASES

Compared with horses, the donkey rarely gets any form of urticaria and contact and systemic skin allergies are seemingly extremely rare.

Insect hypersensitivity, however, occasionally occurs in donkeys but is not often the typical sweet itch syndrome seen in horses. In the author's experience, many of the animals suffer from sensitivity to other biting flies rather than *Culicoides* spp. Nevertheless, many do show a typical distribution and seasonal onset of severe pruritus that is indistinguishable from equine sweet itch. Typically, the affected donkey shows an intense pruritus that becomes worse when they are exposed to the causative insects and show a progressive severity with succeeding years.

Self-trauma causes extensive hair loss, dermatitis, and variable lichenification and thickening of the skin on the neck and withers regions in particular. The rump and tail head are also affected in many cases. The legs can also be involved and again the self-trauma can cause devastating pathology. Secondary infection, further fly irritation, and exposure to ultraviolet light the condition can rapidly become very serious in individual animals.

Although treatment is required in any animal that exhibits signs, it is far better to prevent exposure to the allergen. This may be easier said than done! Most insects do not like windy, cold, or rainy conditions and so this can be a useful way of helping. However, the downside of this is that these conditions are not ideal for donkeys in other respects. Housing during maximal risk periods and turn-out at minimal risk periods (eg, overnight and in the heat of the day) can help; however, because the condition is not always caused by *Culicoides* spp. midges, the effectiveness of this strategy might also vary markedly. The key point is to avoid contact with the causative insect—assuming that this can be established. Insect repellents and other synthetic pyrethroids as well as various natural and other insect repellents will help, but in severe cases the only effective way is to separate the donkey from the allergen. Rugs and blankets are seldom helpful in donkeys and often create more problems than help. Severely excoriated skin can be treated with antibiotic, steroid, and local anesthetic creams and parenteral medication with corticosteroids such as prednisolone may be the only way of reducing the severity of the inflammation. In the author's limited experience, the use of depot steroids such as methylprednisolone acetate is not very useful in donkeys.

NEUROLOGIC DISEASES OF THE SKIN

Primary cutaneous neurologic disease is very rare in donkeys—even more so than in horses. However, importantly one of the most common signs of rabies in donkeys is "pruritus."

A hyperaesthetic (apparently pruritic) skin disorder that resulted in severe self-trauma has been encountered. The donkey had sustained a fracture of a cervical vertebra and the associated dermal segment showed persistent sweating and remained a constant source of irritation to the donkey. The area was traumatized persistently, and topical local anesthetics and steroids applied to the skin site had no material effect.

Rabies is a critical disorder in all species both for the case and for its clear zoonotic potential. Donkeys are liable to rabies like all other mammals and affected animals may show severe (central or paradoxic) pruritus. Often the main presenting sign is pruritus and self-trauma either on perineal or distal limb locations. It is easy to be misled by this finding and, in endemic areas, the possibility of rabies must be considered. The patient will bite, lick, and rub at the site or region of the original inoculation. Usually, there is a history of a bite at the site and so clinicians must always ask before they examine a donkey in an endemic area that shows a focal severe progressive pruritus. The signs of rabies in donkeys can be much subtler, however, and even a failure to "clear" flies at normal fly-worry sites may be a sign. Usually the course of the condition is rapid and so a diagnosis may be assumed or confirmed from the clinical and supportive tests.

TRAUMATIC SKIN DISEASE

Probably the most prevalent and the most dramatic and disturbing skin disease is accidental trauma. Donkeys maintained in poor conditions that are required to work very hard with poor nutrition and with ill-fitting harness (if any is fitted at all!) are commonly afflicted with chronic long-standing open wounds. Traumatic skin diseases are a recurrent and major concern in working donkeys worldwide. Like many of the other skin disorders, this is best regarded as a direct consequence of domestication. Feral populations of donkeys are remarkably free of skin disease of any sort and traumatic injuries usually heal remarkably well.

The geographic locations where donkeys work usually mean that both their nutritional status and the risks of parasitic and bacterial infection of wounds is high.

Although donkeys have a very resilient skin they can react to inappropriate contacts through dirty tack or through chemical injury from inappropriate treatment methods that make matters worse not better. Usually, the clinical features of these dermatoses relate to specific defined areas of application/contact with the irritant material. Saddle or harness oils may be irritants and then, for example, the pattern of contact will be evident from the clinical examination—lesions are usually restricted to contact areas.

CHEMICAL AND TOXIC SKIN DISEASES

Donkeys are liable to the full range of toxic skin disease and perhaps the most alarming is photosensitization arising as a result of chronic or terminal liver failure. Direct (primary) photosensitization does not seem to occur as commonly in donkeys as in horses.

Ragwort (*Senecio jacobaea*) is highly toxic to donkeys (as for horses) but despite its unpalatability, donkeys may eat it in the green state when food is otherwise in short supply. Advanced liver failure signs from pyrrolizidine alkaloid toxicity may be present to guide the clinician, but sometimes photosensitization is the first sign. Extensive exudative inflammatory dermatitis over exposed areas of the skin arises. Interestingly in the donkey it is this author's experience that the eruptions are not necessarily always confined to the white-skinned areas, although the white areas are invariably much worse.

Chemical skin damage is common as result of overly strong chemicals used to treat skin disease. There is a general belief that the skin of the donkey can tolerate every known insult, but in reality, donkey skin is probably one of the most sensitive to chemical insult.

IATROGENIC AND IDIOPATHIC SKIN DISEASE

It is an unfortunate fact that many donkeys are subjected to all manner of mistreatment for trivial skin disease or are inclined to be ignored until the skin is appallingly bad and then subjected to an inappropriate treatment. Engine oil and hot mineral oil have regrettably been used for years to treat lice. Of course, they do kill the lice but the disadvantages are plain!

NEOPLASTIC SKIN DISORDERS

The donkey is liable to several cutaneous tumors including (in order of prevalence) sarcoid, squamous cell carcinoma, fibroma, fibrosarcoma, melanoma, and giant cell tumor (histiocytoma).

Sarcoid

By far the commonest neoplasm is the sarcoid (**Fig. 17**). There is no doubt that donkeys can be severely affected, but the type and distribution of the sarcoid is somewhat different from the disease in horses. Donkeys are more liable to severe invasive and fibroblastic lesions and the occult and verrucose forms are less common in this species. It is also however, easy to overlook the verrucose and occult forms of the disease in donkeys.

A virus has been suggested as the etiology, but the epidemiology in both horses and donkeys is not fully explained by this alone. There is much anecdotal evidence of contagion, but whether this is simply a matter of virus contact is another debate all together.

Predilection sites for sarcoid in donkeys include the face (especially around the mouth and eyes), the groin and sheath regions where aggressive fibroblastic sarcoids are common.

Notwithstanding the diagnostic benefit that can be derived from biopsy, it is probably unwise to biopsy a sarcoid lesion without a plan for its immediate treatment. In any case, the condition in donkeys is easily recognized clinically.

The treatments available are very limited and all have problems of one sort or another and are described in detail by Knottenbelt and colleagues.[5] The reality is that early treatment of any sarcoid may serve at least to limit the long-term severity and improve the long-term prognosis, but ill-advised attempts that lack proper thought may exacerbate the problem. Thus, surgical excision may be an effective option where the limits of the sarcoid can be defined, but simply debriding the bulk of the lesion or failure to include a wide enough margin may result in a dramatic deterioration. It is now well-established that recurrence at the site of a sarcoid excision surgery is a common feature and this can arise either from partial excision or from seeding of the operative site with cells from the lesion itself during surgical procedures. In the authors experience the latter results in a more extensive exacerbation than the former.

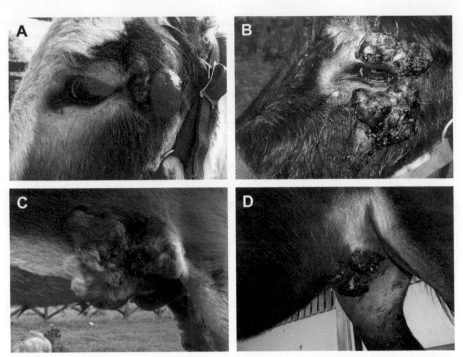

Fig. 17. The sarcoid is by far the commonest skin tumor of donkeys. The donkey and the mule to a lesser extent perhaps seems to have a higher propensity for fibroblastic sarcoid than other equidae. The number and location of sarcoids on an individual animal is extremely variable. They are often found on the face (*A, B*), inguinal area (*C*), and prepuce (*D*). Treatment is very difficult and all options and combinations of treatments should be considered carefully for every individual lesion. Failure to resolve the condition usually causes serious consequences.

Cryosurgery is also possible, but suffers from the same limitations. Cryosurgery is limited in its efficacy to small lesions in convenient sites and to limited numbers. The hitherto recognized remote effects on sarcoids at other sites (suggested to be due to haematogenous cryoantigens released into the blood) does not occur in donkeys in the author's experience. The simple application of liquid nitrogen to the skin of any animal without proper control is totally unacceptable as a veterinary procedure.

Laser surgery and diathermy are logical provided that they are carried out under controlled conditions by experienced surgeons. Burning the lesions with red hot irons and electrically heated wires are totally unacceptable—these measures are illogical, cruel, and do nothing to help the disease.

Immunologic mechanisms may be of value. There are anecdotal reports from Central America of the benefits of autogenous blood injections, but it is very hard to see any immunologic benefit from this approach.

The reality is that a few cases do seem to spontaneously resolve (although this seems to be less common in donkeys than in horses). The use of intralesional BCG has been advocated and this seem to be a useful but by no means certain treatment for localized nodular and fibroblastic lesions around the eyes of the donkey in particular. The critical factors seem to be the true intralesional injection: perilesional injection has no material benefit and risks the development of anaphylaxis. Repeated injections are required but, as the tumor becomes necrotic and decays, true intralesional injections become more difficult.

Topical cytotoxic compounds based on heavy metals and cytotoxic and antimitotic chemicals such as AW5 (Liverpool cream), 5% 5-fluorouracil and blood root/zinc chloride mixtures may all be used with some benefits and are valuable because they are convenient and relatively inexpensive. Often these are the only material options available. They do, however, cause tissue necrosis and some pain is inevitable. The results suggest that some localized lesions and those that have a superficial nature are more responsive to the methods but again there are wide variations in response and some lesions will not respond at all. There are many questionable materials that purport to be effective treatments but most of these (if not all) have no proven efficacy and have not been studied properly. For the most part unproven and nonveterinary treatments should be avoided as far as possible.

Intralesional chemotherapy with aqueous or slow-release (emulsion or bead) forms can be effective also. As is always the case there are health and safety issues with the use of cisplatin, carboplatin, 5-fluorouracil, and mitomycin C.

The gold standard for the treatment of the equine or asinine sarcoid is radiation therapy, but the availably of teletherapy and interstitial brachytherapy is very limited. The expense and practicality are severely limiting factors.

Other Tumors

Melanoma is very rare in donkeys, even though they are commonly grey in color, as with black skin. However, they do occur from time to time around the eye region in particular. There is little correlation with hair coat and skin colors. As with any other nodular skin disease, a biopsy is usually helpful.

Squamous cell carcinoma occurs in donkeys in much the same way and character as in horses. Cutaneous and ocular forms are more common than penile/vulvar forms. Ulcerative and proliferative (and mixed destructive-proliferative) forms occur. Treatment options are effectively limited to surgical excision or cryosurgery. There are no scientific comparative studies on the use of cisplatin, 5-fluorouracil or radiation in donkeys and given the paucity of literature reports it is difficult to predict which treatments are best in any particular circumstances.

Other skin tumors do occur from time to time, but they are all rare and occur sporadically; there is correspondingly little established about the treatment options and their relative prognosis.

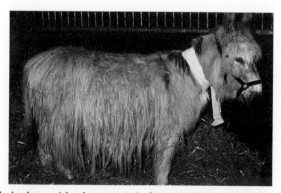

Fig. 18. An aged donkey with characteristic hypertrichosis of pituitary pars intermedia dysfunction/Cushing's disease. The pituitary pars intermedia was grossly enlarged at necropsy. (*Courtesy of* The Donkey Sanctuary, Devon, UK.)

Pituitary pars intermedia dysfunction or Cushing's disease does occur from time to time in donkeys (**Fig. 18**). It is somewhat surprising perhaps that the diagnosis is less common than in horses, because many donkeys live active lives up to age 40 years and older. The cardinal features of the disease are broadly the same as for horses with hirsutism/hypertrichosis. Failure to shed the hair in summer is less obvious in some donkeys because as a species they do not have an identical shedding pattern as horses. Nevertheless, an unexplained long summer coat is probably sufficient to diagnose the disease in a donkey of 15 years or older. They are also liable to the full range of secondary skin infections and infestations that accompany immunosuppression. Laminitis seems less common than in horses. Endocrine tests for horses also to apply to donkeys and consideration should be given to season when testing. Daily pergolide is used to good effect in confirmed donkey cases.

ACKNOWLEDGMENTS

The author is much indebted to my friends and colleagues at the Donkey Sanctuary, the American Fondouk, SPANA, World Horse Welfare and Brooke for their help with this article and to others who have regularly consulted and shared cases with me over the years. Several individuals have helped provide both information and images for this article and particular mention should be given to Michael Crane, Amadou Doumbia and Mariano Hernandez Gill.

REFERENCES

1. Svendsen ED. The professional handbook of the donkey. 4th edition. Yatesbury (England): Whittet Books; 2008.
2. Knottenbelt DC. Pascoe's principles and practice of equine dermatology. Oxford (England): Saunders; 2009.
3. Scott DW, Miller WH. Large animal dermatology. Philadelphia: Saunders; 2003.
4. Liénard E, Nabuco A, Vandenabeele S, et al. First evidence of *Besnoitia bennetti* infection (Protozoa: Apicomplexa) in donkeys (Equus asinus) in Belgium. Parasit Vectors 2018;11(1):427.
5. Knottenbelt DC, Patterson Kane J, Snalune K. Clinical equine oncology. Oxford: Elsevier; 2015.
6. Mohamed FH, Abu Samra MT, Ibrahim KE, et al. Cutaneous habronemiasis in horses and domestic donkeys (Equus asinus asinus). Rev Elev Med Vet Pays Trop 1990;42:535–40.

Anesthesia, Sedation, and Pain Management of Donkeys and Mules

Nora Matthews, DVM[a],*, Johannes P.A.M. van Loon, DVM, PhD[b]

KEYWORDS

- Donkey • Mule • Anesthesia • Analgesia • Pain

KEY POINTS

- There are major differences in behavior and physiology between donkeys, mules, and horses.
- The response to pain is less evident in donkeys and mules compared with horses.
- These differences affect duration and use of sedatives, analgesics, and anesthetics.
- Anesthetic management of donkeys and mules is similar to horses but with subtle differences.

INTRODUCTION

Previous tutorial articles[1,2] have covered some of the differences in physiology, behavior, and pharmacology that exist between donkeys and horses. Although donkeys and mules have a reputation for being "stubborn," recent research carried out at the Donkey Sanctuary showed that donkeys and mules outperformed horses in a test of spatial cognition and perseveration abilities and mules outperformed dogs.[3] These species-related differences have numerous implications for anesthetic and analgesic strategies in donkeys and mules. Numerous publications have discussed differences in pharmacokinetics of anesthetics and analgesics,[4–7] whereas at the same time, much of the available knowledge on donkeys is from clinical experience and does not come from scientific research. However, this empirical and scientific knowledge from equine studies can be used together in order to develop optimal strategies for anesthesia and analgesia in donkeys and mules. Since the last time the authors published a review article of anesthesia and analgesia in donkeys and mules,[1] several new studies have been published emphasizing a need for continued research and information on these "alternative" equines. Furthermore, Grint and colleagues[8]

The authors have nothing to disclose.

[a] Texas A & M University, Freeville, NY, USA; [b] Department of Equine Sciences, Faculty of Veterinary Medicine, Utrecht University, Yalelaan, Utrecht 3584 CM, The Netherlands
* Corresponding author. 157 West Dryden Road, Freeville, NY.
E-mail address: nmatthews@cvm.tamu.edu

published a survey on the current use of analgesics prescribed for donkeys in practice and to collect opinions from veterinary surgeons and donkey owners on the importance of different pain-related behaviors in donkeys.

PREANESTHETIC EVALUATION AND PATIENT PREPARATION

Preoperative evaluation of the donkey or mule should be as thorough as it would be for a horse, including weighing the animal when possible. When weight scales are not available, body weight estimators based on heart girth and height to the withers are available from the Donkey Sanctuary (www.thedonkeysanctuary.org.uk).[9] It is critically important to recognize that normal parameters for temperature, respiratory and heart rates, as well as hematological and biochemical parameters may be significantly different for donkeys than in horses; the number of differences that exist between mules and horses has not been documented. Up-to-date reference ranges can be obtained from the Donkey Sanctuary (www.thedonkeysanctuary.org.uk) and from Erin L. Goodrich and Erica Behling-Kelly's article, "Clinical Pathology of Donkeys and Mules," in this issue of the clinics. Normal values for adrenocorticotropic hormone and insulin differ between donkeys and horses, while other values (eg, cortisol) are not different.[10] Preoperative assessment and treatment of pain should also be diligent; donkeys and mules may not exhibit pain as openly as horses, so more severe pain may be overlooked. Regan and colleagues[11] developed an ethogram to record behavioral expressions of pain in working donkeys and showed improvement in these behaviors after the administration of a nonsteroidal antiinflammatory drug (NSAID; flunixin meglumine). Frequency of changes in head carriage, eye closing, limb shifting, and self-grooming decreased after NSAID administration.[12] These investigators also documented that pain responses to castration were similar to that seen in ponies and horses; therefore, appropriate analgesics should be used in donkeys.

In the opinion and experience of one investigator (NSM), failure to adequately treat pain preoperatively may lead to cardiovascular decompensation after induction of anesthesia. Appropriate NSAID use in donkeys is well reviewed by Grosenbaugh[2]; there is minimal mule-specific information.[4] However, NSAIDs are the mainstay of analgesic drugs used. Although some differences between sizes/breeds of donkeys have been documented for analgesics such as phenylbutazone,[13] as well as injectable anesthetics,[14] there is little information about many other breeds of donkeys or mules throughout the world. As a general rule, NSAIDs have a shorter half-life in donkeys (there is minimal data for mules) so may need to be given at shorter intervals than in horses. Pharmacokinetic properties of flunixin meglumine in mules are similar to horses.[4] Comparative studies of drugs such as tramadol, which has been shown to have low bioavailability in Italian donkeys[15] might show differences in other breeds.

INTRAVENOUS CATHETERS AND PREMEDICATIONS

Jugular catheter placement is facilitated with good restraint (**Fig. 1**), and the catheter must be long enough (the investigator prefers at least 9 cm or more) to penetrate the thicker skin and fascia of the donkey while still remaining in the vein. Although the jugular vein is in the same location as in the horse, it is covered by the cutaneous colli muscle, which is thicker than in the horse,[16] as well as a fascial layer. This may make it more difficult to visualize the vein, and the catheter may need to be introduced at a slightly different angle compared with the horse. This difference may not be as great in the mule (depending on what type of mule it is), but mules may be even less tolerant of needles than donkeys; use of a lidocaine "bleb," placed subcutaneously over the vein, is recommended for increased tolerance to catheter placement. Transdermal

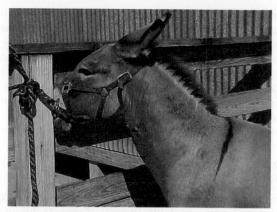

Fig. 1. Restraint and preparation for intravenous catheter placement.

lidocaine can be used to improve patient tolerance; 20 to 30 minutes must be allowed for sufficient transdermal absorption to anesthetize the skin.

Choices for sedation and premedication were previously reported.[17] Since that publication, Latzel[18] reported on the pharmacokinetics of xylazine in mules compared with horses. The half-life of xylazine in mules was 15 minutes shorter than that in the horse, and the horse dose (0.6 mg/kg intravenously [IV]) did not provide sufficient sedation in the mules. They recommended a dose 50% higher in mules compared with that in horses. This is consistent with the authors' practice for sedation of mules but not usually required for donkeys. Alpha-2 agonists (xylazine, detomidine, romifidine, and dexmedetomidine) have all been used in donkeys and mules; these drugs are often combined with an opioid (eg, butorphanol, morphine) to increase the degree of sedation and analgesia provided. The degree of sedation and analgesia achieved is dose dependent with sedation lasting longer than analgesia.[19] For donkeys, all alpha-2 agonistic drugs can be dosed similar to what is used in horses, whereas dosages for mules should be higher. The recent introduction of detomidine oral gel has been found to be useful for donkeys and mules, which may be difficult to inject (NSM. Personal observation); the label oral detomidine dose for horses seems to provide good sedation in donkeys when adequate time (40 minutes) is allowed for absorption (**Fig. 2**). Lizarraga investigated sedation and analgesia with 2 doses of oral detomidine

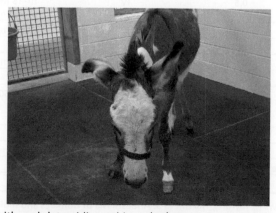

Fig. 2. Sedation with oral detomidine gel in a donkey.

gel and found sedation with both doses, which was deeper with the higher dose (40 μg/kg compared with 20 μg/kg).[20] The investigators do not have experience on the use of this product in mules; a higher dose might be necessary to provide good sedation. As is the case with horses, doses of drugs used for sedation will vary considerably depending on degree of sedation required, temperament and training of the patient, route of administration, as well as other drugs used. Choice of drug used for sedation and premedication also depends on availability and familiarity with that particular drug. As a general rule, intramuscular (IM) administration will require 2 to 3 times the usual IV dose and will take longer to reach maximal effect.

INDUCTION AND SHORT-TERM INJECTABLE ANESTHESIA
Ketamine-Based Anesthesia

Numerous drug combinations with ketamine have been used for induction and short-term maintenance with injectable drugs[17] (**Table 1**). Intermittent boluses of xylazine and ketamine can be used but need to be given more frequently than in horses: approximately every 10 minutes compared with 15 to 20 minutes in

Table 1
Suggested drug doses for sedation, induction, maintenance, and analgesia of donkeys and mules

	Dose (mg/kg)	Route	Expected Duration
Sedation			
Xylazine	1.0 (0.4–1.5)	IV, IM	15–20 min
Romifidine	0.08 (0.05–0.1)	IV, IM	30–60 min
Detomidine	0.01 (0.005–0.02)	IV, IM, sublingual	20–40 min, longer for sublingual
Dexmedetomidine	0.005	IV, IM	20–30 min
Acepromazine	0.03 (0.02–0.05)	IV, IM, sublingual	30 min–2 h
Induction			
Ketamine	2.2–2.5	IV	10–15 min
Diazepam/ midazolam	0.05 (0.02–0.1)	IV	10–15 min with ketamine
Propofol	2.0	IV	10–15 min
Propofol	0.5	IV	10–15 min used with ketamine
Alfaxalone	2.0	IV	10–15 min
Thiopental	6–8	IV	20 min
Telazol	1.0	IV	20–30 min
Maintenance			
Triple drip	Guaifenesin 50 mg/mL, ketamine 2 mg/mL, Xylazine 0.5 mg/mL	IV	Up to 60–90 min
Analgesics			
Butorphanol	0.03 (0.02–0.05)	IV, IM	30–60 min
Buprenorphine	0.006	IV, IM, sublingual	6 h
Morphine	0.1	IV, IM	2–3 h

Data from Matthews N, Taylor T, Hartsfield S. Anaesthesia of donkeys and mules. Equine Vet Educ 2005;7:102-107.

horses because donkeys metabolize ketamine more rapidly than horses.[17] Dar and Gupta[21] evaluated the effect of ketamine and diazepam bolus administration (2.2 mg/kg IV and 0.03 mg/kg IV, respectively) in mules after premedication with xylazine (1.3 mg/kg IV). The mules showed hypertonicity of the pelvic limbs during induction with acceptable levels of anesthesia and antinociception. However, muscle relaxation was deemed incomplete. Duration of anesthesia was short (15.3 ± 1.6 minutes). Because xylazine-ketamine (or similar combinations) may not provide enough time for the surgical procedure, various combinations of guaifenesin with ketamine and xylazine (G-K-X) were evaluated in donkeys.[7] These investigators found that G-K-X (guaifenesin 50 mg/mL, ketamine 2 mg/mL, xylazine 0.5 mg/mL) produced satisfactory anesthesia following premedication with xylazine (1.1 mg/kg IV). Induction was accomplished by rapid gravity administration of the mixture until the donkey became recumbent, then the infusion was slowed and maintained as indicated by monitoring anesthetic depth (approximately 1.5 mL/kg/h of the mixture mentioned earlier). For larger donkeys and mules, where restraint of the patient during induction might be difficult, a xylazine/ketamine induction can be used and then the G-K-X mixture started for maintenance. This mixture can be used when transport of the patient is required. This study was prompted by early experience with guaifenesin in donkeys, which showed that donkeys may be more sensitive to guaifenesin while metabolizing ketamine more rapidly, hence needing higher concentrations of ketamine. Matthews and colleagues[22] showed a mean recumbency dose of guaifenesin of 131 ± 27 mg/kg for donkeys, whereas this dose was 211 ± 8 mg/kg for horses. Although donkeys were more sensitive to guaifenesin, they metabolized it more quickly, based on higher clearances (546 ± 73 mL/h/kg) for donkeys compared with horses (313 ± 62 mL/h/kg).

Molinaro Coelho and colleagues[23] described inductions of general anesthesia in donkeys with a ketamine/propofol combination (1.5 mg/kg and 0.5 mg/kg IV, respectively). Maintenance was performed with a continuous rate infusion (CRI) of ketamine (0.05 mg/kg/min and 0.15 mg/kg/min IV, respectively). This study is further described in the section on propofol. Vullo and colleagues[24] described a G-K-X anesthesia maintenance protocol in mules, which, compared with the G-K-X mixture evaluated by Taylor and colleagues[7] in donkeys, required an increase in xylazine dose from 0.5 mg/mL to 1.0 mg/mL.

Thiopental

Thiopental was used for induction (7 mg/kg IV) and maintenance (8 mg/kg IV) of anesthesia for 100 minutes after premedication with atropine, acepromazine, and xylazine in donkeys.[25] Induction and maintenance quality were reported to be good, but recovery was slow; standing time was 92 minutes after anesthesia was finished. Smooth and uneventful inductions with thiopental (6 mg/kg IV) after premedication with xylazine (1.3–1.6 mg/kg IV) were described in mules.[24] Anesthesia was maintained with triple drip for field castrations.

Propofol

Propofol has been reported for use in donkeys.[17] A recent report compared propofol bolus administration (2 mg/kg IV) with thiopental bolus (10 mg/kg IV) after premedication with xylazine (1 mg/kg).[26] Induction time was slightly faster and of better quality with thiopental, but recovery was better with propofol (less attempts to obtain sternal recumbency and shorter duration of recovery). Induction apnea was seen with thiopental, but not with propofol. Propofol (1 mg/kg IV) was also used with ketamine (2 mg/kg IV) and compared with ketamine alone (3 mg/kg IV) after premedication with xylazine (1 mg/kg IV).[27] The combination of ketamine and propofol produced better induction, better muscle relaxation, longer anesthesia time, and smoother recoveries than with ketamine alone. In this study, the propofol substituted for benzodiazepines, providing better muscle relaxation than was seen without. This was probably because of not only the muscle relaxing effects of propofol but also the lower dosage of ketamine that was used.

In a similar study, donkeys were premedicated with xylazine (1 mg/kg) and induced with either ketamine (1.5 mg/kg) and propofol (0.5 mg/kg) or ketamine (2.2 mg/kg) and diazepam (0.05 mg/kg).[23] Anesthesia was maintained for 60 minutes with a CRI of either ketamine (0.05 mg/kg/min) and propofol (0.15 mg/kg/min) or a mixture of ketamine (2 mg/mL), xylazine (0.5 mg/mL), and guaifenesin (50 mg/mL) given at 2 mL/kg/h. Both combinations led to satisfactory anesthesia procedures but produced hypoxemia (without administration of oxygen). Intermittent shortages of diazepam and midazolam have led to drug substitutions in an attempt to provide balanced anesthesia. In addition, the lack of commercial guaifenesin in some countries has led to its substitution by use of low-dose propofol. Larger doses of propofol usually produce apnea and arterial desaturation in horses, but as demonstrated by the aforementioned studies, apnea does not seem to be a problem with lower doses in combination with ketamine in donkeys. However, one study[28] used 2 mg/kg propofol for induction in donkeys premedicated with acepromazine (0.04 mg/kg IV) followed by propofol infusion for 30 minutes (CRI of 0.2 mg/kg/min). No apnea was reported in this study although very mild hypoxemia did occur. In the investigators' opinion, it is wise to be prepared to intubate and provide short-term ventilation (eg, with a demand valve or Ambu bag and small oxygen tank) whenever propofol is used.

Alfaxalone

A recent study compared midazolam (0.05 mg/kg IV) and alfaxalone (1 mg/kg IV) with midazolam (0.05 mg/kg IV) and ketamine (2.2 mg/kg IV) following premedication with xylazine (2 mg/kg IM, followed by 0.5 mg/kg IV after 60 minutes) in donkeys.[29] Inductions were quicker with alfaxalone but recoveries were smoother and shorter in the ketamine group. Hypoxemia occurred with both drug combinations.[29]

MAINTENANCE WITH INHALANT ANESTHETICS, SUPPORT, AND MONITORING

Maintenance with inhalant anesthesia is recommended for longer procedures (>60 min) and for older or high-risk patients (horses older than 20 years of are considered geriatric).[30] Endotracheal intubation can usually be achieved blindly, although it may be slightly more difficult than in horses, due to anatomic differences in the donkey.[16] Occasional cases of hypoplastic trachea or abnormal conformation (especially in dwarf donkeys) may make the use of a laryngoscope or a flexible endoscope necessary. The donkey's upper airway conformation may need to be considered if the head seems abnormal. Halothane, isoflurane, or sevoflurane can be used; no apparent differences in minimum alveolar concentrations have been noted between horses and donkeys.

Heart and respiratory rates, blood pressure, eye signs (including eyelid reflex and positioning of the eyeball), swallowing reflexes, and muscle relaxation should all be monitored. Respiratory rates are usually higher in anesthetized donkeys than in horses and respiratory depression seen with isoflurane in horses does not seem to be as great a problem in donkeys; that is, the "breath holding" seen in horses rarely occurs in donkeys. A review of the authors' clinical records for a year yielded anesthetic records for 16 miniature and standard donkeys and 19 mules. When allowed to breathe spontaneously on injectable or inhalational anesthetics, respiratory rates for donkeys averaged 19 to 32 bpm and for mules 18 to 27 bpm. No Mammoth asses or draft mules were anesthetized, so it is possible that the higher breathing rate might be associated with smaller body size. When mechanically ventilated, a respiratory rate of approximately 10 bpm was used with tidal volumes adjusted to produce normocapnea.

As in horses, blood pressure seems to be the most reliable indicator of depth of anesthesia in donkeys; rapid increase usually indicates the patient is too light and likely to move. Blood pressure can be measured indirectly (using a cuff placed on tail or limb) or directly using an arterial catheter attached to an aneroid manometer or pressure transducer. The invasive measurement is the gold standard, whereas indirect measurement by means of oscillometric techniques merely enables assessment of trends in blood pressure.[31] Percutaneous placement of the arterial catheter is facilitated by cutting through the skin with a sterile needle before introducing the catheter to prevent "burring" of the catheter by the thick skin and fascia. A branch of the maxillary artery (facial or transverse facial artery) or lateral metatarsal artery is easiest to catheterize, but large auricular arteries are also available (**Fig. 3**).

Administration of intravenous fluids (such as lactated Ringer solution) is recommended at 5 to 10 mL/kg/h, especially during inhalant anesthesia, to support blood pressure. Appropriate positioning to protect radial and peroneal nerves and padding to prevent myositis is also recommended. Myositis seems to be less of a concern in donkeys than in horses (presumably because of smaller muscle mass) but might be a problem in larger donkey breeds or larger mules (ie, draft); therefore prevention of myositis is indicated.

Treatment of other anesthetic complications (eg, hypotension) should be the same as would be done for horses. Donkeys respond very well to dobutamine infusion when being hypotensive and not dehydrated, hypovolemic, or septic.

PERIOPERATIVE ANALGESICS

Butorphanol (CRI, 0.02–0.04 mg/kg/h IV), ketamine (CRI, 0.4–0.6 mg/kg/h IV), or lidocaine (CRI, 1.5 mg/kg/h IV) can be used to provide intraoperative analgesia in combination with inhalant anesthesia when needed, but there is no information specific to the use of these drugs in donkeys compared with horses; clinical judgment must be used. The same is true for alpha-2 agonist CRIs; some (mainly visceral) analgesia may be provided but they may be more helpful to lower inhalant dose needed while providing some support of blood pressure. Local blocks (with lidocaine, mepivacaine, or bupivacaine) can also be used for specific procedures (eg, pastern arthrodesis,

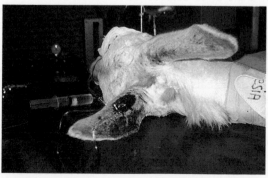

Fig. 3. Arterial catheter placed in ear for direct blood pressure measurement.

castration, ocular or dental surgery) to achieve analgesia. The intraoperative use of intrafunicular lidocaine during castration in donkeys resulted in lower levels of isoflurane required for maintenance of anesthesia. Transdermal fentanyl patches have been used on donkeys and may be effective for some types of pain; however, information specific to absorption of fentanyl and resulting analgesia in donkeys is greatly needed. The pharmacokinetics of tramadol has been reported, but no information about efficacy is available.[15] In general, there is a lack of information on the use of analgesics, especially opioids, in the donkey.

RECOVERY

Donkeys usually recover well from injectable or inhalant anesthesia but often take longer to attempt standing than horses. As with horses, attention must be paid to ensure a patent airway; "snoring" noises may indicate partial airway obstruction, which can be relieved by straightening the donkey's head and neck or passing a small nasogastric tube into the upper airway. Lack of analgesia can produce a rough recovery, but donkeys are not prone to becoming excited or hysterical in recovery as horses. Many donkeys will require a "boost" on the tail and may get up hind end first as a cow, whereas others will get up in the same manner as a horse. Because of their size, most donkeys can be assisted by hand and do benefit from this.

LOCAL ANESTHETIC TECHNIQUES

Similar to human anesthesia and anesthesia of other species, the use of locoregional anesthetic techniques can be beneficial in a modern multimodal approach.[32] Both during general anesthesia and in standing surgical procedures, these techniques can be a valuable additive. Some specific examples of local anesthetics are discussed in the following section.

Epidural Anesthesia

Epidural anesthesia was described in the donkey by Shoukry and colleagues.[33] Most common indications include rectal or vaginal prolapse or to treat melanomas on the tail and in the perineal region, but it can also be used for long-term analgesia after hindlimb surgery or with painful conditions in the hindlimb such as septic arthritis or laminitis. Burnham[34] gives a nice description of the anatomy of the sacral and coccygeal vertebrae. The first intercoccygeal space in the donkey is narrower than the second and therefore, the latter is more suited for caudal epidural puncture. The needle can be directed at an angle of 30 degrees from the horizontal and can be introduced into the vertebral canal, because there are no large tail muscles. The spinal processes of the sacral and coccygeal segments are more easily palpated in the donkey compared with the horse. Correct placement of extradural needles can be supported by means of an acoustic device to identify the extradural space. This technique was described for horses by Iff and colleagues[35] and has also been proved useful in other species, such as dogs and cats.[36] Numerous studies have been published on the use of different types of analgesic drugs for epidural application in horses.[37] Not all of these drugs have been described for donkeys, but in a recent publication, Marzok and El-Khodery[38] described the analgesic and sedative effects of lidocaine, tramadol, and the combination of both drugs for caudal epidural anesthesia in donkeys. They found that epidural combination of tramadol and lidocaine (0.5 mg/kg and 0.2 mg/kg, respectively) produced an antinociceptive effect in the perineum, which was rapid in onset (within 6 minutes) and had a longer duration of action (180 minutes) than lidocaine alone (duration of 75 minutes). Torad and Hassan[39] found the combination of nalbuphine and lidocaine (at dosages of 0.2 and 0.11 mg/kg, respectively) to lead to rapid onset (6.7 minutes) and long duration (147 minutes) of epidural anesthesia in donkeys. Hamed and colleagues[40] described the sedative and analgesic effects of epidural dexmedetomidine and xylazine in donkeys. They administered dexmedetomidine (5 μg/kg) and xylazine (200 μg/kg) in a cross-over design. All donkeys showed mild sedation and ataxia. Dexmedetomidine produced quicker onset (5.8 minutes) and longer duration of analgesia (160 minutes) compared with xylazine (14.2 minutes and 116 minutes, respectively). Although not specifically addressed in donkeys, according to the investigators, epidural morphine (0.1–0.2 mg/kg) would be the first choice for epidural analgesia, because of its good analgesic properties and relatively long duration of effect due to its hydrophilicity.

Local Anesthetic Techniques for Castration

Intrafunicular lidocaine (5 mL of 2% lidocaine) during total intravenous anesthesia has been used for field castration in mules.[24] Suriano and colleagues[41] compared intrafunicular lidocaine (10 mL lidocaine 2% with adrenaline) with saline injection during unilateral castration in 10 donkeys (one side with saline and the other side with lidocaine injection, 1 month apart). In lidocaine-injected castrations, heart rate (but not blood pressure) was lower compared with saline-injected castrations. Furthermore, end-tidal isoflurane requirements were lower during lidocaine-injected castrations. These findings correspond with the studies that have been performed in horses, where lidocaine is most often injected intratesticularly instead of injecting into the spermatic cord.[42]

Local Anesthetic Techniques of the Head

Both in standing and recumbent animals, local anesthetic techniques can be a useful adjunct for surgery of the head. Various studies describe several nerve blocks of the equine head and these techniques can equally be applied in donkeys.[43,44] Hagag and Tawfiek[45] recently described the use of ultrasound-guided maxillary nerve blocks in donkeys on cadavers and in 9 live donkeys (**Fig. 4**). Just as in horses,[46] this technique shows promising results for clinical application in donkeys and mules. In a case report by McCluskie and Tremaine,[47] caudal auricular and auriculopalpebral branches of the trigeminal and facial nerve were desensitized with mepivacaine in a recumbent donkey for surgical removal of an auricular sarcoid with a technique that was described for horses.[48]

In order to perform standing surgery in donkeys, proper sedation is a first requisite. Sedative and analgesic effects of detomidine have been described in donkeys by Mostafa and colleagues.[49] They showed that 5 to 10 μg/kg IV provides adequate sedation, with concurrent good to deep analgesia with doses of 20 to 40 μg/kg IV. Although donkeys seem to have similar clinical response to alpha-2 agonists than horses, mules clinically seem to require approximately 50% more xylazine compared with donkeys and horses.[17] Higher requirements for romifidine were also reported in untamed mules.[50] Protocols for standing surgery can be composed of sedatives in CRIs, combined with systemic opioids and local anesthetic techniques. Such a protocol has been described for horses[51] and used for donkeys as well. Dosages used in horses (romifidine: 80 μg/kg loading dose and 30 μg/kg/h CRI; butorphanol: 18 μg/kg loading dose and 25 μg/kg/h CRI) can be extrapolated to donkeys. The CRI dosages should be used as a guideline and adapted to clinical effect (just as in horses). As an alternative for butorphanol, morphine could be used in premedication at a dosage of 0.1 to 0.2 mg/kg IV. A CRI administration is then not used by the

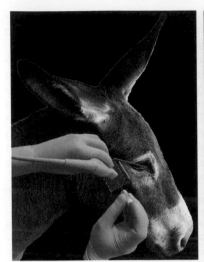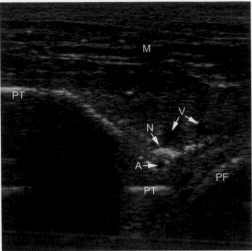

Fig. 4. Ultrasound-guided maxillary nerve block in donkeys. (*Left*) Acoustic window for ultrasound-guided maxillary nerve blockade (*dotted white lines*). The transducer is positioned caudal to the facial crest (*green line*), ventral to an imaginary line connecting the medial and lateral canthi and extending beyond the facial crest (*red line*). The needle is inserted about 1 cm ventral to the probe. (*Right*) Ultrasonogram of the pterygopalatine fossa in a donkey beneath the masseter muscle (M) demonstrating the maxillary nerve (N) related to branches of the deep facial vein (V), the infraorbital artery (A), and bounded by the perpendicular plate of the palatine bone (PT) and fascia of the periorbital cone (PF). (*From* O'Neill H, Garcia-Pereira F, Mohankumar P. Ultrasound-guided injection of the maxillary nerve in the horse. Equine Vet J 2014;46:180-184; with permission.)

investigators because of the longer duration of effect. Aziz and colleagues[52] describe laparoscopic ovariectomy in standing donkeys using xylazine sedation and local infiltration of the laparoscopic portal sides with lidocaine. This protocol could be combined with epidural morphine (0.1 mg/kg), a technique that is described for horses[53] and used by the investigators. Adding epidural morphine to this standing anesthesia protocol led to decreased surgical time, improved patient comfort, and reduced sedation needed to perform ovariectomy.

REFERENCES

1. Matthews N, van Loon JPAM. Anaesthesia and analgesia of the donkey and mule. Equine Vet Educ 2013;25:47–51.
2. Grosenbaugh DA, Reinemeyer CR, Figueiredo MD. Pharmacology and therapeutics in donkeys. Equine Vet Educ 2011;23:523–30.
3. Burden F, Thiemann A. Donkeys are different. J Equine Vet Sci 2015;35:376–82.
4. Coakley M, Peck K, Taylor T, et al. Pharmacokinetics of flunixin meglumine in donkeys, mules and horses. Am J Vet Res 1999;60:1441–4.
5. Mealy K, Matthews N, Peck K, et al. Pharmacokinetics of R(-) and S(+) carprofen after administration of racemic carprofen in donkeys and horses. Am J Vet Res 2004;65:1479–82.
6. Sinclair M, Mealy K, Matthews N, et al. Comparative pharmacokinetics of meloxicam in clinically normal horses and donkeys. Am J Vet Res 2006;67:1082–5.

7. Taylor E, Baetge C, Matthews N, et al. Guaifenesin-ketamine-xylazine infusions to provide anesthesia in donkeys. J Equine Vet Sci 2008;28:295–300.

8. Grint N, Johnson C, Clutton R, et al. Spontaneous electroencephalographic changes in a castration model as an indicator of nociception: a comparison between donkeys and ponies. Equine Vet J 2015;47:36–42.

9. Svendsen ED. Heart girth Nomogram. In: Duncan J, Hadrill D, editors. The professional handbook of the donkey. 4th edition. Wiltshire (United Kingdom): Whittet Books; 2008. p. 400.

10. Dugat S, Taylor T, Matthews N, et al. Values for triglycerides, insulin, cortisol, and ACTH in a herd of normal donkeys. J Equine Vet Sci 2010;30:141–4.

11. Regan F, Hockenhull J, Pritchard J, et al. Identifying behavioural differences in working donkeys in response to analgesic administration. Equine Vet J 2016; 48:33–8.

12. Grint N, Murrell J, Whay H. Investigating the opinions of donkey owners and veterinary surgeons towards pain and analgesia in donkeys. Equine Vet Educ 2015; 27:365–71.

13. Matthews N, Peck K, Taylor T, et al. Pharmacokinetics of phenylbutazone and oxyphenbutazone in miniature donkeys. Am J Vet Res 2001;62:673–5.

14. Matthews N, Taylor T, Sullivan J, et al. A comparison of 3 combinations of injectable anesthetics in miniature donkeys. Vet Anaesth Analg 2002;29:36–42.

15. Giorgi M, Del Carlo S, Sgorbini M, et al. Pharmacokinetics of tramadol and its metabolites M1, M2 and M5 in donkeys after intravenous and oral immediate release (fasted/fed) single-dose administration. J Equine Vet Sci 2009;29:569–74.

16. Herman CL. The anatomical differences between the donkey and the horse. In: Matthews N, Taylor T, editors. Veterinary care of donkeys. Ithaca (NY): International Veterinary Information Service; 2009. Available at: www.ivis.org.

17. Matthews N, Taylor T, Hartsfield S. Anaesthesia of donkeys and mules. Equine Vet Educ 2005;7:102–7.

18. Latzel S. Clinical and pharmacological studies on elimination kinetics of xylazine (Rompun®/Bayer) in mules. Dissertation (thesis). 1st edition. Munich (Germany): Ludwig-Maximilians-University, Faculty of Veterinary Medicine; 2008. Verlag Dr. Hut, Munich.

19. Lizarraga I, Castillo-Alcala F, Robinson L. Comparison of sedation and mechanical antinociception induced by intravenous administration of acepromazine and four dose rates of dexmedetomidine in donkeys. Vet Anaesth Analg 2017;44: 509–17.

20. Lizarraga I, Castillo-Alcala F, Varner K, et al. Sedation and mechanical hypoalgesia after sublingual administration of detomidine hydrochloride gel to donkeys. J Am Vet Med Assoc 2016;249:83–9.

21. Dar K, Gupta A. Total intravenous anaesthesia in adult mules. Vet Anaesth Analg 2016;43:204–8.

22. Matthews N, Peck K, Mealey K, et al. Pharmacokinetics and cardiopulmonary effects of guaifenesin in donkeys. J Vet Pharmacol Ther 1997;20:442–6.

23. Molinaro Coelho CM, Duque Moreno JC, Goulart D, et al. Evaluation of cardiorespiratory and biochemical effects of ketamine-propofol and guaifenesin-ketamine-xylazine anesthesia in donkeys (Equus asinus). Vet Anaesth Analg 2014;41:602–12.

24. Vullo C, Carluccio A, Robbe D, et al. Guaiphenesin-ketamine-xylazine infusion to maintain anesthesia in mules undergoing field castration. Acta Vet Scand 2017; 59:67–75.

25. Emami M, Seifi H, Tavakoli Z. Effects of totally intravenous thiopental anesthesia on cardiopulmonary and thermoregulatory system in donkeys. J Appl Anim Res 2006;29:13–6.

26. Abd-Almaseeh Z. Comparative anesthetic protocols: propofol and thiopental in xylazine premedicated donkeys. J Anim Vet Adv 2008;7:1563–7.

27. Abass B, Al-Hyani O, Al-Jobory A. Anesthesia in xylazine premedicated donkeys with ketamine and ketamine-propofol mixture: a comparative study. Iraqi J Vet Sci 2007;21:117–23.

28. Naddaf H, Baniadam A, Rasekh A, et al. Cardiopulmonary effects during anaesthesia induced and maintained with propofol in acepromazine pre-medicated donkeys. Vet Anaesth Analg 2015;42:83–7.

29. Maney J, Durham H, Goucher K, et al. Induction of anesthesia and recovery in donkeys sedated with xylazine: a comparison of midazolam-alfaxalone and midazolam-ketamine. Vet Anaesth Analg 2018;45:539–44.

30. Seddighi R, Doherty T. Anesthesia of the geriatric equine. Vet Med Res Rep 2012;3:53–64.

31. Yamaoka T, Flaherty D, Pawson P, et al. Comparison of arterial blood pressure measurements obtained invasively or oscillometrically using a Datex S/5 compact monitor in anaesthetised adult horses. Vet Anaesth Analg 2017;44:492–501.

32. Lamont LA. Multimodal pain management in veterinary medicine: the physiologic basis of pharmacologic therapies. Vet Clin North Am Small Anim Pract 2008;38:1173–86.

33. Shoukry M, Saleh M, Fouad K. Epidural anesthesia in donkeys. Vet Rec 1975;97:450–2.

34. Burnham S. Anatomical differences of the donkey and mule. AAEP Proc 2002;48:102–9.

35. Iff I, Mosing M, Lechner T, et al. The use of an acoustic device to identify the extradural space in standing horses. Vet Anaesth Analg 2010;37:57–62.

36. Ertelt K, Turkovic V, Moens Y. Clinical practice of epidural puncture in dogs and cats assisted by a commercial acoustic puncture assist device-epidural locator: preliminary results. J Vet Med Educ 2016;43:21–5.

37. Natalini C. Spinal anesthetics and analgesics in the horse. Vet Clin North Am Equine Pract 2010;26:551–64.

38. Marzok M, El-khodery S. Comparative analgesic and sedative effects of tramadol, tramadol-lidocaine and lidocaine for caudal epidural analgesia in donkeys (Equus Asinus). Vet Anaesth Analg 2015;42:215–9.

39. Torad F, Hassan E. Epidural lidocaine, nalbuphine and lidocaine-nalbuphine combination in donkeys. J Equine Vet Sci 2016;37:1–5.

40. Hamed M, Abouelnasr K, Ibrahim H, et al. Comparative sedative and analgesic effects of epidural dexmedetomidine and xylazine in donkeys (Equus asinus). J Equine Vet Sci 2017;59:104–9.

41. Suriano R, Varasano V, Robbe D, et al. Intraoperative analgesic effect of intrafunicular lidocaine injection during orchiectomy in isoflurane-anesthetized Martina Franca donkeys. J Equine Vet Sci 2014;34:793–8.

42. Haga H, Lykkjen S, Revold T, et al. Effect of intratesticular injection of lidocaine on cardiovascular responses to castration in isoflurane-anesthetized stallions. Am J Vet Res 2006;67:403–8.

43. Tremaine W. Local analgesic techniques for the equine head. Equine Vet Educ 2007;19:495–503.

44. Hermans H, Veraa S, Wolschrijn C, et al. Local anaesthetic techniques for the equine head, towards guided techniques and new applications. Equine Vet Educ 2017. doi: 10.111.eve.12757.
45. Hagag U, Tawfiek M. Blind versus ultrasound-guided maxillary nerve block in donkeys. Vet Anaesth Analg 2018;45:103–10.
46. O'Neill H, Garcia-Pereira F, Mohankumar P. Ultrasound-guided injection of the maxillary nerve in the horse. Equine Vet J 2014;46:180–4.
47. McCluskie L, Tremaine W. Surgical removal of an aural sarcoid in a donkey using ultrasonic shears. Vet Rec 2009;164:561–3.
48. McCoy A, Schaefer E, Malone E. How to perform effective blocks of the equine ear. AAEP Proc 2007;53:397–8.
49. Mostafa M, Farag K, Zomor E, et al. The sedative and analgesic effects of detomidine (domosedan) in donkeys. Zentralbl Veterinarmed A 1995;42:351–6.
50. Alves G, Faleiros R, Gheller V, et al. Sedative effect of romifidine in untamed mules. Cienc Rural 1999;29:51–5.
51. Marly C, Bettschart-Wolfensberger R, Nussbaumer P, et al. Evaluation of a romifidine constant rate infusion protocol with or without butorphanol for dentistry and ophthalmologic procedures in standing horses. Vet Anaesth Analg 2014;41:491–7.
52. Aziz D, Al-Badrany M, Taha M. Laparoscopic ovariectomy in standing donkeys by using a new instrument. Anim Reprod Sci 2008;107:107–14.
53. Van Hoogmoed L, Galuppo L. Laparoscopic ovariectomy using the endo-GI stapling device and endo-catch pouches and evaluation of analgesic efficacy of epidural morphine sulfate in 10 mares. Vet Surg 2005;34:646–50.

Dental Disorders of Donkeys

João B. Rodrigues, DVM, PhD[a,b,*], Gemma Lilly, BAEDT[a]

KEYWORDS

- Donkey • Donkey dentistry • Dental disorders • Prevalence • Dental treatment

KEY POINTS

- Dentistry should be assumed as something prophylactic, through the early diagnosis and treatment of oral and dental disorders in a conservative way.
- Donkeys are very stoic animals and a high number may suffer from apparently asymptomatic dental and oral disorders.
- The self-perpetuating nature of dental disease in addition to the potential for serious juvenile dental pathology means that regular prophylactic treatment from a young age is essential if we are to ever stand a hope of reducing incidence and severity of dental disorders in older animals.
- Dental disease in donkeys is correlated to increasing age, colic, body condition score, hyperlipaemia, sinusitis, quality of life, and mortality.

INTRODUCTION

Dentistry should be assumed as something prophylactic. This is especially important when working with donkeys, which are very stoic animals, and a high number may suffer from apparently asymptomatic dental and oral disorders.[1]

Even if asymptomatic, some oral and dental disorders are among the most painful conditions for donkeys, including those that may affect secondarily related structures such as the sinuses.[2]

Recent studies on donkey dentistry have described anatomic similarities with the horse, the prevalence of dental pathologies through clinical and postmortem reports, and the potential deleterious effect of dental disease on systemic health.[2–8]

The Donkey Sanctuary places dental disease as the second most common veterinary problem encountered in donkeys, after feet disorders. Regular dental examinations and treatment have a positive effect on long-term dental health as well as

Disclosure Statement: The authors have nothing to disclose.
[a] Research and Operational Support Department, The Donkey Sanctuary, Trow Offices, Sidmouth, Devon EX10 0PB, England; [b] CIMO – Mountain Research Center, Polytechnic Institute of Bragança (ESA/IPB), Bragança, Portugal
* Corresponding author. Welfare Assessment, Research and Operational Support Department, The Donkey Sanctuary, Trow Offices, Sidmouth, Devon EX10 0PB, England.
E-mail address: joao.rodrigues@thedonkeysanctuary.org.uk

Vet Clin Equine 35 (2019) 529–544
https://doi.org/10.1016/j.cveq.2019.08.008
0749-0739/19/© 2019 Elsevier Inc. All rights reserved.

general health and welfare. On the other hand, lack of regular examination and preventative treatment in the donkey makes this a welfare issue, where minor problems can cause pain and discomfort.[9]

Most of the donkeys rarely have regular dental examinations. In working donkeys, this may be for economic reasons, but also because of a lack of knowledge and education in remote and poorly educated communities. In the companion donkey, a lack of education and understanding of the need for regular preventive treatment and care is also common.

From the authors' experience, donkeys with good oral conformation may never develop serious problems, whereas donkeys with poor oral conformation (eg, craniofacial abnormalities [CA]) may show a decline in dental health over a few months in the absence of appropriate treatment.

ANATOMIC FEATURES AND ENVIRONMENTAL ADAPTATIONS

Equids present a series of anatomic features in the head and oral cavity related to the need to feed on abrasive diets. The following list describes some of these anatomic features.

- A long preorbital region result from the elongation of the head, leading to a long oral cavity and complex sinus system; these structures are anatomically closed and disorders affecting the oral cavity may also affect the sinuses[10];
- Hypsodont cheek teeth (CT) working as a functional unit of 6 CT per quadrant[7];
- The presence of a rostro-mesial compression from the corner incisors (03s) keeps the arcade to act as a single unit[11];
- Donkeys present a greater degree of anisognathia, that is, the maxilla is approximately 30% wider than the mandible (5%–7% wider than in horses) at its widest point, apparently from a narrower straight mandible rather than a wider maxilla.[7] The authors believe that the higher degree of anisognathia in donkeys may be related to their need for wider lateral excursion movement. Donkeys evolved in very dry regions, and to properly chew poor-quality forage a wider jaw was necessary for lateral excursion; this anatomic feature also raises questions on whether enamel "overgrowths" in donkeys are physiologic or pathologic structures.
- In donkeys, rostral and caudal maxillary sinuses may communicate as they are incompletely divided by a ventrally located low bony ridge that does not extend dorsally enough to divide both sinuses[12];
- The angulation of the rostral and the caudal CT, in addition to the curvature of the last molars (11s), maintains a tight apposition of all CT at the occlusal surface. The curve of Spee is quite noticeable in some donkey breeds and should be treated as a variation of normal conformation, and CT should not be modified to correct the condition[2,13];
- The nasolacrimal duct foramen in donkeys is located in the lateral to dorsolateral aspect of the nostril, near the mucocutaneous junction (**Fig. 1**).[12]

CLINICAL EXAMINATION OF THE HEAD

In donkeys there is little to no correlation between dental abnormalities and clinical signs, so regular clinical examination (not necessarily involving treatment) will allow the identification of oral and dental problems at an early stage, avoiding the development of more serious disorders that may be difficult or even impossible to treat.

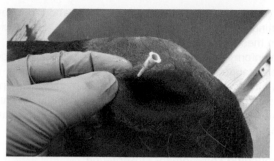

Fig. 1. Anatomic location of the nasolacrimal duct foramen in a donkey.

Periodicity of Oral Examinations

The periodicity of orodental examination may be determined by the age of the animal, individual oral conformation, and the age at which the animal began to be followed by a professional (**Table 1**). Other factors such as pregnancy status or concomitant disease may interfere on dental examination scheduling.

Clinical History, Individual Data

Common clinical signs of dental disease include slow/intermittent eating, complete reluctance, head shaking, quidding, visible changes in shape and symmetry of the head, halitosis, abnormal behavior, protrusion of the tongue, drooling/excessive salivation, oral malodor, abnormal sounds during chewing, blood in the mouth, nasal (and sometimes lacrimal) discharge, weight loss, etc.[2]

Table 1 Periodicity of oral examinations		
Age	**Examination Schedule**	**Comment**
0–5 y	Six monthly	Most dynamic period in equids' oral cavity, with the eruption of deciduous (incisors and premolars) and definitive teeth (canines and molars), as well as the dental exchange process affecting incisors and premolars (from 2.5 to 5 y). Donkeys may exchange the deciduous teeth 2–6 mo later than recorded in horses, so extra care must be taken when deciding to remove apparently retained caps.[4]
5–15/20 y	Annual	Animals with developmental problems, such as CA may need to be followed every 6 mo or even less.
Older than 15/20 y	Six monthly	Teeth may start suffering anatomic changes, related with the conical shape of the reserve crown and apex region, as well as the loss of the infundibula in the maxillary CT. When presented with an aged donkey with poor body condition, it is important to not assume that dental health is the primary or even sole source; in these cases, it is important that a veterinarian carry out a full clinical examination, which may conclude dental pathology as the least of the animal's concerns.

It is important to collect information from the owner about donkey's temperament and behavior, eating and management habits, possible vices, and the presence of recent changes in these aspects.

Other important information such as vaccination status is also important, especially in countries where zoonotic diseases may be prevalent. Always be aware of the possibility rabies infection; dumb rabies can cause hypersalivation in donkeys and precaution should be taken when carrying out oral examination in animals with behavioral changes. All animals receiving dental examination and treatment should be vaccinated against tetanus.

Donkey and Surrounding Environment Observation

Whenever possible, donkeys should be observed in their natural environment, obtaining information about behavioral changes and the surrounding environment. Feeders and drinkers should be assessed, looking for signs of poorly chewed food. Manure should also be observed for undigested grain or increased average fecal fiber length. The optimal average fecal fiber length for donkeys is just under 2 mm (Phillips C. Effects of dental treatment of faecal fibre length in donkeys. Unpublished dissertation, UWE-Hartpury College, 2015).

Extraoral Physical Examination

Examination should always start with a general physical examination.

Regarding the head, a detailed visual, olfactory, and tactile examination should be performed, checking both hard and soft tissues for evidence of pathologic changes, with special emphasis on those structures related with the oral cavity.[14]

The examination should be performed standing directly in front of the donkey's head, evaluating conformation and symmetry of all anatomic structures, using both hands simultaneously to check deformations/enlargements in hard and soft tissues, including salivary glands and regional lymph nodes, muscular tone, atrophy and inflammation, as well as presence of nasal and ocular discharge, mucocutaneous lesions, and fistulas, that may indicate the presence of orodental disorders.

Lateral examination should also be performed, mainly assessing the frontal area of the head. Rostrocaudal movement may also be assessed, extending and raising the head, followed by a forced flexion.[14]

The close contact with the facial region also allows the operator to create a bond with the animal, also facilitating further clinical procedures.

Nociceptive Tests

Manual nociceptive tests (pressure tests) evaluate donkeys' behavioral response to pain. These tests should be part of any clinical examination, being considered by the authors as an effective way to obtain reliable information about oral pain and discomfort (**Table 2**).[15]

Even if behavioral indicators may be less satisfactory for donkeys, in the case of severe and/or acute pain such as the one caused by the pressure tests, donkeys will show a positive response.

The duration that the mouth is open during intraoral examination and treatment must be limited if there is any response to the temporomandibular joint (TMJ) test. In the authors' opinion, this procedure should be adopted in all cases to avoid iatrogenic damage of the TMJ (**Fig. 2**).

Table 2
Nociceptive tests

Nociceptive Test	Description and Comments
Cheek pressure	Digital pressure is exerted bilaterally and simultaneously on the cheeks at the level of the maxillary CT by pressing the cheek against the entire CT row. Signs of discomfort (tossing the head) may be the result of pain from sharp CT enamel overgrowths or any other abnormal wear patterns on the vestibular/rostral aspect of the upper CT (eg, displaced teeth).
Tongue/hyoid pressure	Digital pressure is exerted bilaterally on the intermandibular space, pushing the body of tongue dorsally leading to close contact between the mandibular CT and the lateral aspect of the tongue. Signs of discomfort may be the result of dental trauma at the back of the mouth causing ulcers or lacerations of the tongue, sharp CT enamel overgrowths, or lingual displaced CT.
Temporomandibular joint (TMJ)	Digital pressure is exerted bilaterally and simultaneously in the articular space of the TMJ. Pressure may result in a positive response indicating the presence of disease affecting TMJ or more chronic and severe oral disorders.

From Rodrigues JB, Ferreira LM, Bastos E, et al. Influence of dental correction on nociceptive test responses, fecal appearance, body condition score, and apparent digestibility coefficient for dry matter of Zamorano-leonés donkeys (Equus asinus). J Anim Sci. 2013; 91:4765–4771; with permission.

INTRAORAL EXAMINATION

In order to perform a correct intraoral examination a flush of the oral cavity is mandatory, preferably using a dosing syringe with a blunt ending.

Based on the authors' experience, unsedated donkeys may object to oral rinsing, reacting violently on occasion. The presence of water under pressure in the oral cavity stimulates the soft palate to contract causing a rostral displacement of the

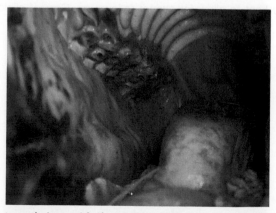

Fig. 2. Donkey's intraoral view, with the tongue pushed dorsally against the third arcade, and the right cheek pushed medially against the first arcade, simulating what happens during the nociceptive tests.

palatopharyngeal arch, leading to a blockage of the entrance of the trachea. The mouth should not be flushed with the gag on and the mouth open, avoiding potential accidents, including aspiration. If necessary, the throat region should be stimulated and donkeys will swallow, relaxing all the adjacent structures.

Until this point of the clinical examination animals should not be sedated, ensuring that the information gathered is not affected by sedation. Dosing for sedatives (eg, xylazine) is similar to horses; however, these drugs have a shorter duration of action in donkeys[2]; mules often require higher doses.

Donkeys should be properly restrained to ensure the safety of the operator, animal, and equipment. The halter should be removed before placing the speculum to avoid excessive pressure of soft tissues against the CT when opening the mouth.

Most of the donkeys allow intraoral examination and nonpainful procedures without sedation.

When working with unsedated donkeys, it helps to keep their head high, using a hanging halter with a quick safety release system (**Fig. 3**). This will reduce donkey's attempts to escape, by counteracting its natural way of escape—head to the floor while trying to move away. While sedated, the donkeys head should be at the same level of back and neck, and not higher than this line.

A detailed examination of the rostral structures of the oral cavity should be performed before fitting the full mouth speculum, including incisors and canines (when present). Alterations to the normal number and position of the teeth, symmetry, and occlusion surface; presence of CA; or diseased incisors may lead the operator to change the procedure, approaching these teeth first.

In the authors' experience, even in donkeys with a few stable incisors or with no incisors, it is better to use ground-out incisor plates than to make use of the traditional "gum" bars, which may inflict marked trauma to the interdental space even when padded.

Regular size donkeys may be treated with standard equine dental equipment. Miniature donkeys may require specialized smaller size tools. The tongue should not be grabbed and manipulated inside the mouth, but left free to avoid serious lesions.

The presence of wolf teeth should be recorded. It is not unusual for donkeys to have up to 4 wolf teeth (one per arcade), which in normal position seldom interfere with the bit and should not be removed (**Fig. 4**).

All orodental disorders present should be recorded in a systematic way and updated records kept to allow for proper follow-ups. Correct clinical language and

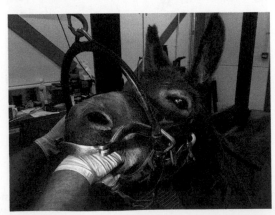

Fig. 3. Unsedated donkey during dental examination, with the head kept in a high position.

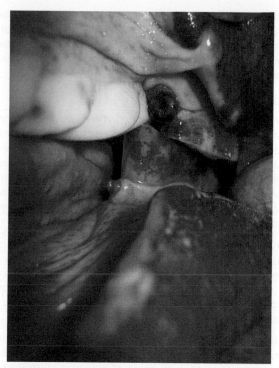

Fig. 4. Presence of maxillary and mandibular wolf teeth in a donkey. When present, the mandibular wolf teeth are usually smaller. Please note the presence of a peripheral caries affecting 205.

the modified TRIADAN system must be used to ensure accurate collection of clinical data.[16] Dental conditions rarely present singularly and a complete treatment plan is needed for donkeys suffering multiple conditions. A good treatment plan is only possible if an accurate diagnosis is achieved. This may require the use of ancillary diagnostic tests.

ANCILLARY DIAGNOSTIC TESTS

Ancillary diagnostics improve the clinical capacity to assess parts of the head that cannot be properly examined with conventional methods.[17] Imaging modalities used in horses are valid for donkeys. It is important to mention that donkeys and some mules have narrow nasal passages than similar size horses, and choosing a proper diameter endoscope as well as lubrication facilitates rhinoscopy and reduces the risk of bleeding.[14]

ORAL AND DENTAL DISORDERS IN DONKEYS

Clinical and postmortem studies in donkeys highlighted the importance of dental health when assessing the health and welfare of these animals.[3–6]

Acquired problems may be secondary to developmental disorders, so where a condition is acquired it may be necessary to address the primary cause as part of the treatment.

One study found a prevalence of incisor disorders in 74% of donkeys, ranging from 56.8% in young animals to 90.3% in the oldest.[3] The prevalence of CT disorders in working and retired donkeys ranged from 62% to 93%, respectively, and further increasing with age, proving the importance of routine dental examination to prevent acquired disorders.[4–6]

Developmental Disorders

- *Craniofacial abnormalities*: donkeys may present alterations in craniofacial bones that may lead to incorrect dental occlusion and function overtime, affecting both incisors and CT. Clinical features of CA include occlusal surfaces of the maxillary incisors rostral to the occlusal surface of the mandibular incisors, with or without contact (overjet and overjet with overbite, or brachygnathism); or vice versa (underjet and underjet with underbite bite, or prognathism). Donkeys may present variable degrees of lateral premaxillary (incisive) and maxillary bone deviation, referred to as "wry nose."[3]

Early detection and treatment of CA can avoid its progression to more severe conditions. Newborn donkey foals with severe CA may not be able to nurse due to the inability to create a vacuum in the oral cavity; this is a life-threatening situation.

One study on endangered breeds of donkeys reported a high prevalence of CA, affecting 49.3% of the population, suggesting loss of genetic variability and inbreeding as responsible factors for these abnormalities.[3]

- *Dental dysplasia*: alterations in the correct gross form of the teeth include dilacerations (abnormal bending of the teeth), alterations in size and shape, connation, and concrescence of teeth, with roots of adjacent teeth joined by cementum. Although this is uncommon (0.50%), because of its potential relation with genetics, animals presenting with these disorders should not be used for breeding purposes.[3]
- *Polyodontia*: presence of teeth in excess of the normal dental formula, as a result of an inappropriate differentiation of dental germinal tissue during gestational development. External trauma may be a factor and dental germs may be affected[3]; supernumerary teeth are uncommon in donkeys but usually located in the caudal aspects of the maxillary CT rows (*distomolars*). A recent study recorded a prevalence of polyodontia in 2.3% of donkeys, but even if uncommon, it should be considered in the differential diagnosis of dental disease.[18] The same study found a higher prevalence of fully erupted supernumerary teeth in older animals, suggesting a delayed eruption process, and therefore, even in donkeys undergoing regular dental prophylaxis, service providers should remain diligent.[18] The presence of abnormal teeth can lead to acquired disorders such as axial displacements, dental overgrowths, dental-related soft tissue damage, diastemata formation, periodontal disease (PD), and development of secondary sinusitis.[8]
- *Retained deciduous teeth*: the presence of deciduous teeth beyond their normal time of shedding, interfering with the normal eruption process of the permanent dentition, is an age-specific disorder, affecting mainly donkeys between 2.5 and 5 years.[3,4] Only caps found to be digitally loose, having partial crown loss, and clear and palpable demarcation between deciduous and permanent teeth should be considered for extraction. Retained fragments should also be extracted. Recent studies showed that teeth fragments are more commonly found in the medial aspect of the arcades in donkeys, so extra care is needed during the extraction of these fragments, avoiding laceration of the great palatine artery.[4,6]

The deciduous 08s are the most common CT affected in donkeys, considering it has to erupt between definitive adjacent 07s and 09s (**Fig. 5**).[4] In the case of incisors, studies focused on donkeys showed that central incisors (01s) tend to be the most common deciduous teeth retained.[3]

- *Eruption cysts*: these are enlarged, focal swellings, beneath young permanent premolars, in the developing apex region, palpable mainly in the mandible region.[4] Eruption cysts are relatively common and usually without complications. In donkeys, only 6.4% of eruption cysts were directly related with retained teeth, and no related cases of apical infection were recorded in a survey.[4] The authors advise that all cases of mandibular and maxillary swellings should be examined for retained deciduous CT.
- *Abnormal dental eruption/displacements/developmental diastemata formation* donkeys may present gross displacements and/or rotations of incisors and CT due to intrinsic developmental reasons, retained deciduous teeth, or because of previous trauma.[4,5] Donkeys present the same mechanisms described in horses for the formation of developmental diastemata in the CT.[19] A similar mechanism may explain the presence of open diastemata in all mandibular IPS in young donkeys, recently described in donkeys.[3]

The significant increase in displaced teeth prevalence with age recorded in several surveys indicates that most of these displacements were acquired rather than developmental.[4,5]

Acquired Disorders of Teeth

- *Hypodontia*: reduced number of teeth when compared with the normal formula (44 in total). This can be developmental, a result of an inappropriate differentiation of dental lamina and tooth germs (agenesia), or may occur during the animal's lifetime, with PD suggested as the main cause of premature tooth loss in adult donkeys.[5,6] Studies showed that nondevelopmental hypodontia is more common than developmental, mainly affecting older animals and directly related with tooth loss due to age, affecting both incisors and CT.[4,5]

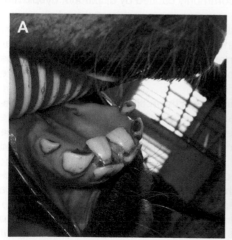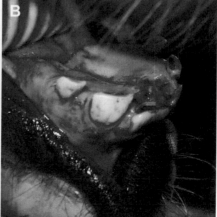

Fig. 5. Retained 701 and 801 displaced lingually, before (*A*) and after (*B*) extraction.

Clinical and postmortem studies in donkeys highlighted a correlation between age and a higher prevalence of missing teeth compared with studies focused in younger populations.[4–6]

- *Abnormalities in occlusal surface*: observed in both incisors and CT and described as any variations affecting the normal wear process/attrition between ipsilateral opposing teeth, leading to potentially restricted mandibular movement and increasing the possibility of soft tissue damage.[3,4]

In one study, ventral curvature (VC) in the incisor arcade was observed in 97% of donkeys, suggesting this is its normal appearance.[2] Although, other studies focused on a younger population of donkeys presented a lower prevalence (20.9%), increasing significantly with age. VC is an acquired age-related disorder, probably secondary to CT disorders, and a combined phased correction is advised, balancing and correcting the disorders at CT, while restoring normal incisor occlusion.[3] Incisor overgrowth may also occur in incisors that have not been exposed to normal wear, usually secondary to CA, or due to disorders affecting the opposing teeth.[2]

Abnormalities of wear in the CT are usually the most common disorders recorded, mainly enamel overgrowths, affecting all arcades.

A clinical study in working equids presented a high prevalence of CT enamel overgrowth (73.13%), despite most of those donkeys having a forage diet, including daily grazing.[4] The higher degree of anisognathia could explain this high prevalence, but interestingly, associated soft tissue lesions (affecting 6.5% of those donkeys) were described mainly affecting the cheeks corresponding to those areas where halters may exert pressure, raising questions about the cause of this disorder. Because a diagnosis of enamel overgrowth is subjective (in the absence of soft tissue lesions), it could be argued that a high level of protruding enamel on the CT is physiologic and is a normal feature for donkeys. The pain response to cheek and tongue/hyoid pressure tests is a very good indicator for the need of dental correction in case of enamel overgrowths.

Focal/partial overgrowths affecting the 06s and the 11s are also common (37.25%), mainly in those donkeys with some degree of CA.[4]

Overgrowths of the complete tooth caused by poor or absent occlusal contact are usually related with maleruption of the opposing CT and are usually bilateral situations. This type of overgrowth may also be less commonly caused by displaced, dysplastic, worn, senile loss, or fractured CT.[4]

These overgrown teeth may remain dominant or even increase in dominance throughout the animal's life, worsening and interfering with normal chewing movement, and may predispose to the development of wave mouth (undulating appearance of the occlusal surface, in a rostrocaudal plane) or even shear mouth, that usually are recorded mainly unilaterally.[4]

Shear mouth is the presence of a steeper angle in the occlusal surface of the CT row (usually >35°) in the palatal-buccal plane[5] and is related with a long-term consequence of an inappropriate management of CT overgrowths and unopposed teeth, and so the age-related increasing prevalence of shear mouth in donkeys is expected as observed in several studies.[4,5,20]

In geriatric donkeys it is also possible to observe smooth mouth, defined as a reduction or complete loss of enamel ridges, which may be defined as worn teeth if only a limited number of crowns are affected.[4–6]

Early detection and treatment of abnormalities of wear can avoid its development to more severe conditions. Service providers are therefore encouraged to make regular check-ups and carry out prophylactic procedures to maintain the correct occlusal table angle, which varies between 12.5° and 30° throughout the length of the arcades and between maxillary and mandibular CT.[7]

- *Dental displacements:* any variation of the normal position; this disorder is more commonly found affecting the molars, both in a vestibular and lingual/palatal sense, dealing to diastemata formation, PD, and soft tissue trauma. Displacements may result from lack of space during the eruption process or due to incorrect orthodontic forces in the oral cavity; for example, in cases of CA, it is normal to find 06s displaced, due to the presence of focal overgrowths in these CT.[4]

If diagnosed early, displaced teeth may be easier to treat; profiling of the clinical crown to the direction of displacement allows for the alignment of the arcade to be improved and may be enough to correct incorrect orthodontic forces and even resolve associated diastemata. Increased scheduling of routine dental treatments in donkeys may be necessary to treat and maintain displaced teeth under control. The authors have successfully utilized radiographs of displacements to provide clues to the causes and likely directions of impending displacements.

If not treated, dental displacements may become severe and if PD has not advanced sufficiently, these teeth may have very solid attachment.

Extraction of severely displaced CT is one course of action, yielding very good results in terms of resolution of tissue trauma and localised PD. It is the authors experience that extreme caution must be used when extracting CT that are very steeply angled (some are virtually horizontal) as incorrect use of molar forceps will readily cause fracture to one or more apices.

- *Diastemata*: abnormal increase of the interproximal space (IPS), with or without food pocketing and including valve and open diastemata.[19] Diastemata with food entrapment and associated PD is a very painful disorder that can be difficult to diagnose, especially in the more caudal mandibular IPS.[5,6] Acquired diastemata were diagnosed in donkeys as a common disorder, affecting mainly mandibular CT. This is an age-related disorder, increasing not only the prevalence of affected animals but also the number of diastemata per donkey; postmortem studies in donkeys found a prevalence of 85% diastema of the CT.[6]

Following diastemata development, a self-perpetuating cycle of food infiltration, degradation, and infection occurs, resulting in tooth loss from severe PD.[1] Despite the suggested stoicism of the donkey, it is likely that affected animals experience considerable pain and it is imperative that a thorough visual and digital oral examination be part of any investigation associated with excessive salivation, oral malodor, inappetence/anorexia, colic (especially impaction), hyperlipaemia, and weight/condition loss.[1]

- *Periodontal disease*: this is a significant disorder in equids affecting the periodontium, ranging from gingivitis without attachment loss (stage 1) to severe, deep periodontal pocketing (stages 2, 3, and 4 with <25%, <50%, and more than 50% of attachment loss, respectively).[21] It may affect all teeth, and it is clearly an age-related disorder, with prevalence increasing with age. Recent studies in donkeys show an age-related increase in number of CT affected per donkey together with an increase in the severity of the disease, whereas in incisors an increase in number of teeth affected per animal was observed, but without increasing the severity of the disease.[3,4] This fact is mainly related with the primary disorders causing PD. In the case of CT, the fact that almost 90% of teeth diagnosed with PD were caused by CT diastemata could explain the age-related increase in severity reported for these teeth. Other less common causes of PD may include peripheral caries, due to damage in the normal tight junction between gingiva and peripheral cementum at the gingival margin, leading to attachment loss in some cases, and retained deciduous CT, presenting usually gingivitis/early stage (grade 2) periodontitis, which may also present halitosis, due to food entrapment beneath the retained deciduous tooth.[4]

- *Caries:* this is defined as a dissolution of the peripheral and infundibular calcified dental tissues, due to demineralization and bacterial infection, affecting only the cementum (stage 1); cementum and enamel (stage 2); cementum, enamel, and dentin (stage 3); or the integrity of the tooth (stage 4) in most severe cases.[22]

Studies focused on donkeys showed that prevalence and severity of this disorder increases with age. The same studies suggest a direct relation between presence of peripheral caries and other severe concurrent dental diseases responsible for the reduction of masticatory movements, thus promoting food stasis around the CT.[4]

- *Calculus:* calculus deposition occurs mainly at dentition local to salivary ducts openings; the pH of the saliva once ejected from the duct serves to calcify the existing plaque (Lilly G. Topography and clinicopathology of equine canine teeth. Unpublished dissertation, UWE-Hartpury College, 2015). There is some suggestion that calculus in equids occurs when saliva and forage are not moving correctly inside the mouth.[4] Therefore, it is hypothesized that calculus may be related with the presence of other concomitant dental disorders. Elderly donkeys may present considerable malodorous deposits not only at the canines and incisors but also around the maxillary premolars, which are adjacent to the ostium of the parotid duct.

The lower canines may erupt in very close proximity to the incisors (displaced rostrally), frequently allowing for mass accumulation of calculus covering canines and typically corner incisors. It is likely that because incisor eruption decelerates and canine eruption is static in mature animals, the opportunity for calculus exfoliation is minimized; hence build up becomes significant in aged animals.[23]

There seems to be less sexual dimorphism (regarding the canines) than demonstrated in horses and so both male and female donkeys may be affected.[23]

When calculus accumulates on the lateral edges of the CT, it may well hinder ingesta enroute to deglutition and cause food stagnation at the IPS and along the free margin of the gingiva. Furthermore, calculus may become very sharp and ulcerate adjacent soft tissues occasionally to a severe extent.[23] The Donkey Sanctuary even has one recorded terminal case of internal gastrointestinal laceration owing to ingestion of calculus dislodged from the CT (Emmett, personal communication, 2010). Calculus regrowth at the premolars may be as rapid as greater than 1 cm thickness in under 6 months, consequently affected patients warranting very regular attention.[23] Calculus deposits should not be underestimated with regard to pathogenesis and traumatic risk to soft tissue (**Fig. 6**).

- *Fractures*: idiopathic or traumatic injury of the teeth, affecting part or all of its components: *uncomplicated fracture*—only external components of the teeth (cementum, enamel, and sometimes, the dentin) are affected; *complicated fractures*—the pulp cavity is exposed.[3]

In donkeys, no fractures were detected in a postmortem study, whereas in live animals the prevalence varied between 2% and 17%, with the higher prevalence possible being related to biting hard objects during daily grazing on poor and stony soils.[3] Nevertheless, the vast fractures in incisors were uncomplicated, affecting only the external components of the teeth. These small fractures, normally located

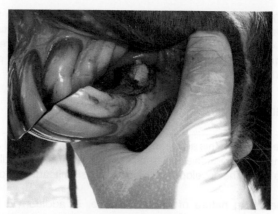

Fig. 6. Calculus formation with food entrapment in 304.

in the transition area between the occlusal surface and the labial aspect of the teeth, can be a predisposing factor to the development of peripheral caries, as previously mentioned.[3]

Idiopathic fractures are more commonly found than traumatic fractures in the CT due to their anatomic protection. Both types of fractures had a low prevalence in donkeys.[4,5]

- *Apical infection:* extension of pulpar disease through the apical foramen into the periapical (apical) periodontal tissues, with infections usually spreading around the apex, causing clinical changes to the alveoli and supporting bones. A peri-oendodontic infection may also occur. These infections are secondary to other disorders (vertical impaction/overcrowding, retained deciduous teeth, fractures, caries, and PD) but mainly occur via anachoresis (blood-born bacterial infection).[23] Pulp exposure may also occur due to iatrogenic damage, so the authors highlight the risks associated with excessive wearing of occlusal surface due to the excessive use of electromechanical instruments.

The clinical signs caused by apical infections are directly related with the site and age of the infected tooth and the duration and the extent of the infection. Infection in the mandibular CT, especially in younger donkeys, may lead to fistula formation with the drainage tract under the affected tooth.[23] In the maxillary CT, infection usually leads to maxillary sinusitis (with unilateral mucopurulent nasal discharge) if the caudal 3-4 maxillary CT are infected.[23] When the more rostral maxillary CT are infected, rostral maxillary swellings and sinus tracts into the nasal cavity may also occur.

Treatment of infected teeth is similar with that described for horses, including secondary sinusitis treatment.

Soft Tissue Lesions

Soft tissues in the oral cavity may also be affected, presenting mainly ulcers and chronic oral scarring, due to direct contact with sharp and abnormal dental structures, both developmental and acquired.[2,24] Periodontal tissues may also be affected, in cases of PD, affecting initially the gum, but progressing and affecting deeper tissues, in case of periodontitis.

Although, it is important to be aware that lesions in the soft tissues may not be only related with dental disorders and may result from incorrect handling procedures, aggressive bits, or traditional restrain systems with tight nosebands and/or other components. A detailed observation of all oral soft tissues is vital during the clinical examination, and if there are signs that lesions are related with incorrect handling equipment and/or procedures, the approach of the problem with the owner/user is advised.

PREVENTION AND TREATMENT

Prevention

As previously mentioned in this article, dentistry should be assumed as being prophylactic, through the early diagnosis and treatment of oral and dental disorders in a conservative way, to avoid the development of clinically significant pathologies previously described.

The self-perpetuating nature of dental disease, in addition to the potential for serious juvenile dental pathology, means that regular prophylactic treatment from a young age is essential if we are to hope at reducing the incidence and severity of dental disorders in older animals.

Treatment

Before proceeding with dental treatment, it is important to consider the general health of the donkey. Successful treatment relies on good-quality prophylaxis and correction of pathologies, preceded by a detailed action plan.

From the authors' experience, regular conservative procedures are preferable than curative treatments, especially in cases of acute/chronic anorexia, dysprehension/dysmastication, colic, and hyperlipaemia, where treatment stress and postprocedural discomfort may adversely affect recovery. Indeed, some malocclusions will never be corrected and consideration must always be given to the amount of reserve crown available. According to the authors' experience, because donkeys typically live longer than horses, it is possible to perform minor reductions and regain occlusion in animals in their late teens/early twenties. However, it is best to occasionally let minor focal overgrowths to remain in order to allow as much occlusion as possible in elderly patients. When worn teeth exfoliate or wear beyond functionality, the dominant teeth may then be reduced to prevent contact with the opposing jaw and to increase jaw motility.[25]

All dental reductions should follow current protocols whereby occlusal tissue is removed in stages, resulting in a reduction but not complete removal of the dark staining of the secondary dentine and preferably with incomplete loss of the transverse ridging. If reductions are continued much past this point there is considerable and unnecessary risk of irritation to the odontoblast processes and/or direct pulp exposure.[25]

It is usual for donkeys with multiple oligodontia/exodontia to require dietary modifications to provide adequate nutrition while minimizing risk of choke, colic, or hyperlipaemia.[9]

Multiple extractions in a singular session should be avoided wherever possible because the sudden reduced function, in addition to stress, and possible pain and potential infection may cause acute inappetence. Consequently there is a likelihood of rapid-onset hyperlipaemia, which is a serious and often fatal problem in donkeys.[9] Extractions should always be staged if the affected teeth are on contralateral arcades, as it is beneficial to leave the donkey with one pain-free side on which to masticate. Pain assessment and subsequent management are very important for success. For veterinarians performing extractions, the use of sedation and regional nerve blocks are mandatory (see Nora Matthews and Johannes P.A.M. van Loon's article, "Anesthesia, Sedation and Pain Management of Donkeys and Mules," in this issue).

Postprocedural care and management changes need to be considered and discussed at length with the owners.

Treatment of diastemata may include profiling of the clinical crown, widening, flushing with or without medication, and application of temporary polyvinyl bridges again with or without the addition of medicaments placed deep into the pockets.[2]

REFERENCES

1. Thiemann A, Barrio Fernandez E, Rickards K, et al. Assessing quality of life and welfare of donkeys in the UK. Practice 2018. https://doi.org/10.1136/inp.k2584.
2. Du Toit N, Dixon PM. Common dental disorders in the donkey. Equine Vet Educ 2012;24:45–51.
3. Rodrigues JB, Araújo S, Sanroman-Llorens F, et al. A clinical survey evaluating the prevalence of incisor disorders in Zamorano-Leonés and Mirandês Donkeys (*Equus asinus*). J Equine Vet Sci 2013;33:710–8.
4. Rodrigues JB, Dixon PM, Bastos E, et al. A clinical survey on the prevalence and types of cheek teeth disorders present in 400 Zamorano-Leonés and 400 Mirandês donkeys (*Equus asinus*). Vet Rec 2013;173(23):581.
5. Du Toit N, Burden FA, Dixon PM. Clinical dental examinations of 357 donkeys in the UK. Part 1: prevalence of dental disorders. Equine Vet J 2009;41:390–4.
6. Du Toit N, Gallagher J, Burden FA, et al. *Post mortem* survey of dental disorders in 349 donkeys from an aged population (2005-2006). Part 1: prevalence of specific dental disorders. Equine Vet J 2008;40:204–8.
7. Du Toit N, Kempson S, Dixon PM. Donkey dental anatomy. Part 1: gross and computed axial tomography examinations. Vet J 2008;176(3):338–44.
8. Du Toit N, Burden F, Dixon PM. Clinical dental examinations of 357 donkeys in the UK. Part 2: Epidemiological studies on the potential relationships between different dental disorders, and between dental disease and systemic disorders. Equine Vet J 2009;41(4):395–400.
9. Burden F, Du Toit N, Thiemann A. Nutrition and dental care of donkeys. Practice 2013;35:405–10.
10. Merkies K, Paraschou G, McGreevy PD. Preliminary investigations into relationships between donkey and horse skull morphology and brain morphology. Proceedings of the 13th International Conference of International Society for Equitation Science. Wagga, NSW, Australia, November 23-25, 2017. p. 88.
11. Dixon PM, Du Toit N. Dental anatomy. In: Easley J, Dixon PM, Schumacher J, editors. Equine dentistry. 3rd edition. London: Elsevier; 2011. p. 51–76.
12. Herman CL. Anatomical differences between the donkey and the horse. In: Matthews NS, Taylor TS, editors. Veterinary care of donkeys. Ithaca (NY): International Veterinary Information Service; 2009. p. 1–5.
13. Easley J, Schumacher J. Basic equine orthodontics and maxillofacial surgery. In: Easley J, Dixon PM, Schumacher J, editors. Equine dentistry. 3rd edition. London: Elsevier; 2011. p. 289–317.
14. Easley J, Tremaine H. Dental and oral examination. In: Easley J, Dixon PM, Schumacher J, editors. Equine dentistry. 3rd edition. London: Elsevier; 2011. p. 185–98.
15. Rodrigues JB, Ferreira LM, Bastos E, et al. Influence of dental correction on nociceptive test responses, fecal appearance, body condition score, and apparent

digestibility coefficient for dry matter of Zamorano-leonés donkeys (*Equus asinus*). J Anim Sci 2013;91:4765–71.

16. Rodrigues JB, Viegas CAA, San Roman F. Applying advanced record techniques for dental charting in the study of oral and dental pathology in endangered breeds of donkeys in field conditions. In European Veterinary Dental Society, ed. Proceedings of the 19th European Congress of Veterinary Dentistry. Nice, France, September 23-25, 2010. p. 88–90.

17. Barakzai S. How to radiograph the erupted (Clinical) crown of equine cheek teeth. Clin Tech Equine Pract 2005;4:171–4.

18. Rodrigues JB, Sanroman-Llorens F, Bastos E, et al. Polyodontia in donkeys. Equine Vet Educ 2013;25(7):363–7.

19. Dixon PM. Cheek teeth diastemata and impactions. In: Proceedings: Focus on Dentistry, American Association of Equine Practitioners, Indianapolis (IN): 2006. p. 68–82.

20. Dixon PM, Tremaine WH, Pickles K, et al. Equine dental disease. Part 3: a long-term study of 400 cases: disorders of wear, traumatic damage and idiopathic fractures, tumours and miscellaneous disorders of the cheek teeth. Equine Vet J 2000;32:9–18.

21. Klugh D. Equine periodontal disease. Clin Tech Equine P 2005;4:135–47.

22. Borkent D, Dixon PM. Equine peripheral and infundibular dental caries: a review and proposals for their investigation. Equine Vet Educ 2017;29:621–8.

23. Dixon PM, Tremaine WH, Pickles K, et al. Equine dental disease. Part 4: a long-term study of 400 cases: apical infections of cheek teeth. Equine Vet J 2000;32: 182–94.

24. Du Toit N, Burden FA, Dixon PM. Clinical dental findings in 203 working donkeys in Mexico. Vet J 2008;178:380–6.

25. Lilly G, Rodrigues JB. The head and oral cavity. In: Evans L, Crane M, editors. The clinical companion of the donkey. Leicester: Matador; 2018. p. 23–38.

Clinical Evaluation and Preventative Care in Donkeys

Elena Barrio, MVDr, Cert AVP, MRCVS[a,b],
Karen J. Rickards, PhD, BVSc, MRCVS[a,b],
Alexandra K. Thiemann, MA, Vet MB, Cert EP, MSc, MRCVS[b,c,*]

KEYWORDS

- Donkey clinical examination • Behavior • Preventative care • Dentistry • Farriery
- Vaccination • Quality of life

KEY POINTS

- Donkeys are physiologically well-adapted to resource poor environments, and management should reflect this to avoid overfeeding, obesity and associated disorders such as equine metabolic syndrome and laminitis.
- Donkeys are frequently neglected in preventative health care programs, including regular hoof care, dentistry, vaccination, and deworming.
- Companion donkeys are not used for hard work, often live into old age, and subtle problems may be overlooked, while working donkeys may be used to exhaustion and are frequently deprived of basic management and veterinary care.
- Quality of life assessment is important to ensure welfare in donkeys and mules, but also facilitates challenging decisions such as euthanasia.
- Due to their prey species behavior and ability to mask pain, recognizing normal and pain-related behavior is critical in the evaluation of sick donkeys.

INTRODUCTION

Donkey are frequently given lower quality care than horses for reasons associated with their use, status, and ownership. This article aims to provide clinicians with the information to use their skills to perform a complete examination of the donkey, taking into account species related differences. The basic format of the clinical examination and relevant preventative care closely follows that required for the donkey's short-eared relation – the horse.

Disclosure Statement: The authors have nothing to disclose.
[a] The Veterinary Department, The Donkey Sanctuary, Sidmouth, Devon EX10 0NU, UK; [b] The Veterinary Hospital, Brookfield, Honiton, Devon EX14 9SU, UK; [c] Education, The Veterinary Department, The Donkey Sanctuary, Sidmouth, Devon EX10 0NU, UK
* Corresponding author. The Veterinary Hospital, Brookfield, Honiton, Devon EX14 9SU, UK.
E-mail address: alex.thiemann@thedonkeysanctuary.org.uk

GENERAL EXAMINATION

Important parameters to consider during clinical evaluation of donkeys are listed in **Table 1**.

Behavior

The donkey's response to a stressful situation is more inclined to freeze, while the horse exhibits flight behavior, and the mule tends to fight. These unique reactions to stress have led to differences in the way these equids are used and perceived. Veterinarians working with donkeys will be more successful if they understand species-specific behaviors, allow donkeys time to work out a problem, and use their cautious trusting behaviors to form good bonds with the owner and companion donkeys. A companion donkey can be invaluable in helping a sick donkey recover, walk into an evaluation room, or follow into a trailer for transportation, and if held close by, it can make clinical examination and routine procedures such as dentistry and farriery much easier.

The term stoic is often used to describe donkey behavior, but it more accurately describes the typical predator-avoidance behavior displayed by a prey species, where remaining strong and behaving normally will reduce the chance of being targeted by a predator. Stoicism is not synonymous with a lack of ability to process pain, though; it just means that the behavioral responses to pain may be more subtle. This is important for the clinician to bear in mind when examining a donkey, as minor changes in behavior reported by the owner or seen on examination may be the only indication of disease and/or pain. Although there are several system-specific responses that donkeys will exhibit, which will be described in more detail later on in this article, often a sick donkey will display nonspecific signs such as dullness, inappetence, and recumbency irrespective of the disease process occurring.

As donkeys can live to advanced age and in many countries are worked near to exhaustion, there is a misconception that all donkeys tend to look dull or quiet. Donkeys express the same normal behaviors as horses, being friendly, inquisitive, and playful, particularly when young. Donkeys have evolved to live in environments with sparse food and limited water access where they will graze and browse on low-energy forage for 14 to 18 hours a day.[1] As a prey species, they spend limited time lying down (15 minute bouts for a total of 2–6 hours). Therefore, it is not normal for animals of any age to lie down for long periods, which should prompt the owner and clinician to investigate the cause.

Physiology

One of the donkey's physiologic adaptations to survive on highly fibrous, low-energy forages is a prolonged gastrointestinal transit time.[2] This has implications for examinations such as gastroscopy, as gastric emptying is longer than in the horse. It is also an important factor to consider in management systems where donkeys have access to energy-rich forage, which may lead to excessive weight gain, obesity, and potential complications (donkey nutrition and malnutrition). Donkeys also tend to be more insulin-resistant than horses, which is part of their evolutionary adaptation to harsh conditions.[3] This, combined with a predisposition to easily gain weight increases their risk for equine metabolic syndrome. Insulin resistance and obesity are also risk factors for hyperlipaemia.[3] Another physiologic adaptation of donkeys is water conservation; they do not hemoconcentrate until they are 20% dehydrated[4] and efficiently recycle water from the large colon, so packed cell volume, pulse quality, and capillary refill time are minimally affected from fluid loss.[5]

Table 1
Important parameters for clinical examination in donkeys

Examination	Parameter	Units	Average	Range	Important Points
Demeanour and behavior Observation history	A dull donkey is very likely to be seriously ill. Treat as an emergency.				Very subtle changes in behavior may indicate severe disease. A dull donkey usually indicates stress or pain (eg, colic, hyperlipemia, laminitis, dental disease, or liver disease). Observe mobility; signs of lameness or increased recumbency.
Body condition Appetite Skin	Weight – important for drug administration Body condition – important for appropriate nutrition, underlying illness Appetite – important for underlying illness	kg	180	90–400	The thick hair coat can hide skin conditions and mask a poor body score; use a donkey-specific body score chart. Watch for sham eating (pretending to eat). 180 kg is average weight of donkey. Palpate and check for skin conditions, lumps, and parasites.
Temperature	Adult donkey	°C	37.1	36.5–37.8	Newborn foal - 37.5–38.5°C, 99.5–101.3°F
		°F	98.8	97.2–100	
	Young donkey	°C	37.6	36.2–38.9	
		°F	99.6	97–102	
Cardiac auscultation and pulse rate	Adult donkey	Beats per minute	44	36–52	>52 indicates stress or pain. >70 could indicate severe pain or hypovolaemic shock without pain. Pulse quality may be less affected by dehydration and fluid loss in the donkey.
	Young donkey		60	40–80	
	Newborn foal			80–120	
Respiratory tract auscultation and respiratory rate	Adult donkey	Breaths per minute	20	12–28	Consider the use of a rebreathing bag to accentuate subtle lung sounds, especially in obese donkeys where fat deposits muffle sounds. The donkey has an insensitive cough reflex. The respiratory rate decreases in the newborn foal after 12 h.
	Young donkey		28	16–48	
	Newborn foal After 12 h			60–80	
				30–40	

(continued on next page)

Table 1
(continued)

Examination	Parameter	Units	Average	Range	Important Points
Mucous membranes color Texture (eg, moist/tacky) Capillary refill time	Capillary refill time	Seconds	1.5	1–2.5	Capillary refill time may remain close to normal despite fluid loss or dehydration.
Abdominal auscultation	Auscultation of borborygmi				Both mixing and propulsive contractions should be auscultated, and sounds should be present in all 4 quarters of the abdomen, where size allows delineation.
Examination of the oral cavity	An essential part of any clinical examination in the donkey				The use of an oral speculum is essential, as the narrow mandibular arcade makes visualization more challenging.
Ocular examination					Note the different location of the nasal opening of the nasolacrimal duct in the donkey.
Rectal examination					This can be safely performed in most donkeys with care and lubrication. A spasmolytic can be used.
Peritoneal tap					A peritoneal tap can be difficult because of adipose deposits along ventral body wall (be aware that fat may be up to 14 cm in depth in obese donkeys).
Ultrasound					Subcutaneous fat may obscure detail from ultrasound imaging.
Blood sample Haematology, biochemistry, and screen for hyperlipemia	Triglycerides	mmol/L mg/dL	1.4 124.6	0.6–2.8 53.4–249.2	>2.8 mmol/L (249.2 mg/dL) indicates mild hyperlipemia. >8 mmol/L (712 mg/dL) indicates moderate disease with increased mortality rates. >15 mmol/L (1335 mg/dL) indicates severe disease with significantly increased mortality rates.

Work Load and Age-Related Factors

Considering that donkeys are nonathletes, subtle signs from musculoskeletal and respiratory conditions can be missed, resulting in a more advanced stage of disease when clinical signs become apparent. This is particularly apparent with the respiratory system, where donkeys with extensive interstitial pulmonary fibrosis can be found dead with little to no history of respiratory signs. A rebreathing bag examination is indicated to accentuate subtle respiratory sounds in situations where exercising the animal is risky or impractical.

Donkeys can live 30 to 40 years, and geriatric conditions such as dental disease, pituitary pars intermedia dysfunction (PPID), laminitis, and degenerative joint disease (DJD) have become more common. It is worth noting that in nonworking donkeys it is more common to find DJD in the upper limb joints such as hips and shoulders (**Fig. 1**), and the extent of cartilage damage and bony changes can be severe relative to the clinical signs exhibited because of their stoic nature and lack of exercise. In the authors' experience, 1 indication of DJD can be a change in the donkey's behavior at farriery, when the donkey can be more difficult to handle and resent having limbs held. If this is reported, the clinician should examine the musculoskeletal system in more detail, as ankylosing spondylitis of the cervical vertebrae, but more often the thoracic spine, can also occur as part of the aging process. In working donkeys, DJD of the lower limb joints is more commonly seen and at a younger age.

Examination of working donkeys requires specific attention to presenting clinical signs, as many conditions are preventable. Wounds may be linked to poorly made/fitting harness, and musculoskeletal injuries could be related to excessive loads and difficult terrain. The environment and improper management, including lack of rest, improper feeding, heavy loads, lack of water, hot weather, and abuse could lead to dehydration, exhaustion, even organ failure. There are many examples of donkey welfare issues seen in both developed and developing countries.

Foals

When examining foals it is important to know that foals of most donkey breeds are considerably lighter than the average horse, with weights ranging from 5 to 40 kg. It

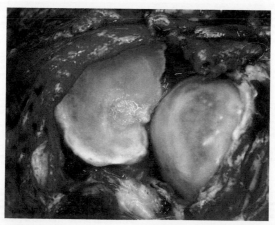

Fig. 1. Severe osteoarthritic changes in the hip joint of a donkey. Note significant erosion of cartilage on both the femoral head and acetabular surface. This donkey presented with a bilaterally shortened cranial phase to the hind limb gait.

is useful to have the following equipment available: male urinary catheter for stomach tubing, small-bore (20–22 gauge) intravenous catheter for administration of hyperimmune plasma or isotonic fluids, and a large dog size thermal rug or blanket. If required, mare's milk replacer can be used for orphan donkey foals, as can equine hyperimmune plasma using the same immunoglobulin G (IgG) concentration ranges to determine the need as is used for horses where there is failure of passive transfer.

NORMAL PARAMETERS - CLINICAL, HEMATOLOGICAL, BIOCHEMICAL, AND ENDOCRINE

When examining donkeys, it is important to note that the normal ranges for temperature, heart rate, and respiratory rate are different from the horse, both in foals and adults (see **Table 1**). The body condition score (BCS) is assessed using a 5-point system, with a condition score of 3 being ideal (**Fig. 2**). Horse weight tapes are inaccurate for donkeys, and there are donkey-specific weight estimators based on heart girth and height at the withers.[6] Miniature donkeys weigh 70 to 100 kg, standard size donkeys weigh 150 to 220 kg, and larger breeds such as the Poitou donkey can weigh up to 400 kg.

There are also differences in hematological and biochemical parameters, with packed cell volume and red blood cell count being lower, but triglycerides higher (0.6–2.8 mmol/L; 53.4–249.2 mg/dL) than horses.[7] Reference ranges for both adrenocorticotropic hormone (ACTH) and insulin also differ, although similar to horses, donkeys exhibit a seasonal ACTH peak in the fall (**Table 2**). In view of the concerns over prolonged fasting and the risk of hyperlipemia, basal insulin concentrations have been measured in donkeys on a basic ration of ad libitum straw.

DONKEY BODY CONDITION SCORE CHART

Accurate body condition scoring is a hands-on process for feeling the amount of muscle and fat that are covering the donkey's bones. Using this chart as a guide, feel the coverage over the bones in five specific areas listed below. Fat deposits may be unevenly distributed especially over the neck and hindquarters. Some resistant fat deposits may be retained in the event of weight loss or may calcify (harden). Careful assessment of all areas should be made and combined, to give an overall score. When deciding on the correct course of action following condition scoring, you might have to take into consideration the age of the donkey and any veterinary conditions they have. Aged donkeys can be hard to condition score due to lack of muscle bulk and tone giving thin appearance dorsally with dropped belly ventrally, while overall condition may be reasonable. If in doubt, get advice from your vet.

Condition score	Neck and shoulders	Withers	Ribs and belly	Back and loins	Hindquarters
1. Poor (very thin) 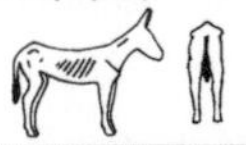	Neck thin, all bones easily felt. Neck meets shoulder abruptly, shoulder bones felt easily, angular.	Dorsal spine and withers prominent and easily felt.	Ribs can be seen from a distance and felt with ease. Belly tucked up.	Backbone prominent, can feel dorsal and transverse processes easily.	Hip bones visible and felt easily (dock and pin bones). Little muscle cover. May be cavity under tail.
2. Moderate (underweight) 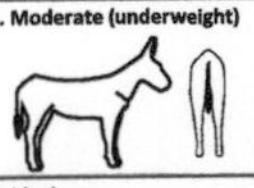	Some muscle development overlying bones. Slight step where neck meets shoulders.	Some cover over dorsal withers, spinous processes felt but not prominent.	Ribs not visible but can be felt with ease.	Dorsal and transverse processes felt with light pressure. Poor muscle development either side of midline.	Poor muscle cover on hindquarters, hip bones felt with ease.
3. Ideal 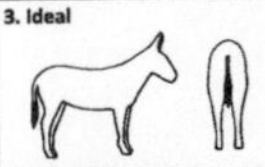	Good muscle development, bones felt under light cover of muscle/fat. Neck flows smoothly into shoulder, which is rounded.	Good cover of muscle/fat over dorsal spinous processes, withers flow smoothly into back.	Ribs just covered by light layer of fat/muscle, ribs can be felt with light pressure. Belly firm with good muscle tone and flattish outline.	Can feel individual spinous or transverse processes with pressure. Muscle development either side of midline is good.	Good muscle cover over hindquarters, hip bones rounded in appearance, can be felt with light pressure.
4. Overweight (fat) 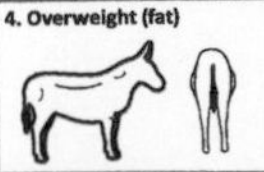	Neck thick, crest hard, shoulder covered in even fat layer.	Withers broad, bones felt with pressure.	Ribs dorsally only felt with firm pressure, ventral ribs may be felt more easily. Belly over developed.	Can only feel dorsal and transverse processes with firm pressure. May have slight crease along midline.	Hindquarters rounded, bones felt only with pressure. Fat deposits evenly placed.
5. Obese (very fat) 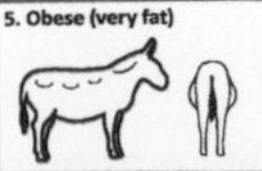	Neck thick, crest bulging with fat and may fall to one side. Shoulder rounded and bulging with fat.	Withers broad, bones felt with firm pressure.	Large, often uneven fat deposits covering dorsal and possibly ventral aspect of ribs. Ribs not palpable dorsally. Belly pendulous in depth and width.	Back broad, difficult to feel individual spinous or transverse processes. More prominent crease along mid line fat pads on either side. Crease along midline bulging fat either side.	Cannot feel hip bones, fat may overhang either side of tail head, fat often uneven and bulging.

Research and Operational Support | © The Donkey Sanctuary | Revised: October 2018

Fig. 2. BCS chart for donkeys. (*Courtesy of* The Donkey Sanctuary, Devon, England.)

Table 2 Reference ranges for resting insulin and adrenocorticotropic hormone for donkeys aged 3 – 20 using the TOSOH AIA-360 analyzer		
Insulin (mU/L)	0–15.1	
ACTH (pg/mL)	2.7–30.4	November - June
ACTH (pg/mL)	9.0–49.1	July - October

From The Donkey Sanctuary. Hyperlipaemia and the endocrine system. In: Evans L, Crane M, eds. Clinical Companion of the Donkey. 1st Ed. Leicestershire, UK: Matador; 2018: 87-98; with permission.

ANATOMIC DIFFERENCES

There are anatomic similarities between donkeys and horses; however, there are also differences to be considered that can impact on management, diagnosis, and treatment. The long ears of the donkey are an evolutionary adaptation to heat dissipation and acute hearing, where small herds need to roam over sparse, resource-poor environments, and their ability to congregate fast and detect predators assures survival.

Head and Neck

The nasolacrimal duct opening is located dorso-laterally in the nares, lateral to the alar fold within the false nostril (**Fig. 3**), as an adaptation to reduce sand/dirt blocking the ostium.

The donkey has relatively narrow nasal passages, and using small-bore nasogastric tubes is advisable to avoid the risk of hemorrhage. The nasopharynx is well developed with deep pharyngeal recesses,[8] which play a role in the development of the characteristic bray but can also prove challenging when attempting nasogastric intubation.

Donkeys have the same dentition as horses with a similar aging pattern; however, there is a larger degree of agnisonathia, which may be related to the need for increased lateral excursion for effective chewing of more fibrous diets.[9] This anatomic difference is important to consider when deciding whether enamel overgrowths are physiologic or pathologic. Donkeys also have a more pronounced curve of Spee, which needs to be taken into consideration when assessing overgrowths of the caudal cheek teeth to ensure that crown height follows the jaw line.[10] The teeth and head are larger in proportion to body size than a horse, which reflects the coarse diet and browsing habits of this species. As a result, the strong neck muscle supporting the

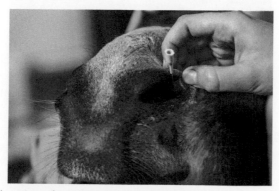

Fig. 3. Anatomic location of nasolacrimal duct foramen in donkeys.

head, the cutaneous colli, is particularly well developed and may obscure the jugular groove in well-muscled donkeys. In view of this, it can be easier to obtain intravenous access in the upper or lower third of the jugular groove.

Body Shape and Condition

Donkeys have a flatter back with poorly developed withers, which has led them to be used primarily as pack rather than riding animals. This also predisposes them to wounds and back pain when poorly harnessed or using tack designed for horses. They also distribute body fat in a different pattern than horses, developing marked regional deposits, particularly along the side and topline (**Fig. 4**), which is why a different BCS chart for donkeys has been developed (see **Fig. 2**). This is also true of internal fat deposition, which occurs prior to accumulation of external fat, meaning that a donkey with a BCS of 3 can still have significant fat deposits around internal organs such as the kidney and the ventral abdomen. This has implications for procedures such as abdominocentesis, as there can be 8 to 10 cm of fat in the ventral midline, and longer needles, catheters, or teat cannulas might be necessary, particularly if carrying out the procedure without ultrasound guidance.

The first coccygeal space is often fused with the sacrum, resulting in occlusion of the sacrococcygeal space, and the first intercoccygeal space is much narrower than the second, making the second space the preferred site for epidural injection. The spinal cord ends at the second sacral vertebral segment, while the dural sheath extends back to the first or second coccygeal vertebrae. Donkeys typically have less musculature over the rump and tail head, so when performing an epidural injection, the angle of needle introduction is shallower than in the horse (approximately 30° from the horizontal plane).[11]

Conformation and Hooves

The donkey is well adapted to be sure-footed in hard terrains and has a tendency to a plaiting gait in front, a narrow chest, and toe-in conformation. The hind limbs may be poorly muscled, and the base narrow. There is generally little muscle in the chest area, making it unsuitable to injections.

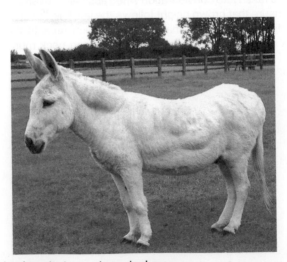

Fig. 4. Regional fat deposits in an obese donkey.

Although the overall structure of the asinine and equine hoof is similar, in the donkey it is more upright with a U-shaped solar surface (**Fig. 5**). The size and number of horn tubules also differ, resulting in a hoof wall that contains 10% more moisture and has a more elastic structure, and a solar surface that does not flake away. This has implications for hoof trimming, as the sole needs to be scalloped out to avoid it becoming load bearing and explains why the donkey's hoof wall continues to grow and curl up like a Turkish slipper when in moist environments rather than crack and break away if left untrimmed as occurs in horses. A combination of the higher moisture content and wet underfoot conditions experienced in temperate climates is also likely to predispose the donkey to white line disease.[12] There are also differences in the radiological parameters associated with the pedal bone, which will have an impact on the diagnosis and treatment of laminitis.[13]

Skin

Although most skin conditions seen in donkeys are similar to those in horses, the donkey's coat tends to be longer and dryer than that of the horse, and studies have shown that the hair density and thickness are less than a similar-sized horse or pony.[14] This means that the requirement for shelter from cold, wind, and rain is more important for donkeys than native ponies, and they will suffer if not provided with relief from the elements. The difference in hair coat also has implications for the effective use of topical preparations, as dispersal may not be so widespread unless larger quantities of the product are used. Likewise, pour-on preparations that rely on the natural oils in the horse's coat for penetration and dispersal may be less effective in donkeys. The longer coat can also make it more difficult to identify ectoparasites such as lice and ticks and can mask poor body condition. It can also mean that wounds may be missed, and skin disease can be in the advanced stages before being visible (**Fig. 6**). When lesions are present, it is therefore advisable to clip the affected areas to ensure the full extent of the lesions is exposed. In temperate climates, lack of shelter can predispose the donkey to skin conditions associated with wet weather. Use of waterproof rugs may help, but it is important to note the large surface area associated with their ears, which can result in significant heat loss and can still be a focus for skin disease such as dermatophilosis. It is useful to map the location of lesions and wounds, as these may give an indication

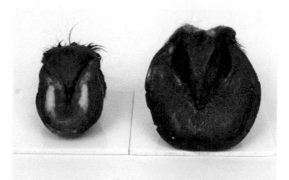

Fig. 5. Comparison of the solar surface of the donkey and horse showing the U-shaped conformation in the donkey.

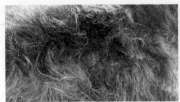
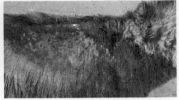

Fig. 6. Superficial areas of dermatitis obscured by long, matted hair prior to clipping (*Top*). The full extent of the skin lesions became evident following clipping (*bottom*).

of the cause, particularly in working donkeys, where wounds are often associated with poor fitting tack/harness, excessive loads, and/or poor handling techniques (**Fig. 7**).

Sarcoid tumors are well recognized in donkeys and may be hidden by a long or poorly maintained coat. Owners and veterinarians should check all areas of the skin regularly, especially high-risk areas such as around the sheath.

PREVENTATIVE CARE

Lack of preventative care is a major concern for donkeys around the world, particularly as donkeys often do not display obvious clinical signs despite suffering from severe or even life-threatening conditions. It is therefore, even more important in this species to ensure appropriate routine care to maintain good health and enable prompt identification of conditions that could have a detrimental effects on welfare if left unmanaged.

Routine care should start at a young age to reduce the risk of developing certain conditions or at least to control them when they occur, avoiding unnecessary suffering and maintaining good welfare. Management changes and preventative care should be effectively planned with the help of a donkey-experienced veterinarian in order to maintain good quality of life throughout the donkey's life.

PREVENTATIVE CARE IN DONKEYS
Routine Dental Care

It is still common to find large populations of adult donkeys that have never received routine dental care or treatment and have moderate-to-severe dental

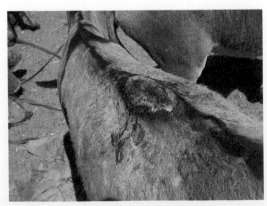

Fig. 7. Wound associated with poorly fitting pack saddle.

disease. Significant dental disease may be present in donkeys that are in good condition and show no clinical signs largely because of being fed calorie-rich diets.[15] An unpublished study at The Donkey Sanctuary identified that 36% of the donkeys admitted in a 30-month period had never received a dental examination (Barrio, 2019). The same study found 72% of geriatric donkeys had moderate-to-severe dental disease on admission.

Major reported conditions in geriatric donkeys included diastemata, missing teeth, overgrown teeth, worn teeth, displaced teeth, and periodontal disease.[10] These conditions may be prevented or more effectively managed if donkeys receive routine dental care from an early age.

Dental disease is a major welfare concern for geriatric donkeys in the United Kingdom as many conditions can be painful, but because of their stoic nature and sedentary lifestyle, clinical signs are often nonexistent or may get missed by owners.

Maintaining dental function when possible and changing the type of diet and bedding if required can maintain a donkey pain free with a good quality of life. The welfare of donkeys with severe dental disease should be closely monitored with end points agreed with the owner to identify when euthanasia is required. End points should include conditions such as progressive weight loss despite correct management, impaction colic, and unmanageable dental pain. Dental treatment may require a staged approach to avoid the risk of inappetence following major dental corrections that would predispose the donkey to hyperlipemia. Dental disease itself is also a risk factor for hyperlipemia.[16]

Farriery

Inadequate foot care and poor farriery are significant welfare issues globally.[17] Donkeys' hooves require regular trimming every 6 to 10 weeks, a clean, dry environment, and a hoof health routine including daily foot picking. Unfortunately, there are still many cases of neglected overgrown hooves, which increase the risk of injury and disease. For example, (Barrio, 2019) from The Donkey Sanctuary found that 41% of donkeys arriving had their last farrier visit more than 12 weeks previous.

Conditions such as white line disease and thrush are common in temperate regions with high rainfall. A donkey-experienced farrier working in conjunction with a veterinarian can advise extensive debridement of white line disease lesions back to healthy horn. This can be successful when combined with the use of disinfectants such as 10% iodine solution and dry underfoot conditions. It can also be helpful to use disinfectants after hoof picking and farrier trims to reduce the risk of development of complications.

Conditions of the musculoskeletal system are one of the main reasons for euthanasia, and a lack of regular foot care frequently contributes to this.

Annual Vaccinations

Donkey owners often keep donkeys isolated from other equines and wrongly believe that their vaccination is unnecessary. Data from The Donkey Sanctuary found that 77% of newly arriving donkeys were not protected against influenza or tetanus. It is important for veterinarians to be aware of the need for tetanus prophylaxis when treating injured donkeys or mules, as many are unvaccinated.

Different countries have their own vaccination recommendations depending on endemic or exotic disease risk. Although few vaccines are licensed for donkeys, they should be included in vaccination programs to enhance herd immunity and reduce individual risk. Donkeys and mules should be vaccinated according to the manufacturer's instructions for horses.

Skin Care

Preventative skin care such as daily grooming helps in the detection of ectoparasites and the early stages of neoplasia such as sarcoids that are commonly seen in donkeys. Sarcoids if left untreated or undetected can be extremely difficult to resolve and can affect the donkey's quality of life and be a reason for euthanasia. Ectoparasites can be a welfare concern because of discomfort, hair loss, and pruritus. Donkeys can develop very thick coats, requiring regular and thorough inspections.

Skin care should include fly control; the use of fly masks, repellents, and stockings to protect the legs can be helpful.

Topical and systemic products to reduce lice burdens are available; however, regular use of certain products can result in parasite resistance. A tea tree oil spray is available that has been shown to reduce louse burdens when used at 2-week intervals for at least 2 treatments (EquineNitNat, AgriEnt Ltd., United Kingdom).[18] The donkey's thick coat can affect penetration of certain products; therefore, clipping may be required before treatment can be applied. If donkeys are clipped, it is important to ensure that their body temperature is maintained appropriately using rugs and/or heat lamps during the winter and by providing shade and sun cream lotion during the spring and summer.

Donkeys with unpigmented skin should have appropriate ultraviolet (UV) light protection applying sun cream lotion as often as required and or UV light protection rugs, muzzle, and head covers. Wet weather and lack of shelter can also cause skin disease, so it is important to ensure appropriate shelter for donkeys, noting that rugs can help to improve thermoregulation; however, significant heat loss can still occur via the ears.

Nutritional Advice, Diet Formulation, and Weight Control

Donkeys are often fed inappropriately by their owners, which, added to their often sedentary lifestyles, increases the risk of obesity and related diseases. Details of donkey nutrition are covered in Faith A. Burden and Nicola Bell's article, "Donkey Nutrition and Malnutrition," elsewhere in this issue. The basis of a healthy donkey diet should be low-calorie, high fiber forage supplemented with micronutrients. Pasture management should include parasite control, removal of toxic plants, and controlled grazing. Regular BCS assessments by owners and veterinarians are part of a good preventative health care program. Major weight loss of over 5% in a month or cumulative weight loss can be a sign of severe or chronic disease and is a risk factor for hyperlipaemia.[16] The BCS (see **Fig. 2**) and weight tape measurements[6] are important to assess and monitor weight changes, including response to therapies and nutritional management.

Parasite Control

The basis of good parasite control is strategic deworming based on fecal worm egg counts (FWECs). Donkeys are susceptible to the same endoparasites as horses and should be screened for strongyles, ascarids, tapeworms, lungworms, liver flukes, and pinworms depending on their regional prevalence. It should be noted that donkeys with large burdens of endoparasites may not exhibit signs such as weight loss, diarrhea, colic, or poor condition. It is also important to note that donkeys with persistently high strongyle counts can have underlying conditions such as PPID. Donkeys are asymptomatic hosts for lungworms (*Dictyocaulus arnfieldi*), can contaminate clean pastures when introduced without prior deworming and quarantine, and indirectly can infect horses and ponies.

Pregnancy Diagnosis and Follow-Up Care of the Mare

It is common for mating to occur in an uncontrolled manner, meaning that service dates are often unknown for the owner and veterinarian. Early pregnancy diagnosis can be done by rectal ultrasonography or measurement of estrone sulfate (over 120 days of pregnancy). It is important for pregnant jennies to be appropriately vaccinated and dewormed. Late-stage pregnancy and lactation are major risks factors for hyperlipemia, so it is essential to ensure adequate caloric intake during these periods.[3] Attention should also be paid to routine health care, including dentistry and farriery.

Castration

Castration is recommended for behavioral and management reasons, but also as population control, to avoid unwanted foals that are neglected, cause welfare concerns, increase feral populations, and add pressure to equine charities. Ideally, donkeys should be castrated between 6 and 12 months of age when a closed technique via a scrotal approach can be used, which can be safely carried out under field conditions.[19] In mature jacks (4 year old and older or over 150 kg body weight), the recommended approach is via an inguinal route, which requires general anesthesia in a hospital environment. Delaying castration in donkeys will increase the risk of postoperative complications, the anesthetic risk, and the costs of surgery.

Geriatric Management

Donkeys are classed as geriatric over the age of 20, and in many cases management changes are required as they get older. Regular monitoring of dental disease and appropriate treatment plans will minimize the risk of complications such as impaction colic; however, changes such as the use of short chopped fiber products and bedding change to prevent the ingestion of long fibers may be helpful.

Regular health assessments, including evaluation of quality of life should be carried out to inform owners of chronic conditions that will likely deteriorate over time, such as DJD and dental disease. Long-term analgesic medications may be required to reduce pain, and efficacy should be regularly assessed.

Geriatric donkeys are at a higher risk of age-related disorders such as liver disease, PPID, and laminitis, so these conditions should be screened when suspected, based on clinical findings of dullness, weight loss, poorly healing wounds, recurrent infections, laminitis, or high FWECs. Routine care such as dentistry and hoof trimming may be required more frequently in geriatric donkeys.

QUALITY-OF-LIFE ASSESSMENT

In addition to identifying specific conditions during a clinical examination, it is also important to assess the impact of these disorders on the donkey's quality of life. This can enable the implementation of strategies to reduce the risk of additional complications. It can guide decisions on medications, interventions, and treatment monitoring. It also allows for discussions with owners about deterioration in quality of life and to ensure that animal welfare is not compromised.[20] A recent project looking at equine end of life found that veterinarians serve an important role in supporting owners when making the decision to euthanize their donkeys at the most appropriate time. Although quality-of-life assessments are often done by owners with their veterinarians, objective evaluations are necessary to monitor deterioration of chronic conditions. The project also highlighted that there can be a lack of understanding by owners about the objectives of quality-of-life assessment and owners were keen to receive more information and education on this topic and on geriatric care.[21] **Fig. 8** gives an example of

MONITORING YOUR DONKEY'S QUALITY OF LIFE

Name of donkey: Date:

Heart girth measurement (refer to nomogram):

Feeding	Yes	No	Comments
Change in diet			
Enthusiastic to eat			
Dropping food			
Choking on food			
Drooling			
Behaviour	**Yes**	**No**	**Comments**
Alert (frequently moving ears or is head and ear carriage lower)			
Responsive			
Interacting with friends			
Lying down more			
Lying down less			
Difficulty in getting up			
Difficulty getting down			
Enjoying a daily roll			
Locomotion	**Yes**	**No**	**Comments**
Walking and trotting easily			
Turning without difficulty			
Hooves same shape and size			
Walking as much as before			
A bit slower/pottery/taking shorter strides			
Using all of the paddock			
Enjoying walks			
Breathing	**Yes**	**No**	**Comments**
Breathing with ease			
Carrying out normal activities without getting out of breath or exhibiting flared nostrils			
Laboured or noisy breathing			
General	**Yes**	**No**	**Comments**
Any lumps			
Bad breath			
Any eye discharge			
Any nasal discharge			
Passing faeces normally			
Wounds on hocks/knees - indicates difficulty rising			

Fig. 8. Parameters to monitor quality of life in donkeys. (*Courtesy of* The Donkey Sanctuary, Devon, England.)

an easy-to-use quality-of-life guide that owners can complete on a regular basis that may help them to track changes over time.

There are several tools available to assess equine welfare; however, none specifically focuses on quality of life and end-of-life decision making. Parker and Yeats[22] describe the 6 steps involved in decision making on how to enhance quality-of-life assessment in equine patients, which include identifying what factors are important to evaluate, what information can be useful to assess these factors, and the need to develop an appropriate assessment method. The Donkey Sanctuary has developed a quality-of-life scoring chart (see **Fig. 8**) that allows clinicians and owners to work together to assess a range of parameters associated with the most common chronic conditions that afflict donkeys and set end points to facilitate end-of-life decision making.[20] However, these parameters and end points can be adjusted to reflect particular donkey disorders. Using a formal scoring system and repeated observations at appropriate intervals improves decision making and encourages owners to work with their veterinarians to develop an end of life plan for their donkey. It is important to note that quality of life is not only related to the presence of medical conditions, but also takes into consideration mental well-being, so use of validated assessments such as qualitative behavior assessment should also be considered.[23] This type of assessment can provide valuable information on the emotional state of the donkey, which may be affected both by medical conditions and environmental factors.

WELFARE ASSESSMENTS

These can be done on individuals or groups of donkeys kept in the same environment, and there are several recognized methods that can be used depending on the conditions in which the donkeys to be assessed are kept. In many countries, for prosecution cases, the Universities Federation for Animal Welfare (UFAW) Five Freedoms are used to assess failure of duty to care. The animal welfare indicators network developed a donkey welfare assessment protocol primarily designed for donkeys used in production,[24] and there is a specific assessment tool for working equids.[25] All these methods follow a similar principle of assessing a variety of factors about the animal's health, its interaction with people, and the environment in which it is kept to identify any areas of concern. This information can serve to show a failure of care or can act as a baseline to enable the effectiveness of interventions to be objectively monitored.

SUMMARY

Donkeys can often be perceived to be a challenge to examine and diagnose and frequently fall through the net when it comes to routine health care. This article has described some of the key points to be aware of when examining donkeys and has highlighted the importance of developing a preventative health care program to include quality-of-life assessment where appropriate.

REFERENCES

1. Smith D, Pearson RA. A review of the factors affecting the survival of donkeys in semi-arid regions of sub-Saharan Africa. (Special issue: nutrition and health of donkeys in the tropics). Trop Anim Health Prod 2005;37(Suppl 1):1–19.
2. Pearson RA, Merritt JB. Intake, digestion and gastrointestinal transit time in resting donkeys and ponies and exercised donkeys given ad libitum hay and straw diets. Equine Vet J 1991;23(5):339–43.
3. Durham AE, Thiemann AK. Nutritional management of hyperlipaemia. Equine Vet Educ 2015;27(9):482–8.
4. Yousef MK, Dill DB, Mayes MG. Shifts in body fluid during dehydration in the burro, *Equus asinus*. J Appl Physiol (1985) 1970;29(3):345–9.
5. Sneddon JC, Boomker E, Howard CV. Mucosal surface area and fermentation activity in the hind gut of hydrated and chronically dehydrated working donkeys. J Anim Sci 2006;84(1):119–24.

6. Evans L, Crane M, editors. The clinical companion of the donkey. 1st edition. Leicestershire (UK): Matador; 2018. p. 257. Appendix 2.
7. Burden FA, Hazell-Smith E, Mulugeta G, et al. Reference intervals for biochemical and haematological parameters in mature domestic donkeys (Equus asinus) in the UK. Equine Vet Educ 2016;28(3):134–9.
8. Flores P, Lopez J, Rodriguez A, et al. Endoscopy of the upper airways and the proximal digestive tract in the donkey (Equus asinus). J Equine Vet Sci 2001; 21(1):17–20.
9. du Toit N, Dixon PM. Common dental disorders in the donkey. Equine Vet Educ 2012;24(1):45–51.
10. du Toit N, Burden FA, Dixon PM. Clinical dental examinations of 357 donkeys in the UK. Part 1: prevalence of dental disorders. Equine Vet J 2009;41(4):390–4.
11. Matthews N, van Loon JPAM. Anaesthesia and analgesia of the donkey and the mule. Equine Vet Educ 2013;25(1):47–51.
12. Thiemann AK, Rickards K. Donkey hoof disorders and their treatment. Practice 2013;35:135–40.
13. Collins SN, Dyson SJ, Murray RC, et al. Radiological anatomy of the donkey's foot: objective characterisation of the normal and laminitic donkey foot. Equine Vet J 2011;43(4):478–86.
14. Osthaus B, Proops L, Long S, et al. Hair coat properties of donkeys, mules and horses in a temperate climate. Equine Vet J 2018;50(3):339–42.
15. Evans L, Crane M, editors. The clinical companion of the donkey. 1st edition. Leicestershire (UK): Matador; 2018. p. 24. The head and oral cavity.
16. Burden FA, Du Toit N, Hazell-Smith E, et al. Hyperlipaemia in a population of aged donkeys: description, prevalence, and potential risk factors. J Vet Intern Med 2011;25:1420–5.
17. Evans L, Crane M, editors. The clinical companion of the donkey. 1st edition. Leicestershire (UK): Matador; 2018. p. 113. The Musculoskeletal system.
18. Ilse L, Sands B, Burden FA, et al. Essential oils in the management of the donkey louse Bovicolla ocellatus. Equine Vet J 2016;48(3):285–9.
19. Sprayson T, Thiemann AK. Clinical approach to castration in the donkey. Practice 2007;29:526–31.
20. Thiemann A, Barrio Fernandez E, Rickards K, et al. Assessing quality of life and welfare of donkeys in the UK. Practice 2018;40:249–57.
21. AESE Equine end of life collaborative project. 2017. Available at: www.bef.co.uk/repository/EquineDevelopment/AESE_EEoL_Executive_Summary_FINAL_110917.pdf. Accessed October 19, 2018.
22. Parker RA, Yeates JW. Assessment of quality of life in equine patients. Equine Vet J 2012;44:244.
23. Minero M, Dalla Costa E, Dai F, et al. Use of qualitative behaviour assessment as an indicator of welfare in donkeys. Appl Anim Behav Sci 2016;174:147–53.
24. AWIN Welfare assessment protocol for donkeys. 2015. Available at: https://air.unimi.it/retrieve/handle/2434/269100/384805/AWINProtocolDonkeys.pdf. Accessed October 19, 2018.
25. Brooke Standardised equine based welfare assessment tool (SEBWAT). 2012. Available at: www.thebrooke.org/sites/default/files/Professionals/SEBWAT.pdf. Accessed October 19, 2018.

Respiratory Disorders of the Donkey

Karen J. Rickards, PhD, BVSc, MRCVS[a,b],
Alexandra K. Thiemann, MA, Vet MB, Cert EP, MSc, AFHEA, MRCVS[b,c,*]

KEYWORDS

- Lungworm • Strangles • Pulmonary fibrosis • Infectious respiratory disease
- Asinine herpes virus

KEY POINTS

- Donkeys are generally nonathletes, so respiratory disease can present at a later stage with more severe pathology and a poorer prognosis.
- Certain respiratory diseases have a different presentation in the donkey compared with the horse, resulting in a variation in clinical signs. In some cases disease will be less severe as with African horse sickness.
- Owing to their longevity, geriatric respiratory conditions can occur such as pulmonary fibrosis, tracheal collapse, and pulmonary neoplasia.
- Certain equine diagnostic tests for respiratory infections need to be interpreted with caution in the donkey because they may not have been validated or may be complicated by nonspecific reactivity.

CLINICAL EXAMINATION

In general, the same principles for clinical examination of the respiratory tract in horses should be followed in donkeys; however, there are certain factors to consider that might influence clinical signs, differential diagnosis, and management. Additionally, there are anatomic adaptations the clinician will encounter during examination that enable the donkey to produce its characteristic loud bray.

Before examining the patient, attention should be paid to the environment in which the donkey lives or works because it may have an impact on respiratory health. In temperate climates, many donkeys are bedded on straw and straw is the mainstay of their diet. The quality of this product should be assessed to ensure it does not present a risk to inhalation of fungal spores and dust. In certain working

Disclosure Statement: The authors have nothing to disclose.
[a] The Veterinary Department, The Donkey Sanctuary, Sidmouth, Devon EX10 0NU, UK; [b] The Veterinary Hospital, Brookfield, Honiton, Devon EX14 9SU, UK; [c] Education, The Veterinary Department, The Donkey Sanctuary, Sidmouth, Devon EX10 0NU, UK
* Corresponding author. The Veterinary Hospital, Brookfield, Honiton, Devon EX14 9SU, UK.
E-mail address: alex.thiemann@thedonkeysanctuary.org.uk

environments, donkeys maybe exposed to high levels of dust that could lead to the development or exacerbation of lower airway disease. Many donkeys do not receive the same level of routine health care as their equine counterparts, so it is important to ascertain vaccination status; many donkeys are not vaccinated against respiratory pathogens such as influenza. Likewise, their parasite status and worming history is important, particularly if they co-graze with horses owing to the risk of lungworm infection. The age of the animal also needs to be taken into account, because many nonworking donkeys live well into old age predisposing them to certain geriatric respiratory conditions such as tracheal collapse, pulmonary fibrosis, and neoplasia[1] (**Figs. 1–3**).

Owing to their stoic nature and relatively insensitive cough reflex,[2] subtle changes in the early stages of disease progression may go unnoticed. This factor, combined with their nonathletic lifestyle, can mean that conditions present relatively late and at a severe stage, resulting in a poorer prognosis. It is also important to note that certain respiratory diseases present differently in the donkey when compared with the horse. It has been reported that donkeys can be more severely affected by equine influenza and are more susceptible to glanders, whereas subclinical infection with equine viral arteritis may occur and African horse sickness is less severe and rarely fatal in donkeys.[3] Donkeys also tolerate parasitic infections with lungworms (*Dictyocaulus arnfieldii*), showing minimal clinical signs.

External clinical examination should follow similar principles to the horse and include an assessment of systemic health because tachypnoea and/or pyrexia can be associated with systemic diseases such as hyperlipidemia and can occur as a result of any painful condition that may be unrelated to the respiratory system. Body condition score should be measured using the 5-point scale developed specifically for donkeys[4] and appetite should be carefully assessed owing to the risk of secondary hyperlipidemia. It is important to note the difference in normal range for clinical parameters such as heart rate (36–52 bpm), respiratory rate (12–28 breaths per minute) and temperature (36.5°C–37.8°C). In addition to increased respiratory frequency, donkeys have increased pulmonary resistance and decreased dynamic compliance.[3] Landmarks for auscultation of lung fields are identical to the horse and the smaller size of their thorax makes lung sounds easier to hear; however, this can be hampered in obese animals, where significant fat deposits can muffle respiratory sounds. In view of this and the challenge of increasing respiratory effort

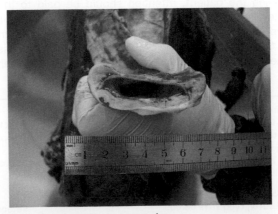

Fig. 1. Tracheal collapse showing airway narrowing.

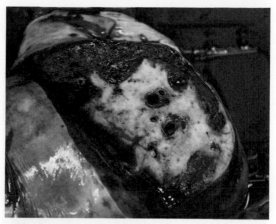

Fig. 2. Post mortem examination of a lung from a donkey with pulmonary fibrosis, white areas show the extent of the fibrosis.

through exercise, a rebreathing bag can be used to accentuate subtle respiratory sounds (**Fig. 4**).

Further diagnostic tests that may be required after the initial examination depend on the clinical signs. Routine hematology can be helpful to identify and monitor response to treatment in infectious or inflammatory diseases, as can measurement of acute phase proteins such as albumin, fibrinogen, and serum amyloid A. The main risk factor for the development of hyperlipidemia is concurrent disease, so if there are any concerns over systemic illness and/or appetite, then biochemistry, including triglycerides, can be useful. The clinician should be aware that normal reference ranges for certain hematologic and biochemical parameters are different in donkeys.[5] If infectious agents are suspected, the use of nasal or nasopharyngeal swabs or nasal washes may be required. In view of the donkey's narrow nasal passages, it is helpful to discuss with your referral laboratory the most appropriate sized nasopharyngeal swab to use.

If endoscopy is indicated, there are certain anatomic variations that clinicians need to be aware of when examining the upper respiratory tract. The nasal passages are narrow, so insertion of the endoscope requires care and good lubrication with small-bore endoscopes being preferable to avoid damaging the fragile, vascular mucosa covering the conchae. The middle meatus can be difficult to examine, making it challenging to assess the maxillary sinus drainage angle.[6] The pharynx is narrower,

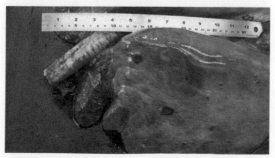

Fig. 3. Neoplastic nodules on the pulmonary surface of a donkey.

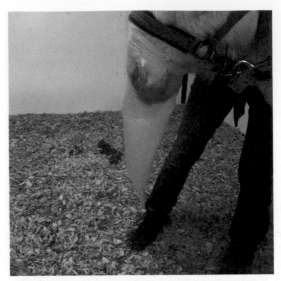

Fig. 4. Use of a rebreathing bag in a donkey.

which predisposes to collapse during endoscopy, and the pharyngeal recess is much deeper, extending 4 to 6 cm caudally from the guttural pouch openings, and forming a deep membranous pouch (**Fig. 5**). The guttural pouch openings may sit more horizontally (**Fig. 6**), however, the technique to enter the pouches is identical to the horse and the anatomy is the same.[2]

The epiglottis is shorter and more pointed, and the apex is found closer to the corniculate process of each arytenoid cartilage (see **Fig. 6**). These anatomic differences mean that the *aditus laryngis* faces in a more caudal direction in the donkey and has a narrower dorsoventral diameter, which makes visualization of the tracheal opening through the *rima glottidis* much more difficult. This anatomic arrangement also means that the openings of the lateral laryngeal ventricles and vocal folds are difficult to visualize in donkeys.[6] It may also increase the risk of acute dyspnea in conditions affecting the nasopharynx or guttural pouches.[2] A

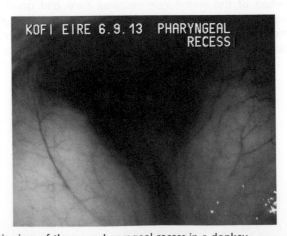

Fig. 5. Endoscopic view of the nasopharyngeal recess in a donkey.

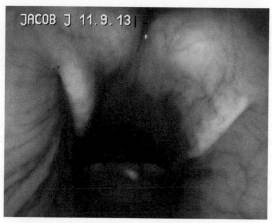

Fig. 6. Endoscopic view of the epiglottis and guttural pouch ostia.

study by Powell and colleagues[7] identified a dorsoventral flattening of the tracheal rings, which was most marked in the distal cervical and rostral thoracic portions of the trachea. This finding correlates with a previous report, where tracheal collapse in a donkey was found to occur at the thoracic inlet,[8] making the diagnosis of this condition through external palpation more challenging and suggests that the oval shape of the trachea in this region is more compressible and susceptible to collapse.[7]

Techniques for bronchoalveolar lavage and transtracheal wash are the same as in horses; however, bronchoalveolar lavage samples from healthy donkeys contain a higher percentage of macrophages and transtracheal wash samples show higher neutrophil and eosinophil counts.[3] Thoracic ultrasound examination can be useful in the diagnosis of conditions such as pulmonary fibrosis and is valuable when performing lung biopsies. Because many donkeys have thick coats, patient preparation is required to obtain high-quality images. In view of their small size, thoracic radiographs can be obtained with standard portable generators used in equine practice **(Fig. 7)**.

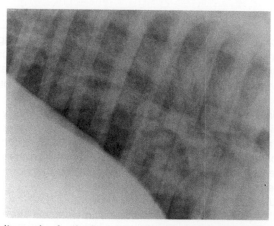

Fig. 7. Thoracic radiograph of a donkey showing mixed interstitial and alveolar pulmonary patterns.

CONDITIONS OF THE UPPER RESPIRATORY TRACT

In general, conditions of the upper respiratory tract can be diagnosed and managed in a similar way to the horse, although the incidence and presentation may vary. Donkey foals can be affected by a number of congenital abnormalities of the palate and mandible.

Sinus

The most common cause of sinusitis in older donkeys is secondary to poorly managed dental disease, which also predisposes them to hyperlipidemia and weight loss. Any proposed treatment plan requires a full evaluation of the animal's systemic health.

Other documented causes include primary inflammation, cysts, neoplasia, and infection. The sinus anatomy is broadly similar to the horse, but the rostral and caudal maxillary sinuses are divided by an incomplete bony septum, and the smaller size of the sinus compartments necessitates a careful surgical approach.

Guttural Pouch Disease

The guttural pouches in the donkey are located in the same relative position as in the horse and can be examined with standard endoscopic equipment. Anatomic variations in the carotid arterial tree has been reported and proposed to account for the reduced incidence of guttural pouch mycosis in donkeys.

Infection with *Streptococcus equi* ssp. *equi* can result in empyema and chondroid formation, severe enough to obstruct the airways. Newly arrived donkeys should be isolated and screened for *S equi* if there is any chance of prior exposure. At present, commercial serology tests for *Streptococcus* A and C antigens are not validated for donkey use, and gold standard screening requires endoscopy with a polymerase chain reaction (PCR) test and bacterial culture of nasopharyngeal or guttural pouch content or lavage.

S equi ssp. *zooepidemicus* occasionally causes empyema and chondroids in donkeys, which may be secondary to immunosuppression, and has been diagnosed as a coinfection with equine/asinine herpesviruses (AHVs).

Owing to the narrowness of the nasal passages, donkeys have a greater risk of hemorrhage during upper airway endoscopy. They should be well-restrained and suitably sedated.

Trachea

Tracheal collapse is a recognized problem in donkeys, becoming more prevalent with aging. There is a gradual age-related decline in tracheal cartilage integrity, which predisposes to this condition. Initiating factors include underlying respiratory disease that increases respiratory effort, and external trauma typically from raised feeder troughs.

Clinical signs include a chronic cough, inspiratory and expiratory dyspnea, excessive tracheal noise and even vibrations on auscultation. In severe cases, distress with nostril flare and attempted mouth breathing can be appreciated.[8]

Radiography can confirm the diagnosis; endoscopy may provoke extreme respiratory distress. The location of the collapse is most often in the thoracic inlet where the tracheal rings are at their most dorsoventrally flattening.

Treatment is usually aimed at decreasing respiratory effort by improving general airway health with the use of environmental modification to minimize dust and allergen inhalation and medication to improve airflow including bronchodilators and corticosteroids where appropriate.

PARASITIC INFECTIONS
Lungworm

The donkey is well-adapted to the lungworm (*Dictyocaulus arnfieldi*) and as parasites reach sexual maturity they lay eggs that are coughed up, swallowed, and passed out in feces. In contrast, in horses this parasite does not develop to sexual maturity, but it causes a severe pulmonary inflammatory response that provokes chronic coughing and dyspnea. Considering that donkeys rarely cough when infected with high numbers of lungworms, they are often seen as a problem when co-grazing with horses and ponies.

Lungworm larvae can remain viable for long periods on moist pasture and can spread widely; the prepatent period is between 8 and 13 weeks. Infective L3 larvae migrate via the lymphatics to the lungs, the adult worms grow up to 8 cm in the small airways.

In donkeys, the diagnosis of lungworm infection can be made by fecal examination using the Baermann technique.[9]

Although it is reported that lungworm in the donkey is less pathogenic than in the horse, post mortem examination of lungs from affected animals will show hyperinflation and inflammation around bronchi, especially in the caudal lung lobes.

Donkeys should be screened for lungworm and treated if necessary using ivermectin (200 µg/kg) orally. It is good practice to screen new arrival donkeys and to confirm the efficacy of treatment using fecal egg count reduction tests.

Pulmonary Hydatidosis

Echinococcus granulosus, the small intestine tapeworm of domestic dogs, cats, and foxes can infect donkeys, mules, and horses if they graze pastures contaminated by infective eggs, in the UK and Europe. A variant of this parasite, *Echinococcus equinus*, has been identified by genetic analysis. This parasite is endemic in some regions of Africa and the Middle East. Once inside the intermediate host small intestine, the embryonated eggs hatch releasing oncospheres that penetrate the intestinal mucosa and migrate via the circulatory system to various organs, especially the liver and lungs. In these organs, large fluid-filled cysts (hydatid cysts) develop lined with protoscolices and daughter cysts that can reinfect a carnivore If they eat the infected offal.

The cysts are usually asymptomatic unless they develop to such a size or number that they compromise organ function. Thoracic and abdominal ultrasound examination in donkeys where this parasite is highly prevalent frequently shows large hydatid cysts associated with the pulmonary parenchyma or liver. It is contraindicated to drain cysts owing to the risk of releasing further infective protoscolices. Treatment has been attempted with long-term albendazole and/or praziquantel. Prevention of infection is achieved by regular deworming of canines with a product effective against tapeworms of domestic carnivores and not permitting feeding of infected offal to canines.

Parascaris Equorum—Ascarids

Ascarids or roundworms (*Parascaris equorum*) infect equally donkey and horse foals. Owing to their migratory lifecycle, the presence of infection is often associated with coughing in young animals, as the larvae pass via the lungs to the pharynx, and then are swallowed and become established as adults in the small intestine. Donkeys seem to not develop such strong immunity as the horse, and adult donkeys can harbor significant ascarid burdens. Diagnosis and treatment should follow best practice guidelines for horses, remembering that few products are licensed for donkeys.[9]

CONDITIONS OF THE LOWER RESPIRATORY TRACT

Typically in donkeys, lower airway respiratory disease has a late presentation of clinical signs, often with accompanying comorbidities. Clinical history, previous diseases, sick animals at the farm, vaccination, deworming, and management practices, as well as a complete clinical examination and response to treatment are important.[10] Blood work, transtracheal wash, or bronchoalveolar lavage results are useful. Thoracic ultrasound examination and radiography can be performed, although obese donkeys can be difficult to image successfully. Donkeys are rarely included in good preventative health programs and vaccinations may not be current. Screening for lungworm is suggested in cases with poor anthelmintic use records.

Treatment regimes follow the same principles as for the horse, using known variations in drug metabolism. Early and aggressive treatment of infections is recommended with close monitoring of appetite and general well-being.

Recurrent Airway Obstruction—"Donkey Asthma"

In donkeys this is usually due to an allergic response to allergens in dried forage or pasture. Soaking straw and hay is required along with rigorous dust free environmental management. Soaking forage leaches out vitamins and minerals, and donkeys should have these supplemented with a forage balancer. Where available, short chopped straw based, low calorie products may be more suitable than straw for feeding and low dust bedding can be used.

On clinical examination there is expiratory dyspnea, abdominal exertion, and nasal flare. Severe cases may progress and precipitate tracheal collapse or lead to the development of right sided heart failure. A rebreathing bag examination is useful to detect mild respiratory sounds in the unexercised donkey.

Pulmonary Fibrosis

Pulmonary fibrosis is becoming more widely recognized, although its exact etiology has not been defined.[11] Clinically, these donkeys show inspiratory and expiratory dyspnea (which differentiates this condition from the expiratory dyspnea of recurrent airway obstruction) that can becomes severe. Generally, these cases present after conventional treatment for recurrent airway obstruction has failed. There may be episodes of pyrexia and nasal discharge consistent with secondary bacterial infection. On auscultation the areas affected have a decreased or absent movement of air, and sound abnormally quiet. Areas adjacent to fibrotic lesions may have increased adventitial lung sounds. There are no characteristic hematologic or biochemical features apart from a response to infection and inflammation.

Ultrasound examination is the most useful diagnostic tool if the fibrosis is subpleural; comet tail artifacts can be seen extending away from the pleura at areas of fibrosis. Radiographically, there could be a generalized nonstructured interstitial pattern or a structured pattern consistent with localized pulmonary fibrosis.

Fibrosis can occur throughout the lungs, from mild to severe focal areas, through to the involvement of whole pulmonary lobes and subpleural thickening secondary to fibrosis. At gross post mortem examination, the lungs are consolidated and can weigh up to twice as much as normal lungs. Histologically, there are giant syncytial cells with lymphohistiocytic and suppurative bronchiolitis.

AHVs 4 and 5 have been isolated from lungs of donkeys affected by pulmonary fibrosis.[12] Pulmonary fibrosis in donkeys resembles equine multinodular pulmonary fibrosis in horses, which has been proposed to be caused by equine herpesvirus 5.

There is no specific treatment for this condition and the aim of therapy is to minimize further airway compromise by a combination of clean air management, regular vaccinations, and medications, including bronchodilators and steroids administered by inhalation or systemically. Donkeys with the condition need regular monitoring with the aim of defining a suitable time for euthanasia, avoiding a respiratory crisis and possible sudden death. There is no evidence that antiviral drugs provide any benefit.

Pulmonary Neoplasia

Neoplasia of the thorax is rare in the donkey, but should be considered as a differential diagnosis in animals with respiratory disease that is not responsive to treatment. Neoplasia is more common in elderly animals. The clinical signs expected would include dullness, weight loss, dyspnea, tachypnoea, lymphadenopathy, potentially pleural effusion, and blood parameter changes consistent with chronic inflammation. Diagnosis may not be reached until post mortem because the tumors can be hard to diagnose and image.

INFECTIOUS RESPIRATORY DISEASES

Donkeys are susceptible to a similar range of bacterial and viral respiratory disease as horses, however, their clinical presentation may vary owing to a number of factors:

- Relative susceptibility to certain pathogens is different resulting in variations in severity of presentation.
- Donkeys can live to an older age so can suffer from concurrent age-related diseases that affect immune status.
- Donkeys are usually nonathletic and thus are less likely to show early subtle signs.
- Donkeys are more likely to show nonspecific signs such as dullness and anorexia

EQUINE INFLUENZA

Equine influenza virus subtype H3N8 has been isolated and characterized from donkeys showing clinical signs similar to the horse, including pyrexia, depression, coughing, and nasal discharge.[10] However, donkeys have been reported to be more severely affected and at a higher risk of secondary bronchopneumonia. Therefore, prompt antibiotic and anti-inflammatory treatment is recommended.[13] Diagnosis is similar to the horse by detection of virus or viral nucleic acid from nasal or nasopharyngeal swabs or via serologic testing. In 2010, during an outbreak of a highly pathogenic avian influenza virus H5N1 in Egypt, the same virus was isolated from donkeys exhibiting respiratory signs, which was the first evidence of an interspecies jump of this virus into a member of the *Equidae* family. This transfer highlights the importance of surveillance in a number of species when dealing with influenza outbreaks.[2] Although none of the commercially available equine influenza vaccines have been evaluated in donkeys, current recommendation would be to use an equine licensed vaccine containing relevant influenza strains. It is important to note, however, that many donkeys are not routinely vaccinated and owner education is essential to highlight the importance of routine vaccination both to the individual animal and the equine population as a whole.

EQUINE AND ASININE HERPES VIRUSES

Donkeys can be infected by both the alpha (EHV-1 and 4) and gamma (EHV-2 and 5) equine herpesviruses, showing similar clinical signs to the horse. In addition, there are several AHV that have been linked with respiratory disease, including AHV-3, -4, and -5. Clinical signs have been described as ranging from a mild rhinitis to interstitial pneumonia. AHV-2 was isolated from the nasal secretions of a mule after an outbreak of respiratory disease.[10] As mentioned, AHV-4 and -5 were isolated from donkeys with pulmonary fibrosis in donkeys.[3,11] Latent infections are also common with stressors such as transport and the introduction of new animals being potential risk factors for recrudescence.

Serologic methods for diagnosis of EHV-1 and -4 infection include the complement fixation test, virus neutralization, and enzyme-linked immunosorbent assay. These tests are based on titer increases, the complement fixation test and virus neutralization do not differentiate EHV-1 and EHV-4, but the enzyme-linked immunosorbent assay does.[14] Detection of viral nucleic acid from nasal or nasopharyngeal swabs via PCR is becoming widely used for EHV-1 and EHV-4; however, few laboratories are set up for AHVs, which have positive cytopathic effect on cell culture monolayers.[2] In the UK, the Irish Equine Center can run an AHV-3–specific PCR.

There are no vaccines available for AHVs and no studies have investigated the efficacy of equine herpesviruses vaccines in donkeys or their cross-protection against asinine strains. As such, a risk–benefit analysis would need to be carried out to decide on the value of vaccination with commercially available equine herpesviruses vaccines.

AFRICAN HORSE SICKNESS

African horse sickness is caused by an arthropod-borne virus (orbivirus) endemic in sub-Saharan Africa where 9 serotypes have been identified. African horse sickness virus is transmitted by various species of *Culicoides* midges and is a major health threat for equidae outside of Africa. The virus can also be transmitted by some species of mosquitoes and ticks. Horses are the most vulnerable to this virus, followed by mules and donkeys. Of interest, donkeys outside Africa are highly susceptible and develop acute and subacute forms of the disease, whereas in endemic regions of Africa infection is often asymptomatic, and donkeys are considered as reservoir hosts.[10] However, they can become viremic after inoculation with a virulent serotype and can exhibit a mild form of the disease known as horse sickness fever, which is characterized by fever and general malaise for 1 to 2 days. The cardiac or subacute form of the disease is characterized by swelling of the supraorbital fossa, eyelids, neck, thorax, and shoulders (**Fig. 8**). The pulmonary or acute form is the most severe and is associated with dyspnea, spasmodic coughing, and frothy fluid oozing out from the nostrils. Mixed infections can also occur and mortality rates in susceptible donkeys range from 5% to 10%.[15] Vaccine development has been hampered by the large number of virus serotypes; however, a polyvalent live attenuated vaccine is licensed in South Africa; a live attenuated vaccine against serotypes 2, 4, and 9 in Ethiopia; and a killed bivalent vaccine against serotypes 4 and 9 in Egypt.

EQUINE ARTERITIS VIRUS

Equine arteritis virus is usually subclinical, but mild clinical signs may be seen in the donkey, which typically include fever, depression, ocular and nasal discharge, and conjunctivitis. Transmission of equine viral arteritis through the respiratory as well as venereal route has been reported in donkeys.[13]

Streptococcus equi ssp. Equi (Strangles)

Donkeys and mules are susceptible to strangles; however, the clinical presentation tends to vary from fever, purulent nasal discharge, and abscessation of mandibular

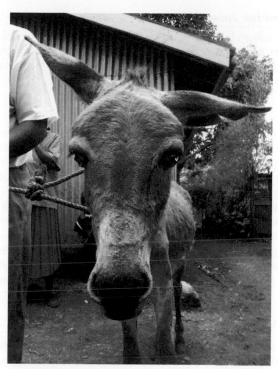

Fig. 8. Donkey with African horse sickness demonstrating severe conjunctival swelling.

and retropharyngeal lymph nodes to mild persistent nasal discharge. They can also act as carriers by establishing a chronic asymptomatic infection in the guttural pouches or present with intermittent nasal discharge.

In the acute phase, diagnosis is by PCR and culture from nasopharyngeal swabs or washes from purulent abscess material. Diagnosis of carriers is more challenging as the serologic test available for detection of S equi antigens A and C has not been validated in donkeys and in the authors' experience, the cut-off values reported for horses are not applicable to donkeys. Serology to M protein indicates exposure, but is not diagnostic. For definitive diagnosis, a guttural pouch wash is required. Upper airway endoscopy in affected animals is highly recommended to assess laryngeal involvement, available lumen, and to identify whether empyema is present in the guttural pouches. Systemically ill animals need additional supportive therapy with particular attention paid to appetite to avoid the risk of hyperlipidemia. Antibiotic instillation into the pouches such as penicillin gel may be required to control the infection, in particular in animals with empyema. Neglected cases of empyema can progress relatively rapidly to acute airway obstruction, so it is advisable to rapidly and thoroughly investigate persistent nasal discharge because limited access makes surgical treatment challenging.[2] Guttural pouch chondroids may develop from inspissated pus. Tracheostomy may be necessary in animals with severe airway obstruction and distress. Complications such as purpura hemorrhagica are unusual in donkeys; however, metastatic infections (bastard strangles) may occur.

The efficacy of strangles vaccines has not be investigated in donkeys so a risk–benefit analysis would need to be carried out to determine the value of vaccination.

Streptococcus equi ssp. Zooepidemicus

Although this bacterium is considered an opportunistic commensal in horses, it has been identified in the guttural pouches of systemically ill donkeys with empyema and chondroids (**Fig. 9**). This suggests that in donkeys, *Streptococcus zooepidemicus* can be a primary pathogen in certain circumstances.

GLANDERS

Donkeys are the most susceptible equidae to this contagious and life-threatening disease caused by *Burkholderia mallei*; mules are less susceptible. Acute disease is usually characterized by nasal or pulmonary forms of the disease. Clinical signs include fever, ulcerating nodules in the nasal passages, decreased appetite and weight loss, depression, coughing, and progressive dyspnea.

Lung abscesses and bronchopneumonia often develop and cases are fatal within a few days to weeks of infection. A latent form of glanders has also been described with clinical signs limited to nasal discharge and dyspnea.

Diagnosis of glanders usually requires bacterial culture, however, the mallein test and serologic assays are available for surveillance. It is also important to note that this disease is a zoonosis so care needs to be taken when handling suspect cases.[10]

MYCOBACTERIAL INFECTIONS

Mycobacterium avium and *Mycobacterium bovis* have been identified in donkeys in pulmonary and disseminated forms.[16] The route of transmission is likely to be oral, where there is strong exposure to the organism. Immunosuppression owing to age and concurrent illness may lead to establishment of the disease or recrudescence of dormant infections. Affected animals may display pyrexia, weight loss, dyspnea, cough, and a number of signs related to the location of infection. Lung disease consists of miliary and caseous lesions with likely involvement of lymph nodes. Although a rare disease in equines, the disease has serious zoonotic implications and humans in contact with potential cases should be screened by appropriate medical authorities.

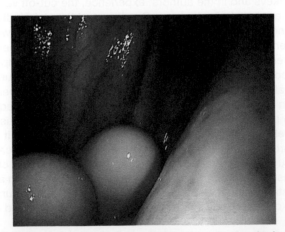

Fig. 9. Endoscopic view of chondroids in the guttural pouch of a donkey affected with *S equi* infection.

SUMMARY

Respiratory disease in the donkey requires a careful diagnostic and therapeutic approach, using knowledge of donkey specific parameters and presentation. Donkeys can present with mild signs but this can mask severe illness owing to their stoicism and lack of athleticism. Donkeys should be included in preventative health programs such as vaccination, for their own welfare and the well-being of equine populations. Donkeys that are inappetant owing to respiratory disease are at high risk of hyperlipidemia and should be managed carefully.

REFERENCES

1. Morrow LD, Smith KC, Piercy RJ, et al. Retrospective analysis of post-mortem findings in 1,444 aged donkeys. J Comp Pathol 2010;144(2–3):145–56.
2. Thiemann AK. Respiratory disease in the donkey. Equine Vet Educ 2012;24(9): 469–78.
3. Mendoza FJ, Toribio RE, Perez-Ejica A. Donkey internal medicine-part II: cardiovascular, respiratory, neurologic, urinary, ophthalmic, dermatology, and musculoskeletal disorders. J Equine Vet Sci 2018;65:86–97.
4. Evans L, Crane M, editors. Clinical companion of the donkey appendix 3. 1st edition. Leicestershire: Matador; 2018. p. 258.
5. Burden FA, Hazell-Smith E, Mulugeta G, et al. Reference intervals for biochemical and haematological parameters in mature domestic donkeys (Equus asinus) in the UK. Equine Vet Educ 2016;28(3):134–9.
6. Fores P, Lopez J, Rodriguez A, et al. Endoscopy of the upper airways and the proximal digestive tract in the donkey (Equus asinus). J Equine Vet Sci 2001; 21:17–20.
7. Powell RJ, DuToit N, Burden FA, et al. Morphological study of tracheal shape in donkeys with and without tracheal obstruction. Equine Vet J 2010;42(2):136–41.
8. Mair TS, Lane JG. Tracheal obstruction in two horses and a donkey. Vet Rec 1990;126:303–4.
9. Burden FA, Getachew AM. Donkeys - a unique and challenging endoparasite host. J Equine Vet Sci 2016;39:S102–3.
10. Barrandeguy ME, Carossino M. Infectious diseases in donkeys and mules: an overview and update. J Equine Vet Sci 2018;65:98–105.
11. Miele A, Dhaliwal K, Du Toit K, et al. Chronic pleuropulmonary fibrosis and elastosis of aged donkeys: similarities to human pleuroparenchymal fibroelastosis. Chest 2014;145(6):1325–32.
12. Kleiboeker SB, Schommer SK, Johnson PJ, et al. Association of two newly recognized herpesviruses with interstitial pneumonia in donkeys (Equus asinus). J Vet Diagn Invest 2002;14(4):273–80.
13. Holland RE, Tudor LR, Timoney JF, et al. Equine influenza in donkeys: severe bronchopneumonia owing to clonal invasion by Streptococcus zooepidemicus. In: Proceedings of the 8th International Conference on Equine Infectious Diseases. March 23-26, 1998. p. 548–9.
14. Hartley CA, Wilks CR, Studdert MJ, et al. Comparison of antibody detection assays for the diagnosis of equine herpesvirus 1 and 4 infections in horses. Am J Vet Res 2005;66(5):921–8.
15. Evans L, Crane M, editors. Clinical companion of the donkey. 1st edition. Leicestershire: Matador; 2018. p. 131–43.
16. Bryan J, den Boon P, McGuirk J, et al. Tuberculosis caused by *Mycobacterium bovis* infection in a donkey. Equine Vet Educ 2018;30(4):172–6.

Donkey and Mule Behavior

Amy Katherine McLean, PhD, MSc[a],*,
Francisco Javier Navas González, DVM, MSc, PhD[b],
Igor Federico Canisso, DVM, MSc, PhD[c]

KEYWORDS

- Donkeys • Mules • Hinnies • Behavior • Cognition

KEY POINTS

- Donkeys and mules behave differently from horses and require more patience.
- Studies and practical experiences suggest that donkeys and mules/hinnies should be trained, handled, and restrained differently from horses.
- High pain tolerance increases the difficulty to recognize and diagnose disease in donkeys and mules if horse standards are considered.
- Ingestive, social, and reproductive behavior is unique to the donkey.

 Video content accompanies this article at http://www.vetequine.theclinics.com.

INTRODUCTION

The donkey was the first domesticated equid more than 5000 years ago. This domestication was likely because of its gentle nature even though its natural defense is to fight and not to flee like horses and other equids (Video 1). Mules (jack × mare) and hinnies (stallion × jenny) inherit a combination of behavioral traits from both species. Based on the type of work and environment, some owners prefer mules and others prefer hinnies. However, there is no evidence than one hybrid is more suited than another for work. The historical importance of mules and donkeys brings up the question especially for mules, "How such an important beast of burden can be so challenging for so many people, yet still prove to be such an important thread in society?"

Disclosure Statement: No relationship or anything to disclose.
[a] Animal Science Department, UC Davis Animal Science, University of California Davis, 2251 Meyer Hall, 1 Shields Avenue, Davis, CA 95616, USA; [b] AGR218 PAIDI Group, Department of Genetics, Faculty of Veterinary Sciences, University of Córdoba, C5 Building (Gregor Mendel), Ground Floor, Rabanales University Campus, Córdoba 14071, Spain; [c] Department of Veterinary Clinical Medicine, College of Veterinary Medicine, University of Illinois Urbana-Champaign, Urbana, IL 61802, USA
* Corresponding author. UC Davis Animal Science, University of California Davis, 2131A Meyer Hall, 1 Shields Avenue, Davis, CA 95616.
E-mail address: acmclean@ucdavis.edu

Vet Clin Equine 35 (2019) 575–588
https://doi.org/10.1016/j.cveq.2019.08.010
0749-0739/19/© 2019 Elsevier Inc. All rights reserved.

vetequine.theclinics.com

Behavior has been a defining trait for both the donkey and its hybrids in terms of its appeal or lack of for professionals and owners. For example, mules tend to exhibit some behaviors that the owner or clinician must work around, such as being hard to catch or ear shy. Such behavior in horses would be less tolerated and generally overcome, whereas with a mule such behavioral differences may require years to overcome or a behavior that may never change. Establishing trust with mules may take years as well as shown in studies comparing their reaction or acceptance of routine procedures by familiar and unfamiliar people.[1] The steady increase in donkey and mule ownership has been raising awareness on their unique behavior and physiology, increasing the demand for knowledge and specialized veterinary care.[2]

Behavior of donkeys and mules is very different from horses; mistakes are made by owners and practitioners when assuming that all these equids behavior similarly. There are many misconceptions about donkeys and mules; for example, stubbornness is often misunderstood when these animals are actually being cautious.[2,3] Working with donkeys and mules can teach patience and recognizing that the slightest variation in behavior could mean major health issues (Video 2). A new owner or practitioner should be aware of the distinctive demeanor of the donkey and its hybrids when compared with horses and learn how to deal with these behavioral differences and not against them.[2–4]

In general, most owners have acquired a great sense of patience in dealing with donkeys and mules,[2,3] and they may help practitioners provide veterinary care by translating the different nuances in behavior when compared with horses. It is a common consensus among owners and professionals that early intensive handling of newborn foals allows them to gain the trust and facilitate routine handling when adults (Video 3). Furthermore, modifying their behavior at later ages may not be an option once they have learned a particular behavior or fear of something. Understanding mule and donkey behavior could be the difference between life and death, as their demonstration of pain is less evident than in horses. Thus, the present review outlines the current state of knowledge and points out differences and similarities among donkeys, horses, and their hybrids, and offers guidelines on how to work with these animals and recognize key behaviors associated with diseases.

NORMAL BEHAVIOR: DONKEY, MULE, HINNY

Mules and donkeys are creatures of habit and do not react well to changes in daily routines.[2,4] For example, a change in the feeding schedule can dismay the animal and create abnormal behavior.[2] More importantly, unfamiliar personnel may prevent a very gentle and friendly mule or donkey from being caught until the stranger leaves the premises.[2,5] These animals tend to bond with their caregiver(s) once trust has been established. Anecdotally, treats can be used as positive reinforcements along with a calm, soothing voice and/or tactile contact (eg, scratches or gentle touch with finger tips).

Donkeys, in general, are easier to work with than mules, even if they have not been handled from an early age. In many developing countries it is not uncommon to observe women and children working with donkeys. The gentle nature of the donkey is often taken advantage of, which results in poor welfare. On the other hand, although mules tend to be more challenging for owners/handlers and practitioners, they are subjected to harsher treatments.

Human interactions with mules tend to vary from excellent to very bad. In many cases, each partner seems only to tolerate the other, although interviews with mule handlers and owners suggested that those who seem to understand mule behavior generally prefer mules over horses and sometimes donkeys.[1,6] Participatory research has indicated that owners and handlers who understand mules typically have worked with them from an early age[1,4,7] (**Figs. 1** and **2**). In addition, mules handled properly from early ages are more tolerant interacting with unfamiliar personnel compared with those who are not handled.[7] Collectively, this is relevant for clinical practice, as while providing veterinary care to mules, these animals may require a familiar handler during approaching or treatment.

Owner preference, perceptions, and attitudes toward mules and donkeys vary according to their use and cultural differences and beliefs. Many mule owners have reported the most challenging routine care is administering an oral anthelmintic or trimming hooves.[1] Most owners have responded to survey questions that they would like more information on training mules and donkeys, and handlers have responded that all mules are aggressive.[1,4,8] Many mules are unruly because of poor handling and mistreatment.

Differentiating between normal and abnormal behavior is paramount to provide professional servicing to these animals. The stoic nature of donkeys and mules could mask pain. It has been suggested they have a higher tolerance to pain, but also it has been suggested that they may feel the same intensity of pain as horses. However, it is possible that disguising pain is a mechanism to prevent predatory attacks. For example, there is a misconception in the lay community that mules and donkeys do not have colic or lameness, but this is obviously inaccurate. However, these animals will show clinical signs of disease when the condition is often in advanced stages[2] (Video 4).

Rolling is normal donkey and mule behavior that could be misinterpreted as a colic sign. These animals appear to enjoy rolling in sandy/dirt areas, but excessive rolling or lying down can be abnormal. It is interesting that mules typically roll in an arbitrarily designated spot and when kept in a group, the different animals of the group tend to roll in the same spot. Again, the duration and frequency of rolling can tell us more about its behavior.

Key Concepts

- Mules tend to exhibit more signs of pain compared with donkeys, but still, those signs may be subtle in comparison to horses.
- One of the most critical elements to managing the health and husbandry of mules and hinnies is knowing their behavior.

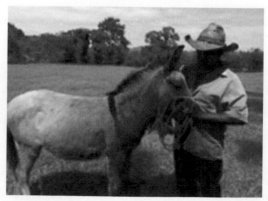

Fig. 1. Mule owner's foal is easy to handle and approach, handled from day one.

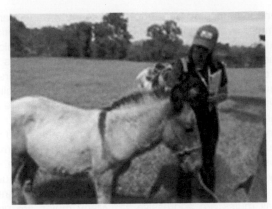

Fig. 2. Mule foal easily approached by unfamiliar person.

- Mules and hinnies, like donkeys, are very stoic animals; and an intuitive owner will be able to pick up on any behavioral changes and inform the practitioner (**Fig. 3**).

HOW TO APPROACH MULES AND DONKEYS

Behavior assessments can be conducted to evaluate the overall behavior, but often research has shown that mules especially are more likely to trust a familiar person compared with an unfamiliar person. When approaching a mule for the first time, approaching them head-on, meaning walking to the face versus the left side of their neck, resulted in more successful approaches.[1,4,7] Donkeys tend to be most tolerant of unfamiliar people and easier to approach than mules or horses.[1] Approaching the donkey's face and then the side after the animal has recognized and accepted the approaching person appears to be useful. A healthy donkey and mule will spend most of its day browsing or grazing, possibly part of it taking dust baths and grooming one another. A mule or donkey that is seen lying on the ground more than normal, not eating, or away from the other donkeys or mules is a reason to be concerned and to check on the animal (Video 5).

Key Concepts

- Often mules and hinnies are perceived to be challenging to work with, especially among professionals and para-professionals working in the field on a routine basis with these animals.
- Mules and hinnies will often trust their familiar handler/owner and are less trusting of unfamiliar handlers.

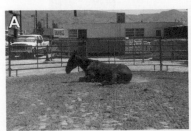
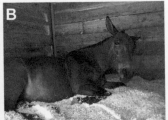

Fig. 3. (*A, B*) Natural for mules and donkeys to express grooming behavior or rolling but excessive rolling is an indicator for abdominal discomfort.

- Read the body language from the posture of the head, eyes, nostrils, neck, and body, and watch the tail and uneven weight distribution on the hind limbs (**Figs. 4–6**).
- Mules have a higher reasoning ability when compared with horses.[6]
- Mules tend to prefer more open areas rather than be confined.
- Owners may find a stronger preference for various stalled or confined areas compared with horses that tend to be more tolerant of small areas.
- Owners may find mules to display some behaviors that more or less need to be dealt with or accepted versus corrected (eg, ear shyness, hard to catch) (Video 6).

SOCIAL BEHAVIOR

Donkeys and mules are social animals and prefer to have companion animals of the same species or not.[4,9] However, mules can become so attached to their companion that it can create an unmanageable situation when separating them from their companion (see Video 6). On the other hand, donkeys when losing a companion or mate will often become depressed, and the stress can trigger metabolic and endocrine imbalances, including fat mobilization and the risk of hyperlipemia.[5,9]

The gentle nature and social flexibility of donkeys make them an ideal companion for horses, foals, goats, sheep, and cattle.[9,10] Donkeys are often seen accompanying newly weaned foals as well as traveling partners for performance horses to reduce stress related to transportation and competition(s).

Playing and socialization are important in domestic donkeys and mules because it establishes a social hierarchy as well as aids in the development of dominating strategies such as learning to fight, biting in key locations such as the throat latch, and knees.[9,10] Excessive play resulting in fighting type behavior is not uncommon in male mules (Video 7); however, some jacks may become too aggressive toward other animals and castration may be required.

ABNORMAL BEHAVIOR

The slightest change in behavior could be indicative of compromised health or disease in a mule or donkey. Learning to read their face from ear position to eyes to nostrils as

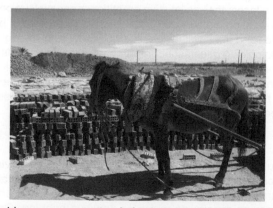

Fig. 4. Painful, avoidance, or aggression behaviors may present in similar ways with ears back and tense body, read the body language before proceeding and have familiar person on hand to assist.

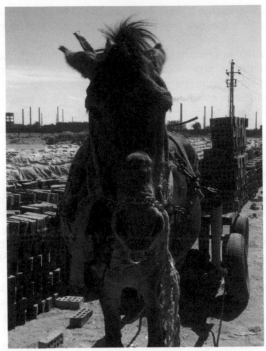

Fig. 5. Mules and doneys are better approached face on as this way we can read their body language on how to proceed. Note the ears are back and nostrils tightened. This is not a welcoming response which maybe caused by pain, discomfort, or fear.

well as head, neck, body, and tail movement can be more informative about the current status in these animals (Video 8). A mule or donkey lying on the ground for an extended period or with reduced food consumption along with superficial lesions from thrashing are indicative signs of discomfort. Identifying the source of discomfort is another challenge (see Video 8).

Donkeys tend to be even more challenging to detect signs of colic, but if one pays attention to the facial grimace by observing ear, head, and neck position, as well as the expression on their faces, then an intuitive practitioner can pick up on signs of abdominal pain. When using some diagnostic tools, such as hoof testers, practitioners have reported that mules and donkeys are less likely to show signs of foot pain, but the use of ancillary technologies (eg, ultrasonography, radiography) to assist with diagnosing lameness and other orthopedic conditions may prove useful.[2] Physiologic parameters should be taken into consideration and the differences between species. For example, the heart rate of the donkey is generally higher than that of a horse, and the mule's heart rate has been reported to be in the mid-40s.[11]

STEREOTYPIES

It seems that mules are more likely to display stereotypic behavior than donkeys. Mules may frantically paw, and walk back and forth in a stall especially when a buddy, mate, or companion has been taken away, bray excessively, and/or weave (see Video 6). There are no reports on mules or donkeys cribbing. One of the authors (AKM) encountered one donkey cribbing before it was given a cookie by the owner each time it displayed the behavior. So, the cribbing behavior was being reinforced

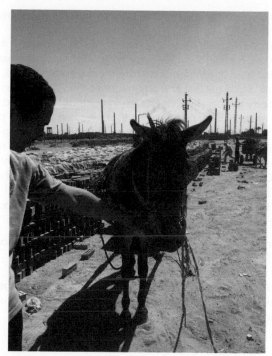

Fig. 6. Consider approaching mules at the face, touch the forehead, chin and then work your way to the neck.

by the food reward. Mules that weave or stall walk tend to express the behavior when they are alone, tied, or in a trailer, but generally this behavior will cease once another equid is brought nearby.

BEHAVIOR ASSOCIATED WITH PAIN

Pain is an unpleasant sensory and emotional experience. Stress is associated with a response to discomfort, such as pain. Identifying behavior associated with pain that is linked with various diseases is key to moving forward with diagnostic and prognostic assessments. When diagnosing pain in mules and donkeys, one will have to look for subtle signs, such as a slight twitch of the tail, the body leaning in one direction or the other, or slight changes in facial expression. The face of a mule will tell the story by focusing on several key areas known as facial action units: ear position, orbital tightening, tension and expression above the eyes, prominent strained chewing muscles, mouth strained, pronounced chin, strained nostrils, and flattening of the lips (see Video 8; Videos 9 and 10).

Attempts to define facial assessments in donkeys with acute pain are being developed, but most often advanced conditions are first noted in donkeys, such as chronic laminitis.[12] No attempts for pain scales or ethograms have been developed for mules yet, but the parameters created for other domestic animals, such as horse can be considered as a possible reference. Other behaviors to evaluate regarding pain include the overall body posture, sweating (which is more challenging to detect in donkeys), movement or lack of locomotion, appetite, response to an auditory stimulus, along with physiologic parameters, such as heart rate, respiratory rate, gut sounds, and body temperature. Video 9 shows a donkey in dystocia showing moderate to severe pain (see Video 9).

Stressful conditions (eg, disease processes) are systemically manifested by increases in heart rate, respiratory rate, body temperature, and behavioral changes,[13] which if severe also alter tissue perfusion (dry mucous membranes, prolonged capillary refill time, weak digital pulses) and organ function[14,15] (see Video 10 colic case). In healthy animals, body temperature, heart rate, respiratory rates, and behavior are also influenced by the environment, circadian rhythm, age, gender, and physiologic status (eg, pregnancy).[16–18] Young donkeys (<4 years old) have an average rectal temperature of 37.4°C (99.32°F), heart rate of 42.6 beats per minute, and respiratory rate of 21.8 breaths per minute, and older donkeys (≥10 year old) have an average body temperature of 37.4°C (99.3°F), heart rate of 43.2 beats per minute, and respiratory rate of 20.5 breaths per minute.[17]

When trying to identify the source of pain, the entire scenario should be considered and the following questions could be asked:

a. Is this a working mule or donkey, or animal used in production or for competition/ recreation?
b. How long has the animal been worked?
c. How often and how long is the animal ridden in preparation for the trail or showing?
d. Are other donkeys and mules in the same area displaying signs of illness by not eating or standing alone?

Key Concepts

- Look for focal points on the face of a donkey and mule for pain, such as ear position, blinking, and nostril flares.
- Consider the posture and presentation of the animal's body in relationship to pain or source of pain.
- Watch for tail swishing and movement in donkeys or mules in pain.
- When conducting a complete physical examination, move slowly and confidently and get to know your long-eared patient before beginning the examination; gaining trust from the mule or hinny will be key in proceeding.
- During clinical examinations that require lifting a limb, it is not uncommon for mules and donkeys to push back or apply weight toward you.
- When trying to identify the source of pain, consider the entire scenario (use of the animal, hours worked, conditions it is working or riding in, equipment and tack being used).

DIGESTIVE BEHAVIOR

Donkeys are well-adapted to consume poor quality forages and maintain good body condition scores even in water-deprived conditions. They are regarded as browsers (ie, ingestion of leaves and bushes) and grazers (ie, ingestion of vegetation at or near the ground level). The narrow muzzle and prehensile-type lips of donkeys and mules is believed to make them able to be more selective when grazing.[18] Donkeys can take larger bites and drink water for a longer period compared with horses. They will often consume plants that are high in tannins, which produce a bitter taste and most livestock avoid.[18] When consuming forage, the donkey will chew food approximately 10 times before swallowing.[18] They do not chew faster than horses, but can consume fiber at a faster rate than most ruminants of similar size because of a more efficient dental and jaw apparatus that permits the ingestion of larger feed particles.[18] Even though donkeys can swallow large feed particles, esophageal obstruction is rarely seen in these animals.[2,18] However, proper dental care for mules and donkeys should not be neglected, as is often the case (see Video 8).

On water restriction, donkeys will fully rehydrate at the rate of 17% to 20% of their body weight when offered water.[19] In general, donkeys are thought to have a lower water requirement when compared with other mammals, except the camel.[19] Water consumption in donkeys is dependent on the type of forage fed.[20]

The donkey's ability to thermoregulate and still provide enough saliva for mastication is essential for its ability to consume food after being dehydrated.[21] Often donkeys will consume hay before drinking water, even when dehydrated, to maintain feed and energy intake.[21] Donkeys can adapt to desert conditions and tolerate 20% of dehydration and continue to work.[21] Due to its ability to rehydrate quickly, regulate plasma volume despite reduced water intake, and rapid energy turnover rate, the donkey has been compared with other desert animals like the camel.[21,22] One study found that donkeys will drink enough water in 5 to 10 minutes to restore 95% to 98% of the water lost.[21] The same study found that donkeys that defecated immediately after drinking had feces containing 66% of water content, which was only 5% less than when the donkeys were hydrated (71%).[21] These traits make it possible for donkeys to live and survive in places such as Death Valley in the United States or the sub-Saharan regions of Africa.[21–24] The donkey's behavior also may play an important role in their efficiency.[21]

Most equid owners judge the health of their animals based on appetite; however, considering that donkeys have a strong appetite even at times of dehydration and disease, this behavior is not a reliable parameter to assess their health status.

Rarely, donkeys, mules, and hinnies overeat to the point to have an overloaded gut, but as previously discussed, they can develop metabolic conditions, laminitis, and gastrointestinal disorders.[1] Laminitis often occurs in all 4 feet and sometimes only in the rear.[4] Because of their ability to mask pain, signs of colic may not be evident, which could reduce survival.[4,13] Donkeys going off feed for days may have abdominal discomfort, resulting in stress and subsequent lipid mobilization and hyperlipemia.[2]

Feeding behavior of mules and hinnies is mostly based on observations and anecdotal experiences. It has been suggested that these donkey-horse hybrids can survive on less forage and nutrients than horses of comparable size. Laymen in Baja California claim that hinnies, like donkeys, can survive for a longer period without water. More information is still needed on feeding and water behavior of mules, hinnies, and donkeys.

Key Concepts

- Donkeys are considered to be both browsers and grazers; they will seek out plants with higher nutrient qualities.
- Donkeys take larger bite sizes and will rehydrate in a shorter amount of time with longer drinking sessions.
- Donkeys continue to eat despite dehydration.
- Information on feeding behavior of mules and hinnies is limited.
- It appears that donkeys more commonly develop laminitis in all 4 feet, less commonly in the hind feet.

TRAINING, MODIFYING, AND RESTRAINING BEHAVIOR

Worldwide, it is a common belief among mule and hinny owners and handlers that these animals should be handled from an early age to facilitate their training. Similar to horses, mule and hinny newborn foals seem to benefit from the imprinting techniques (ie, scratching, petting, working with the legs while picking up the hooves, and rubbing from ears to tail) (see **Figs. 1** and **2**, Video 3). Mules and hinnies attending mobile veterinary clinics with early foal training tended to allow unfamiliar people to more easily approach them and provide treatment.[7,25]

When first approaching a mule, it is recommended to approach their face versus their neck, where they will often flee.[25] Mules tend to be at more ease with verbally provided commands compared with no sound.[25] Consider a plan of action for maintaining mules in the area of treatment, which may include snubbing to a post, keeping a companion animal close by, or the use of chutes or stocks. Mules and hinnies often respond well to treats, petting and scratching the neck and inside of ears, and verbal. If a routine health check or procedure cannot be safely performed, nose twitches can be used for restraining, especially a twitch with a long handle to hold or a string twitch.

Blindfolds to cover the eyes is effective to calm mules and hinnies during varied interventions from vaccinations and deworming to farrier work. Lifting an opposite leg and tying the leg up with a safety knot to a loop made around the neck of the mule that does not slip is another form of restraint may work but must be done by trained personnel.[1,4] When applying a restraint, especially to a mule, it must be applied slowly and correctly. Otherwise, this will incentivize the mule's fearful behavior.[2] Sedation with α2-adrenoreceptor agonists (eg, xylazine, detomidine) alone or in combination with opioids (eg, butorphanol) can be used as ancillary chemical restraint methods. Protocols for the use these drugs in donkeys and mules are outside the scope of this review and are discussed in the article by Nora Matthews and Johannes P.A.M. Van Loon's article, "Anesthesia, Sedation and Pain Management of Donkeys and Mules," elsewhere in this issue.

Key Concepts

- Mules and hinnies are creatures of habit, and changes in routines will make them wary of the situation and become harder to handle at times.
- Restraints may actually decrease the stress placed on the mule/hinny or donkey when they are resisting strongly.
- Nose twitches, not ear twitches, are effective on mules and hinnies for administering injections and are somewhat effective on donkeys.
- For mules or donkeys resisting treatment, consider blindfolds, tying up a front limb or hind limb, or the use of hobbles.
- Remain calm and use your voice, scratching, or positive tactile contact when working with mules and hinnies.
- Mules and hinnies are not for everyone; it takes a very patient person to work with them.

REPRODUCTION BEHAVIOR

Under natural conditions, jacks are territorial breeders, they remain in a self-designated territory and will leave this territory only in case of lack of food and water.[26,27] However, as jennies are migratory animals, they are attracted to the jack's territory typically rich in water and food supply and shade in warm climates. In addition, contrary to stallions, jacks do not form harems and display no herding behavior.[28,29] Jennies, like jacks, defend their territory ferociously against intruders, particularly against other jacks; thus, this may explain the intermale aggression under domesticated situations.[30] On rare occasions, a jack may allow a subordinate jack to live in its territory; however, this is not common.[31] The subordinate donkey may help with the defense of the territory.[27]

Jennies congregate into a sexually active group like cows and mount one another while in estrus, and this is thought to play a role stimulating the jack.[28,32] It is interesting that mouth clapping is the most typical estrus sign in jennies, whereas the clitoral eversion and frequent micturition and expansion of the hindlimbs are less frequent and more discreet than in mares.[29,31,33]

The precopulatory interactions between donkeys and jennies are intense and of short duration. Vocalization, olfaction, naso-nasal, and body parts, particularly the perineal area, and strong bits in the neck, hindlegs, flank, and vulva, is followed by a Flehmen response and a mount without an erection of 10 to 30 seconds[31] (Video 11). Another frequent observation is the rapid and slow withdraw, where the jack remains distant from the female, grazing and gazing around, and appears not interested in the female and then suddenly the penis is exposed, the jack starts masturbating and then approaches the female to copulate.[27,31,33] Other key behavioral signs that the jack is ready to expose the penis include clear liquid dropping from the nasal cavity, lowering his head and neck, a slight jerk upward, and oftentimes a kick with one hind limb straight back. The knowledge of this copulatory behavior can be explored in the controlled breeding situation, as the donkey can be brought near a teaser or female being mated (mare or jenny), then pulled away and kept distant until the penis is exposed and ready to be washed, and then the jack can be conducted to mount the female or dummy.[27–30,32,34]

Naturally, donkeys are more attracted to jennies than mares, partially because estrus mares are less receptive to jacks and the estrus signs are different.[30,32,34] A jack was able to identify estrus in all mares under pasture situation; however, only 31% to 41% of mares displayed estrus to the jack.[34] Mare receptivity to jacks while in estrus can be improved with time and constant exposure to jacks; however, some mares may violently refuse the jack's approach and may require sedation and physical restraining (ie, hock hobbles or twitch) if they are used as mounting females or natural cover.[33] When breeding jacks to mares or jennies, a quiet environment with familiar people and objects is generally best. Some jacks can be very shy and an unfamiliar person or place may increase the time it takes for the jack to show any interest in the mare or jenny or display signs of erection.

Female mules can display signs of estrus that are similar to mares and to a certain extent to jennies. One survey carried out with 100 mule owners in the United States showed that most owners did not have any concerns about their mules displaying estrus behavior, but some may elect to ovariectomize their mare mules to eliminate estrus behavior, especially those being used for competitions or shows.[35] Male mules and hinnies are commonly castrated to presumable suppress aggressive behavior.

Key Concepts

- Jennies will mount one another when in estrus, display mouth clamping, and exhibit behavioral signs of estrus all year.
- Seasonality tends to have less of an effect on donkey reproduction behavior compared with horses.[36]
- Teasing behavior of jacks usually includes vocalization and mounting without an erection.
- Jacks that have been trained to breed only mares may not breed jennies vice versa.

- Behavior before a jack begins to extend his penis includes clear liquid from the nasal passage, lowering of the head and neck, a slight jerk upward, and often a kick with a single hind limb, this natural behavior should not be discouraged.
- Jacks take a longer time to reach an erection and ejaculate compared with horses.[36]
- Breeding area should be quiet and only familiar people should handle the jack, as strangers, noise, or excitement may discourage some jacks from breeding.
- Jacks can be trained to be collected off a phantom.[37]
- Female mules and hinnies will exhibit signs of estrus similar to a mare.
- Male mules can show signs of aggression and play fight with other males, and castration may decrease these behaviors.

SUPPLEMENTARY DATA

Supplementary data related to this article can be found online at https://doi.org/10.1016/j.cveq.2019.08.010.

REFERENCES

1. McLean A, Badr A, Heleski C. Mule behavior a mirror image of human behavior and handling techniques. Animals for Asia Conference - Facilitating human change to improve animal welfare. Kathmandu, Nepal. December, 2017. Available at: http://afakathmandu.com/. Accessed March 20, 2018.

2. Taylor TS, Matthews NS. Donkey and mule scenarios: when to stop, think, read or call. Proc Am Assoc Equine Pract 2002;115–6.

3. Burnham SL. Anatomical differences of the donkey and mule. Proc Am Assoc Equine Pract 2002;48:102–9.

4. Mclean A, Heleski CR, Ali AB, et al. A husbandry guide for mules and hinnies: a method to improve understanding through participatory approaches. Working Animal Conference. Marrakech, Morocco: SPANA; 2017. Available at: https://spana.org/. Accessed March 10, 2018.

5. Miller R. Understanding the differences. Western Mule Magazine 2007; 12(11):28–9.

6. Proops L, Burden F, Osthaus B. Social relations in a mixed group of mules, ponies and donkeys reflect differences in equid type. Behav Processes 2012;90(3): 337–42.

7. Bott R, McLean A, Heleski C. Community-based participatory research interfaced with equine welfare assessment to learn about working equids and their owners in Vera Cruz, Mexico. 7th International Colloquium on Working Equid 2014; Royal Holloway, University of London, London, United Kingdom. p. 28. Available at: http://www.worldhorsewelfare.org/Files/9bd99215-338d-4b29-acb9-a3c4010f75bd/7th-colloquium-on-working-equids-proceedings.pdf. Accessed March 14, 2018.

8. Ali AB, El Sayed MA, McLean AK, et al. Aggression in working mules and subsequent aggressive treatment by their handlers in Egyptian brick kilns-cause or effect? J Vet Behav 2018. https://doi.org/10.1016/j.jveb.2018.05.008.

9. Svendson E. The professional handbook of the donkey. 3rd edition. Suffolk (United Kingdom): Whittet Books Limited; 1997. p. 400.

10. McGreevy P. Chapter 5 - Social behavior. In: Equine behavior. Oxford (United Kingdom): W.B. Saunders; 2004. p. 119–50.

11. McLean AK, Wang W, Navas-Gonzalez FJ, et al. Reference intervals for hematological and blood biochemistry reference values in healthy mules and hinnies. Comp Clin Path 2016;25(4):871–8.

12. Escudero A, González JR, Benedito JL, et al. Electrocardiographic parameters in the clinically healthy Zamorano-leones donkey. Res Vet Sci 2009;87(3):458–61.

13. Matthews NS, Taylor TS. Veterinary care of donkeys: IVIS international veterinary information service. 2004. Ithaca (NY). Available at: https://www.ivis.org. Accessed March 2018.

14. Mueller P, Hintz H, Pearson R, et al. Voluntary intake of roughage diets by donkeys, vol. 13. Rabat (Morocco): Actes Editions; 1994. p. 137–48.

15. Ayo JO, Dzenda T, Zakari FO. Individual and diurnal variations in rectal temperature, respiration, and heart rate of pack donkeys during the early rainy season. J Equine Vet Sci 2008;28(5):281–8.

16. Minka NS, Ayo JO. Effects of shade provision on some physiological parameters, behavior and performance of pack donkeys (*Equus asinus*) during the hot-dry season. J Equine Sci 2007;18(2):39–46.

17. Lemma A, Moges M. Clinical, haematological and serum biochemical reference values of working donkeys (Equus asinus) owned by transport operators in Addis Ababa, Ethiopia. Livest Res Rural Dev 2009;21. Available at: http://lrrd.org/lrrd21/8/lemma21127.htm. Accessed March 20, 2018.

18. Mueller P, Protos P, Houpt K, et al. Chewing behaviour in the domestic donkey (*Equus asinus*) fed fibrous forage. Appl Anim Behav Sci 1998;60(2–3):241–51.

19. Aganga A, Tsopito C. A note on the feeding behaviour of domestic donkeys: a Botswana case study. Appl Anim Behav Sci 1998;60(2–3):235–9.

20. Mueller P, Houpt K. A comparison of the responses of donkeys (Equus asinus) and ponies (Equus caballus) to 36 hours of water deprivation. In: Donkeys, mules & horses in tropical agricultural development. Edinburgh (United Kingdom): D. Fielding; R.A. Pearson; 1991. p. 7.

21. Yousef M, Dill D, Mayes M. Shifts in body fluids during dehydration in the burro, *Equus asinus*. J Appl Physiol 1970;29(3):345–9.

22. Schmidt-Nielsen K. Desert animals: physiological problems of heat and water. 1st edition. Oxford (United Kingdom): Oxford Press; 1964. p. 277.

23. Dill D, Yousef M, Cox CR, et al. Hunger vs thirst in the burro (*Equus asinus*). Physiol Behav 1980;24(5):975–8.

24. Nengomasha E, Pearson RA, Wold AG. Empowering people through donkey power into the next millennium. Proceedings of the workshop of the Animal Traction Network for Eastern and Southern Africa (ATNESA). 2000. Mpumalanga, South Africa, September 20–24, 1999. p. 23–31.

25. McGreevy P. Equine behavior: a guide for veterinarians and equine scientists. 2nd edition. Exeter (United Kingdom): Saunders Ltd.; 2012. p. 378.

26. Havard M, Njoya A, Roland P, et al. Empowering farmers with animal traction. Proceedings of the workshop of the Animal Traction Network for Eastern and Southern Africa (ATNESA). 2000. Mpumalanga, South Africa, September 20–24, 1999. p. 18–21.

27. McDonnell SM. Reproductive behavior of donkeys (*Equus asinus*). Appl Anim Behav Sci 1998;60(2–3):277–82.

28. Canisso I, Morel MD, McDonnell S. Strategies for the management of donkey jacks in intensive breeding systems. Equine Vet Educ 2009;21(12):652–9.

29. Canisso IF, Coutinho da Silva M, Davies-Morel M, et al. How to manage jacks to breed mares. Proc Am Assoc Equine Pract 2009;55:5–9.

30. Canisso I, Carvalho G, Morel MD, et al. Sexual behavior and ejaculate characteristics in Pêga donkeys *(Equus asinus)* mounting estrous horse mares *(Equus caballus)*. Theriogenology 2010;73(1):56–63.

31. Henry M, McDonnell S, Lodi L, et al. Pasture mating behaviour of donkeys *(Equus asinus)* at natural and induced oestrus. J Reprod Fertil 1991;44:77–86.

32. Canisso I, McDonnell S. Donkey breeding behavior with an emphasis on the Pêga breed. Veterinary Care of Donkeys: IVIS International Veterinary Information Service. 2010 Ithaca. 2010. Available at: https://www.ivis.org. Accessed March 10, 2018.

33. Henry M, Figueiredo A, Palhares M, et al. Clinical and endocrine aspects of the oestrous cycle in donkeys *(Equus asinus)*. J Reprod Fertil Suppl 1987;35:297–303.

34. Lodi L, Henry M, Paranhos da Costa M. Behavior of donkey jacks *(Equus asinus)* breeding horse mares *(Equus caballus)* at pasture. Biol Reprod Mono 1995;52:591–8.

35. Heaton K, Ragle C, Godderidge MT, et al. Estrous behavior in mules—an owner's perspective. J Equine Vet Sci 2018;60:109–12. e102.

36. Gastal M, Henry M, Beker A, et al. Sexual behavior of donkey jacks: influence of ejaculatory frequency and season. Theriogenology 1996;46(4):593–603.

37. Pugh D. Donkey reproduction. 48th Annual Convention of the American Association of Equine Practitioners. Proc Am Assoc Equine Pract 2002;48:113–4.

Clinical Pharmacology in Donkeys and Mules

Francisco J. Mendoza, DVM, PhD, MSc[a],*, Alejandro Perez-Ecija, DVM, PhD, MSc[a],
Ramiro E. Toribio, DVM, MS, PhD[b]

KEYWORDS

- Anesthesia • Analgesia • Antibiotics • Anthelmintics • Equus asinus
- Non-steroidal anti-inflammatory drugs • Sedatives

KEY POINTS

- Donkeys and mules have faster metabolic rates and higher cellular water content than horses.
- For most drugs, donkeys and mules need higher doses and/or shorter dosing intervals compared with horses.
- Extrapolating doses and dosing intervals from horses to donkeys or their hybrids could be ineffective (subdosing) or result in side effects (overdosing).
- When doses or pharmacologic information are unavailable for donkeys or mules, and equine dosing is used, close monitoring is indicated.
- Pharmacokinetic and pharmacodynamic studies are lacking for most drugs prescribed for donkeys and mules.

INTRODUCTION

Compared with horses, donkeys and mules have a higher metabolic rate and cellular water content, which could impact the pharmacokinetic and pharmacodynamic properties of drugs used in horses. Clinicians should be aware that for a number of drugs there are pharmacologic differences between donkeys and horses that may influence dose, dosing intervals, or efficacy, but could also lead to side effects.[1]

A concept rarely considered when choosing or extrapolating drug doses in veterinary medicine is allometric scaling. In simple terms, it means that basal metabolic rate is negative to body mass (mass to a power of 0.75), which together with total body water content could influence drug distribution, metabolism, and excretion. This calculation is clearly relevant to donkeys, in particular when most dosing protocols are from horses.

Disclosure Statement: The authors have nothing to disclose.
[a] Department of Animal Medicine and Surgery, University of Cordoba, Campus Rabanales, Road Madrid-Cadiz km 396, Cordoba 14014, Spain; [b] Department of Veterinary Clinical Sciences, The Ohio State University, 601 Vernon Tharp Street, Columbus, OH 43210, USA
* Corresponding author.
E-mail address: fjmendoza@uco.es

In addition to the therapeutic implications of understanding the pharmacology of drugs used in donkeys and mules, there are also economic, cultural, religious, and geographic factors to consider regarding drug fate. For example, donkey byproducts (meat, milk) are consumed in developing countries, but information on drug distribution, excretion, and accumulation is lacking and could be detrimental to human health.

Nonsteroidal Anti-inflammatory Drugs

A number of nonsteroidal anti-inflammatory drugs (NSAIDs) used in horses are metabolized faster in donkeys, mainly owing to higher clearances and shorter half-lives.[1] This indicates that to reach therapeutic levels, for many of these drugs, dosing will have to be increased or dosing intervals reduced. This finding should not be generalized to all NSAIDs.

Phenylbutazone mean residence time (MRT) is shorter and clearance is faster in donkeys compared with horses.[2] Breed differences have been reported, with miniature donkeys clearing phenylbutazone faster than average size donkeys, which in part has been attributed to a faster hepatic oxidative metabolism.[3] Based on this information, miniature donkeys need shorter dosing intervals, because higher doses could theoretically lead to renal and gastrointestinal injury, such as observed in a previous study in miniature donkeys.[4] No phenylbutazone toxicity studies have been performed in mules.

Flunixin meglumine area under the curve (AUC) and MRT were lower, but clearance was higher in donkeys compared with horses.[5] Using a subcutaneous tissue cage model, one study found the opposite results.[6] Flunixin meglumine showed faster tissue penetration in donkeys compared with horses.[6,7] No information on the oral pharmacokinetics of flunixin meglumine is available for donkeys or mules. Flunixin meglumine seems to have fewer side effects compared with phenylbutazone in long-term administration.[4]

Meloxicam, cimicoxib, and firocoxib are selective cyclo-oxygenase-2 inhibitors that have been evaluated in donkeys,[8–10] although they are not marketed for this species. Meloxicam oral suspension is used off-label in donkeys,[11] powder formulations have not been investigated, and pharmacokinetic properties could be different, specifically for the oral presentation because intestinal absorption is different between species. Pharmacokinetic parameters are different between donkeys and horses, with AUC, MRT, clearance, and half-life lower in donkeys.[8] Firocoxib has excellent oral bioavailability but a much shorter half-life in donkeys compared with horses,[10] suggesting that frequent dosing intervals are necessary in donkeys to achieve adequate analgesia. Similar to meloxicam, cimicoxib also has lower pharmacokinetic parameters in donkeys compared with horses, including a smaller AUC.[9]

Within NSAID classes, there are pharmacokinetic differences. For example, intravenous carprofen has a slower clearance and larger AUC in donkeys,[12] whereas intravenous ketoprofen, another propionic acid derivative NSAID, has faster clearance in donkeys than in horses.[13,14]

Except for flunixin meglumine,[5] no NSAID pharmacokinetic study has been carried out in mules. The pharmacokinetic properties of NSAIDs investigated in donkeys and mules are listed in **Table 1**.

Sedation, Analgesia, and Anesthesia

Donkeys and mules are considered stoic and hard-to-read animals. Their response to pain may go unnoticed, which could have serious consequences (eg, hyperlipidemia, laminitis) owing to activation of the hypothalamic–pituitary–adrenal axis as well as somatic and autonomic neural networks that alter metabolic, endocrine, and immune

Table 1
Dose and pharmacokinetic properties of NSAIDs in donkeys, mules and horses

Drug	Animal	N	Dose (mg/kg)	AUC (μg/mL h)	Clearance (mL/kg/h)	MRT (h)	$t_{1/2}$ (h)	V_d (mL/kg)	Reference
Carprofen	D	5	0.7, IV	148.7 ± 30.8	4.9 ± 0.9	—	—	214.1 ± 18.9	Mealey et al,[12] 2004[a]
	H	3		22.5 ± 10.5	36.6 ± 18.4	—	—	517 ± 208.9	
Cimicoxib	D	3	2, PO	0.13 ± 0.1	13861 ± 7147	3.1 ± 0.8	2.7 ± 1.4	46639 ± 8379	Kim et al,[9] 2014[a]
	D	6	5, PO	0.14 ± 0.1	32402 ± 22358	3.9 ± 0.9	5.3 ± 3.5	175005 ± 18814	
Firocoxib	D	3	0.1, PO	0.35	—	—	1.5	—	Matthews et al,[10] 2009
			0.1, IV	0.49	—	—	0.85	604	
	H	12	0.1, PO	1.8 ± 0.74	—	—	29.6 ± 7.5	—	Kvaternick et al,[71] 2007[a]
		11	0.1, IV	2.3 ± 0.81	36.7 ± 13.3	—	33.8 ± 11.2	1695 ± 531	
Flunixin meglumine	D	3	1.1, IV	23.6 ± 5.0	50.3 ± 9.4	3.4 ± 0.5	4.5 ± 0.1	171.1 ± 12.6	Cheng et al,[6] 1996[b]
	D	5	1.1, IV	33.8 ± 8.9	108 ± 30	0.9 ± 0.1	0.75	85 ± 27	Coakley et al,[5] 1999[a]
	M	5		51.6 = 20.6	84 ± 30	1.5 ± 0.5		127 ± 79	
	H	3		58.6 ± 10.1	66 ± 12	1.8 ± 0.4	—	117 ± 16.4	
Ketoprofen	D	8	3, IV	17.1 ± 7.4	200 ± 70	2.4 ± 0.5	2.2 ± 0.5	610 ± 160	Anwer et al,[72] 2012[b]
	D	4	2.2, IV	—	414.1 ± 98.7	0.7 ± 0.2	1.3 ± 0.7	263.1 ± 55.4	Oukessou et al,[14] 1996[a]
	H	8	3, IV	9.6 ± 2.7	300 ± 95	2.7 ± 1.1	2.7 ± 1.1	1250 ± 825	Rehman et al,[73] 2012[a]
Meloxicam	D	8	0.6, IV	6.01 ± 0.1	90 ± 0.01	1.4 ± 0.05	1.0 ± 0.0	130 ± 0.01	Mahmood & Ashraf,[8] 2011[b]
	D	5	0.6, IV	4.5 ± 2.5	187.9 ± 147.3	0.6 ± 0.3	—	93.2 ± 33.7	Sinclair et al,[74] 2006[a]
	H	5		18.8 ± 7.3	34.7 ± 9.2	9.6 ± 9.2	—	270 ± 160	
Phenylbutazone	D	3	4.4, IV	19.2 ± 2.1	214.2 ± 18.1	0.7 ± 0.1	0.6 ± 0.1	146.7 ± 17.6	Cheng et al,[75] 1996[b]
	D	6	4.4, IV	12.6 ± 2.6	360 ± 66	1.4 ± 0.9	—	545 ± 358	Matthews et al,[2] 2001[a]
	D	4	4.4, IV	28.3 ± 9.5	170.3 ± 54.4	1.7 ± 0.7	—	242 ± 97.6	Mealey et al,[3] 1997[a]
	H	6		118.32 ± 12.4	29 ± 4.6	3.6 ± 0.2	—	174 ± 12.4	

Abbreviations: D, donkey; H, horse; IV, intravenously; M, mule; N, number of animals sampled; PO, orally; V_d, volume of distribution;
[a] Data expressed as mean ± standard deviation.
[b] Data expressed as mean ± standard error.
Data from Refs.[2,3,5,6,8–10,12,14,71–75]

function. For this reason, as in other species, analgesia is very important to ameliorate the pain–stress cycle. Drug doses are summarized in **Table 2**.

Sedatives and tranquilizers used in horses are routinely administered to donkeys and mules; however, assuming that donkeys will respond to these drugs in similar ways as horses can lead to problems. The dose of α2-adrenoreceptor agonists (eg, xylazine) often needs to be increased by 50% above the equine dose in mules, miniature donkeys, and feral or excited animals. The pharmacokinetics of xylazine have been studied in mules,[15] but not in donkeys. One study evaluating the hypoalgesic effect of 4 xylazine doses found no difference between donkeys and horses. It was suggested that xylazine doses required to achieve analgesia in donkeys and horses are similar.[16] Owing to its prolonged action and antinociceptive effects, detomidine and romifidine have been proposed as the α2-adrenoreceptor agonists of choice for pain management in donkeys.[17] Hypoalgesia induced by xylazine and dexmedetomidine in donkeys is less intense and of shorter duration than for detomidine and romifidine.[17] Sublingual administration of detomidine gel (40 μg/kg) provides effective sedation in donkeys.[18] Acepromazine at standard doses (0.04–0.05 mg/kg, IV) induces satisfactory tranquilization in donkeys. However, to achieve optimal effect, donkeys may require twice the acepromazine dose used in horses. The pharmacokinetic properties of acepromazine differ between donkeys and horses.[19]

Butorphanol enhances the sedative and hypoalgesic effects of α2-adrenoreceptor agonists in donkeys.[20] Tramadol and flupirtine are also effective analgesics in donkeys.[21,22] Despite donkeys having thicker skin than horses, transdermal fentanyl patches seem to provide good pain relieve.[23]

Metamizole (dipyrone) is an analgesic, antipyretic, and spasmolytic drug with minimal anti-inflammatory properties. The pharmacokinetics of metamizole and its metabolites has been investigated in donkeys, showing shorter half-lives than horses.[24]

Ketamine in donkeys has a shorter half-life and faster clearance than mules and horses, but these variables are similar between mules and horses.[25] This effect could translate into shorter anesthesia duration with ketamine. Guaifenesin (glyceryl guaiacolate) has a longer half-life in donkeys compared with horses, and recovery time could be prolonged in some donkeys.[26] Owing to its suppressive effects on the respiratory system, guaifenesin requires close supervision in donkeys.[27] In miniature donkeys, intravenous propofol is a safe and economical option for anesthesia induction and maintenance. In large donkeys, a combination of propofol and ketamine permits lower dosing, which is also cheaper and safer.[28] Thiopental is a good induction agent in donkeys and mules,[29] although rarely used these days. In 1 study, alfaxalone in combination with midazolam had a shorter time to lateral recumbency compared with ketamine and midazolam; however, time to sternal position was longer for alfaxalone.[30] In mules, the xylazine, diazepam, and ketamine combination is effective and safe for short-term field anesthesia.[31,32] Anesthetic combinations such as tiletamine and zolazepam have been replaced with newer drugs, although they may be used in feral donkeys.

Inhaled anesthetics such as halothane, isoflurane or sevoflurane have similar minimal alveolar concentrations in donkeys and horses.[26,33–37] However, no minimal alveolar concentration data for these anesthetic are available for mules. Additional details on donkey and mule analgesia and anesthesia can be found in Nora Matthews and Johannes P.A.M. van loon's article, "Anesthesia, Sedation and Pain Management of Donkeys and Mules," elsewhere in this issue.

Epidural administration of lidocaine to donkeys provides good regional analgesia, but morphine and fentanyl do not.[38,39] Local anesthetic drugs are used in similar

Table 2
Doses of sedatives, analgesic, tranquilizers and anesthetic drugs used in donkeys and mules

| | Preanesthetics | | | Anesthetics | | | |
	Sedatives (mg/kg)	Analgesic (mg/kg)	Tranquilizer (mg/kg)	Induction (mg/kg)	Maintenance	Observations	Reference
Donkeys							
Acepromazine	—	—	0.03–0.10	—	—		Lizarraga et al,[19] 2017; Grint et al,[35] 2014; Suriano et al,[37] 2014
Alfaxalone	—	—	—	1	—		Maney et al,[30] 2018
Butorphanol	—	0.02–0.04 0.05 IM	—	—	—		Matthews & van Loon,[36] 2013; Evangelista et al,[76] 2018
Detomidine	0.005–0.020 0.06 IM	0.02–0.04	—	—	—		Lizarraga & Janovyak,[17] 2013; Evangelista et al,[76] 2018; Mostafa et al,[77] 1995
Dexmedetomidine	0.003–0.005		—	—	—		Lizarraga & Janovyak,[17] 2013; Lizarraga et al,[19] 2017
Diazepam	—	—	0.02–0.03	—	—		Kalchofner et al,[34] 2006; Suriano et al,[37] 2014
Flupirtine	—	1 (IV) 5 (PO)	—	—	—		Giorgi et al,[22] 2015
Guaifenesin	—	—	—	20–30	1 L 5% GGE + 500 mg xylazine + 2 g ketamine at 1–2 mL/kg/h		Matthews et al,[27] 1997

(continued on next page)

Table 2
(continued)

| | Preanesthetics | | | Anesthetics | | | |
	Sedatives (mg/kg)	Analgesic (mg/kg)	Tranquilizer (mg/kg)	Induction (mg/kg)	Maintenance	Observations	Reference
Ketamine	—	—	—	2.2	—	IV bolus at 0.1 mg/kg can be used for depth anesthetic plane.	Matthews,[40] 2009
Medetomidine	0.007–0.009	—	—	—	—		Lizarraga & Janovyak,[17] 2013; Kalchofner et al,[34] 2006; Suriano et al,[37] 2014
Metamizole (Dipyrone)	—	25	—	—	—		Aupanun et al,[24] 2016
Midazolam	—	—	0.05–0.06	—	—		Maney et al,[30] 2018; Matthews,[40] 2009
Propofol	—	—	—	2	0.2 mg/kg/min	Propofol + ketamine: 0.5 + 1.5 mg/kg (induction)	Coelho et al,[28] 2014; Naddaf et al,[78] 2015
Romifidine	0.1	—	—	—	—		Lizarraga & Janovyak,[17]; Matthews,[40] 2009
Thiopental	—	—	—	5–10	—	Bolus at 1 mg/kg can be used for depth anesthetic plane	Matthews & van Loon,[36] 2013
Tiletamine-zolazepam	—	—	—	1.1	—		Matthews,[40] 2009
Tramadol	—	2.5	—	—	—		Giorgi et al,[21] 2009
Xylazine	0.5–1.1	—	—	—	—	Wild donkeys: 2–2.2 mL/kg/h Double dose if given IM	Lizarraga & Janovyak,[17]; Matthews & van Loon,[36] 2013

					Comments	References
Miniature donkey						
Butorphanol	0.044	—	—	—	—	Matthews et al,[79] 2002
Ketamine	—	—	2.2	—	—	Matthews et al,[79,80] 2002
Propofol	—	—	2–2.2	0.2–0.3 mg/kg/min	Risk of apnea: intubation and oxygen could be required	Matthews et al,[79,80] 2002
Tiletamine-zolazepam	—	—	1.1	—	—	Matthews et al,[79,80] 2002
Xylazine	0.8–1.1	—	—	—	—	Matthews et al,[79,80] 2002
Mule						
Acepromazine	0.03–0.1	—	—	—	—	Grint et al,[35] 2014
Azaperone	0.8	—	—	—	IM	Carmona et al,[81] 2007
Butorphanol	0.02–0.04	—	—	—	—	Matthews,[40] 2009
Detomidine	0.01–0.03	—	—	—	—	Matthews,[40] 2009
Diazepam	—	0.03	—	—	—	Dar & Gupta[32] 2016
Guaifenesin	—	—	20–50	1–2.2 mL/kg/h	—	Vullo et al,[29] 2017
Ketamine	—	—	2–2.2	—	Shorter dosing interval than horses	Dar & Gupta[32] 2016
Midazolam	—	0.06	—	—	—	Matthews,[40] 2009
Romifidine	0.15	—	—	—	—	Matthews,[40] 2009
Thiopental	—	—	5–10	—	—	Vullo et al,[29] 2017; Grint et al,[35] 2014
Tiletamine-zolazepam	—	—	0.5	—	—	Matthews et al,[82] 1992
Xylazine	1–1.6	—	—	—	—	Matthews,[40] 2009

Abbreviation: IM, intramuscularly.
Data from Refs. 17,19,21,22,24,27–30,32,34–37,40,76–82

manner in donkeys, mules, and,[37,40] although specific pharmacokinetic and pharmacodynamic studies are not available for donkeys and mules.

Other drugs used during anesthesia such as vasopressors and inotropes are administered using equine protocols.

Antimicrobials

Despite their relevance in animal health, few studies have been published on the pharmacology of antimicrobial drugs in donkeys and mules. Most studies have been focused on off-label drugs or on antimicrobial doses that are not used clinically. Similar to NSAIDs, compared with horses, donkeys and mules have a faster metabolism for a number of antimicrobial drugs, with higher clearances, lower MRTs, and shorter half-lives. For these antimicrobials, donkeys and mules would need higher doses or shorter dosing intervals. Aminoglycosides (amikacin and gentamicin) are the exception.[41] Information on antimicrobial side effects is scarce and caution should be taken with their use.

Table 3 shows antimicrobial doses and pharmacokinetic properties in donkeys and mules. Most studies used doses different from those recommended for horses. Updated information on antimicrobial dosing for donkeys and their hybrids is necessary for clinical success, but also to implement better antimicrobial stewardship practices.

As other equids, donkeys are susceptible to the toxic effects of ionophores.

Anthelmintic Drugs

Dosing and indications for most antiparasitic drugs are compiled in **Table 4**. As with other drugs, extrapolation from horses to donkeys and mules could lead to undesired effects. Prudent use of macrocyclic lactones (ivermectin, moxidectin, abamectin, eprinomectin) is advised because asinine animals are more likely to develop signs of neurotoxicity.

Piroplasmosis, caused by *Babesia caballi* and *Theileria equi*, is a major donkey and horse disease worldwide. Imidocarb dipropionate is the most effective treatment for this condition; however, donkeys and mules are overly sensitive to this drug and hepatic side effects can be observed similarly to horses.[42] For this reason, donkeys and mules should be treated with lower doses than horses. To avoid imidocarb dipropionate toxicity, which results from acetylcholinesterase inhibition, premedication with anticholinergic drugs such as glycopyrrolate (0.0025 mg/kg intravenously) or N-butylscopolammonium bromide (01–0.2 mg/kg intravenously) 5 to 10 minutes before imidocarb dipropionate administration is advised.[43,44] Buparvaquone, where available, is safer but less effective than imidocarb dipropionate. Oxytetracycline, although not as effective, can be administered at 5 to 7 mg/kg intravenously once or twice a day for 2 to 7 days, in particular against *T equi*.[42]

Deworming practices in recent years have led to the development of anthelmintic resistance,[45] prompting novel approaches to helminth control based on parasite biology combined with strategic deworming.[46] For example, prewinter treatment with moxidectin reduced fecal egg count by 100%, with egg reappearance periods of 42 to 55 days, and low fecal egg count lasting for up to 8 months.[47] Mebendazole resulted in a 95% reduction in fecal strongyle egg counts, with no residues found in the milk of treated jennies.[48] At equivalent doses (10 mg/kg, by mouth), oxfendazole reached higher plasma concentrations than fenbendazole and albendazole in donkeys.[49] Owing to less parasite resistance, available efficacy studies, and safety, fenbendazole is the most commonly used benzimidazole against strongyles in horses, donkeys, and mules. No benzimidazole has been specifically approved for parasite

Table 3
Dose and pharmacokinetic properties for antimicrobials in donkeys and mules compared with horses

Drug	Animal	N	Dose (mg/kg)	AUC (µg/mL/h)	Clearance (mL/kg/h)	MRT (h)	$t_{1/2}$ (h)	V_d (mL/kg)	Reference
Amikacin	D	3	6, IV	—	58	2.8	1.9	150.2	Horspool et al,[83] 1994
	H	3	6, IV	—	45.2	4	2.8	206.6	
Ampicillin	D	3	10, IV	24.5 ± 4	418.8 ± 69.1	0.7	0.71	422.5 ± 214.1	Horspool et al,[84] 1992[b]
	H	3	10, IV	42 ± 3.9	240.5 ± 21.8	0.7	0.75	210.8 ± 16	
Amoxicillin	D	4	10, IV	20.6 ± 12.6	288 ± 78	0.8 ± 0.1	0.79	113 ± 26	Lavy et al,[85] 1995[a]
	D	3	15, IV	—	333	—	—	—	Oukessou et al,[86] 1994
	H	5	—	63.7	239	—	—	—	
Danofloxacin	D	6	1.25, IV	1.3 ± 0.2	1000 ± 170	6 ± 0.3	7.2 ± 0.9	5950 ± 1000	Kum et al,[87] 2009[a]
	D	6	1.25, IM	1.3 ± 0.1	—	9.1 ± 1.3	6.4 ± 0.7	—	
Enrofloxacin	D	6	5, IV	22.7 ± 9.9	249.5 ± 90	7.5 ± 2.3	9.5 ± 0.9	1700 ± 200	Sekkin et al,[88] 2012[a]
	D	6	5, IM	16.5 ± 4.2	—	17.8 ± 2.5	12.1 ± 1.9	—	
	H	6	5, IV	13.2 ± 3.1	510 ± 110	5.1 ± 0.7	4.4 ± 0.6	2300 ± 500	Kaartinen et al,[89] 1997[b]
	H	6	5, IM	25.2 ± 2.5	—	15.0 ± 0.8	9.9 ± 0.5	—	
Gentamicin	D	3	2.2, IV	30.3 ± 4.2	73.2 ± 10.8	2.6 ± 0.2	2.03	127 ± 25.5	Miller et al,[90] 1994[a]
	D	4	2.2, IV	28.6 ± 1.43	77.4 ± 4.2	2.6 ± 0.1	0.84	88 ± 28.1	
	D	3	2.2, IV	22 ± 5.8	100.2 ± 28.8	2.1 ± 0.3	1.87	203 ± 58	Welfare et al,[91] 1996[a]
	D	3	2.2, IV	28.4 ± 1.8	76.2 ± 4.8	2.9 ± 0.3	0.78	220 ± 9.8	
	H	7	2.2, IV	30.8 ± 6.4	71.5 ± 16.8	3.2 ± 0.3	4.4	240 ± 50	Whittem et al,[92] 1996[a]
Marbofloxacin	D	6	2, IV	19.1 ± 3.4	100 ± 20	10.6 ± 2.5	8.9 ± 2.2	1150 ± 90	Gonzalez et al,[93] 2007[a]
	H	5	2, IV	11.3 ± 2.4	190 ± 40	6.3 ± 1.1	4.7 ± 0.8	1170 ± 180	Carretero et al,[94] 2002[a]

(continued on next page)

Table 3
(continued)

Drug	Animal	N	Dose (mg/kg)	AUC (µg/mL/h)	Clearance (mL/kg/h)	MRT (h)	t1/2 (h)	Vd (mL/kg)	Reference
Norfloxacin	D	5	10, IV	15.2 ± 1.5	65.5 ± 7.4	3.6 ± 0.75	3.5 ± 0.6	1934 ± 353	Lavy et al,[95] 1995[a]
	D	6	10, IM	1.5 ± 0.2	—	4.3 ± 0.2	3.31	—	
	D	6	10, PO	4.8 ± 0.33	—	4.5 ± 0.2	3.40	—	
	D	4	20, IM	5.7 ± 0.5	—	5.1 ± 0.8	3.48	—	
	D	4	20, PO	1.9 ± 0.3	—	4.5 ± 0.4	2.75	—	
	H	6	4, IV	35.6 ± 9.3	490 ± 60	4.3 ± 0.9	5.4 ± 1.4	2190 ± 530	Park & Yun,[96] 2003[a]
	H	6	4, IM	4.7 ± 1		29.5 ± 9.5	9.5 ± 2.2		
Penicillin	D	3	10, IV	21.9 ± 0.5	462.9 ± 40.04	0.4 ± 0.03	0.52	204.5 ± 3	Horspool & McKellar,[97] 1995[b]
	D	5	20,000 IU		393			84	Oukessou et al,[86] 1994
	H	3	10, IV	22.4 ± 5.3	514.5 ± 145.6	0.6 ± 0.08	0.65	362.3 ± 106.5	Horspool & McKellar,[97] 1995[b]
Oxytetracycline	D	3	10, IV	96.9	91.4	—	6.46	649.3	Lizarraga et al,[98] 2004
	H	3	10, IV		39.5	—	3.72	348.8	
Sulfadimidine	D	5	20, IV		67.8 ± 10.8	9.5 ± 1.15	8.3 ± 1.5	680 ± 80	Oukessou & Alsouss,[99] 1998[a]
Sulfadiazine	D	5	20, IV		102 ± 8.4	5.8 ± 1.05	7.9 ± 2.2	630 ± 70	
Sulfadimethoxine	D	5	20, IV		45 ± 2.4	9.9 ± 1.4	11.8 ± 1.5	460 ± 50	
Sulfamethoxypyridazine	D	5	20, IV		66 ± 5.4	6.7 ± 0.9	5.0 ± 0.7	470 ± 60	
Sulfamethoxazole	D	5	12.5, IV	96 ± 9	132 ± 12	2.7 ± 0.4	—	335 ± 46	Peck et al,[100] 2002[a]
	M	5	12.5, IV	216 ± 54	60 ± 18	5.9 ± 1.3	—	337 ± 94	
	H	3	12.5, IV	138 ± 6	90 ± 6	3.9 ± 0.1	—	301 ± 20	
Trimethoprim	D	5	2.5, IV	1.8 ± 0.6	1680 ± 540	1 ± 0.5	—	1426 ± 209	
	M	5	2.5, IV	2.4 ± 0.18	942 ± 66	1.4 ± 0.4	—	1351 ± 358	
	H	3	2.5, IV	2.4 ± 0.3	1224 ± 180	1.5 ± 0.1	—	1819 ± 189	
	D	5	2.5, IV		261.6 ± 36	0.5 ± 0.1	0.9 ± 0.4	2210 ± 860	Oukessou & Alsouss,[99] 1998[a]

Abbreviations: D, donkey; H, horse; IM, intramuscularly; IV, intravenously; M, mule; PO, orally; Vd, volume of distribution.
[a] Data expressed as mean ± standard deviation.
[b] Data expressed as mean ± standard error.
  Data from Refs.[83–100]

Table 4
Dose and indications of the antiparasitic drugs evaluated in donkeys

Drug	Indication	Investigated Dose	Reference
Albendazole	Roundworms D arnfieldi	10 mg/kg, PO	Gokbulut et al,[49] 2006
Closantel	Fasciola hepatica	20 mg/kg, PO	The Donkey Sanctuary,[60] 2018
Doramectin	Roundworms D arnfieldi	0.2 mg/kg, PO	Gokbulut et al,[101] 2005
Eprinomectin	D arnfieldi Lice	0.5 mg/kg, pour on	Veneziano et al,[54] 2011; Veneziano et al,[68] 2013
Fenbendazole	Roundworms	30–60 mg/kg, PO	Grosenbaugh et al,[1] 2011
Imidocarb diproprionate	Babesia caballi; Theileria equi	<2.2 mg/kg, IM q24h (B caballi) and 2.2 mg/kg, IM q48h (T equi)	Kumar et al,[102] 2009
Ivermectin	Roundworms D arnfieldi Arthropods	0.2 mg/kg, PO	Gokbulut et al,[101] 2005
Mebendazole	Roundworms D arnfieldi	10 mg/kg, PO 15–20 mg/kg, PO once daily for 5 d	Gokbulut et al,[48] 2017 Clayton & Neave,[51] 1979
Moxidectin	Roundworms D arnfieldi	0.2 mg/kg, IM 400 µg/kg, PO	Trawford et al,[103] 2005 Thiemann et al,[53] 2012
Oxfendazole	Roundworms D. arnfieldi	10 mg/kg, PO	Grosenbaugh et al,[1] 2011
Praziquantel	Cestodes	1 mg/kg, PO	Getachew et al,[104] 2013
Pyrantel pamoate	Roundworms Cestodes	19 mg/kg, PO	Gokbulut et al,[50] 2014
Secnidazole	Balantidium coli	10 mg/kg, PO	Khan et al,[61] 2013
Triclabendazole	F hepatica	18 mg/kg, PO	The Donkey Sanctuary,[60] 2018
		12 mg/kg, PO	Kinabo et al,[58] 1989

Abbreviations: IM, intramuscularly; PO, orally.
Data from Refs.[1,48–51,53,54,58,60,61,68,101–104]

control in donkeys. Pyrantel pamoate in paste and granule formulations have poor intestinal absorption in donkeys, but good efficacy (>95%) until day 28 after treatment against intestinal strongylidae.[50]

Donkeys are considered asymptomatic hosts of lungworms (*Dictyocaulus arnfieldi*) and can spread the parasite to clean pastures and infect more sensitive species such as horses and ponies. Oral mebendazole powder (6 mg/kg) has no apparent effect on lungworms, but a paste formulation (15–20 mg/kg by mouth once daily for 5 days) was effective in some animals.[51] Oral fenbendazole (7.5 mg/kg) is ineffective at eliminating lungworms in donkeys and horses.[52] Moxidectin (400 µg/kg by mouth) is the treatment of choice for lungworms in donkeys.[53] A 100% efficacy in eliminating fecal larvae was documented with a pour-on formulation of eprinomectin, a new generation avermectin.[54]

Anoplocephala perfoliata, *A magna*, and *Paranoplocephala mamillana* infest donkeys.[55] Visceral hydatid cysts (*Echinococcus granulosus*) can be incidentally found in post mortem examinations of donkeys in developing countries.[56] Donkeys can be infested by *Fasciola* spp. in regions where this parasite is endemic. These animals may have eosinophilia and increased liver enzymes.[57] Oral triclabendazole has been used successfully in horses and donkeys to treat *Fasciola hepatica*.[58,59] The kinetics of triclabendazole sulfoxide is similar between horses, ponies, and donkeys; however, triclabendazole sulfone has shorter half-life as well as lower maximal concentration and AUC in donkeys compared with horses and ponies.[58] It has been proposed that donkeys are more efficient eliminating the sulfone metabolite. When triclabendazole is ineffective, closantel may be considered.[60]

Secnidazole seems to be effective against *Balantidium coli*, a protozoan frequently found in donkeys in developing countries.[61] Besnoitiosis (*Besnoitia bennetti*) is an apicomplexan highly prevalent in donkeys around the world, regardless of weather, season, or breed.[62] Trimethoprim-sulfamethoxazole may control clinical signs of besnoitiosis in some donkeys.[63] However, trimethoprim-sulfamethoxazole and ponazuril were ineffective in 2 affected donkeys.[64]

Psoroptic and chorioptic mange in donkeys is treated similar to horses, with topical solutions (pyrethroids, sulfur) or oral macrocyclic lactones (ivermectin, moxidectin, or eprinomectin). Pyrethroids such as cypermethrin and permethrin in topical or pour-on formulation are effective against mites, flies, ticks, and lice.[65,66] Macrocyclic lactones are effective at reducing *Chorioptes* spp. number, but rarely cure the infestation owing to the superficial feeding habits of this mite. Fipronil has not been evaluated in donkeys, but it has been effective in horses.[67] Eprinomectin is effective against the donkey-sucking louse (*Haematopinus asini*).[68]

Habronema spp., *Draschia megastoma*, *Gasterophilus* spp., and *Trichostrongylus axei* have minimal effect on the development of gastric ulcers in donkeys.[69] Rectal prolapse may develop in donkeys with severe infestation by *Gasterophilus* spp. larvae.[70]

Other Drugs

Prokinetic drugs such as lidocaine, metoclopramide, and cisapride are occasionally used in donkeys under protocols similar to horses, but pharmacologic information, including efficacy studies are lacking.

Endocrinopathies such as pituitary pars intermedia dysfunction and insulin dysregulation are managed as horses and ponies. Pergolide is the drug of choice to control signs of pituitary pars intermedia dysfunction. Levothyroxine is used to promote weight loss and enhance insulin sensitivity in donkeys with clinical and laboratory evidence of insulin dysregulation (eg, laminitis, hyperglycemia, hypertriglyceridemia); however, its efficacy has not been critically evaluated.

REFERENCES

1. Grosenbaugh DA, Reinemeyer CR, Figueiredo MD. Pharmacology and therapeutics in donkeys. Equine Vet Educ 2011;23:523–30.
2. Matthews NS, Peck KE, Taylor TS, et al. Pharmacokinetics of phenylbutazone and its metabolite oxyphenbutazone in miniature donkeys. Am J Vet Res 2001;62:673–5.
3. Mealey KL, Matthews NS, Peck KE, et al. Comparative pharmacokinetics of phenylbutazone and its metabolite oxyphenbutazone in clinically normal horses and donkeys. Am J Vet Res 1997;58:53–5.
4. Mozaffari AA, Derakhshanfar A, Alinejad A, et al. A comparative study on the adverse effects of flunixin, ketoprofen and phenylbutazone in miniature donkeys: haematological, biochemical and pathological findings. N Z Vet J 2010; 58:224–8.

5. Coakley M, Peck KE, Taylor TS, et al. Pharmacokinetics of flunixin meglumine in donkeys, mules, and horses. Am J Vet Res 1999;60:1441–4.
6. Cheng Z, McKellar Q, Nolan A, et al. Preliminary pharmacokinetic and pharmacodynamic studies on flunixin meglumine in donkeys. Vet Res Commun 1996; 20:469–72.
7. Landoni MF, Lees P. Comparison of the antiinflammatory actions of flunixin and ketoprofen in horses applying PK/PD modeling. Equine Vet J 1995;27:247–56.
8. Mahmood KT, Ashraf M. Pharmacokinetics of meloxicam in healthy donkeys. Pak J Zool 2011;43:897–901.
9. Kim T-W, Della Rocca G, Di Salvo A, et al. Pharmacokinetics of the novel cyclooxygenase 2 inhibitor cimicoxib in donkeys. J Equine Vet Sci 2014;34:923–5.
10. Matthews NS, Grosenbaugh DA, Kvaternick V. Pharmacokinetics and oral bioavailability of firocoxib in donkeys. In: 10th World Congress of Veterinary Anaesthesia, Glasgow, UK, August 31-September 4, 2009. p. 13.
11. Regan FH, Hockenhull J, Pritchard JC, et al. Identifying behavioural differences in working donkeys in response to analgesic administration. Equine Vet J 2016; 48:33–8.
12. Mealey KL, Matthews NS, Peck KE, et al. Pharmacokinetics of R(-) and S(+) carprofen after administration of racemic carprofen in donkeys and horses. Am J Vet Res 2004;65:1479–82.
13. Owens JG, Kamerling SG, Barker SA. Pharmacokinetics of ketoprofen in healthy horses and horses with acute synovitis. J Vet Pharmacol Ther 1995;18:187–95.
14. Oukessou M, Bouljihad M, Van Gool F, et al. Pharmacokinetics of ketoprofen in the donkey (Equus asinus). Zentralbl Veterinarmed A 1996;43:423–6.
15. Latzel ST. Subspecies studies: pharmacokinetics and pharmacodynamics of a single intravenous dose of xylazine in adult mules and adult Haflinger horses. J Equine Vet Sci 2012;32:816–26.
16. Lizarraga I, Beths T. A comparative study of xylazine-induced mechanical hypoalgesia in donkeys and horses. Vet Anaesth Analg 2012;39:533–8.
17. Lizarraga I, Janovyak E. Comparison of the mechanical hypoalgesic effects of five alpha(2)-adrenoceptor agonists in donkeys. Vet Rec 2013;173:294.
18. Lizarraga I, Castillo-Alcala F, Varner KM, et al. Sedation and mechanical hypoalgesia after sublingual administration of detomidine hydrochloride gel to donkeys. J Am Vet Med Assoc 2016;249:83–9.
19. Lizarraga I, Castillo-Alcala F, Robinson LS. Comparison of sedation and mechanical antinociception induced by intravenous administration of acepromazine and four dose rates of dexmedetomidine in donkeys. Vet Anaesth Analg 2017;44:509–17.
20. Lizarraga I, Castillo-Alcala F. Sedative and mechanical hypoalgesic effects of butorphanol in xylazine-premedicated donkeys. Equine Vet J 2015;47:308–12.
21. Giorgi M, Del Carlo S, Sgorbini M, et al. Pharmacokinetics of tramadol and its metabolites M1, M2, and M5 in donkeys after intravenous and oral immediate release single-dose administration. J Equine Vet Sci 2009;29:569–74.
22. Giorgi M, Laus F, De Vito V, et al. Flupirtine: preliminary pharmacokinetics in the donkey. J Equine Vet Sci 2015;35:309–14.
23. Matthews NS. Donkey anesthesia and analgesia - not just small horses. In: NAVC conference. Orlando, Florida, USA, January 16-20, 2010.
24. Aupanun S, Laus F, Poapolathep A, et al. Pharmacokinetic assessment of the marker active metabolites 4-Methyl-amino-antipyrine and 4-Acetyl-amino-antipyrine after intravenous and intramuscular injection of metamizole (Dipyrone) in healthy donkeys. J Equine Vet Sci 2016;47:55–61.

25. Matthews NS, Taylor TS, Hartsfield SM, et al. P Pharmacokinetics of ketamine in mules and Mammoth asses premedicated with xylazine. Equine Vet J 1994;26: 241–3.

26. Matthews NS, Taylor TS, Hartsfield SM. Anaesthesia of donkeys and mules. Equine Vet Educ 1997;9:198–202.

27. Matthews NS, Peck KE, Mealey KL, et al. Pharmacokinetics and cardiopulmonary effects of guaifenesin in donkeys. J Vet Pharmacol Ther 1997;20:442–6.

28. Coelho CMM, Moreno JCD, Goulart DD, et al. Evaluation of cardiorespiratory and biochemical effects of ketamine-propofol and guaifenesin-ketamine-xylazine anesthesia in donkeys (Equus asinus). Vet Anaesth Analg 2014;41: 602–12.

29. Vullo C, Carluccio A, Robbe D, et al. Guaiphenesin-ketamine-xylazine infusion to maintain anesthesia in mules undergoing field castration. Acta Vet Scand 2017; 59:5.

30. Maney JK, Durham HE Jr, Goucher KP, et al. Induction of anesthesia and recovery in donkeys sedated with xylazine: a comparison of midazolam-alfaxalone and midazolam-ketamine. Vet Anaesth Analg 2018;45:539–44.

31. Dar KH, Gupta AK, Bhadwal MS, et al. Evaluation of xylazine-diazepam-ketamine anaesthesia in mules: anaesthetic, haemato-biochemical, and blood gas studies. Indian J Anim Sci 2014;84:130–5.

32. Dar KH, Gupta AK. Total intravenous anaesthesia in adult mules. Vet Anaesth Analg 2016;43:204–8.

33. Mercer DE, Matthews NS. Minimum alveolar concentrations of halothane and isoflurane in donkeys and minimal alveolar concentrations -sparing effect of butorphanol. In: Proceedings of the Fifteenth PanVet Congress, Campo Grande, Brazil, October 21-25, 1996. p. 129.

34. Kalchofner KS, Ringer SK, Boller J, et al. Clinical assessment of anesthesia with isoflurane and medetomidine in 300 equidae. Pferdeheilkunde 2006;22:301.

35. Grint NJ, Johnson CB, Lorena SD, et al. Electroencephalographic responses to a noxious surgical stimulus in mules, horses, and ponies. J Equine Vet Sci 2014; 34:955–62.

36. Matthews N, van Loon J. Anaesthesia and analgesia of the donkey and the mule. Equine Vet Educ 2013;25:47–51.

37. Suriano R, Varasano V, Robbe D, et al. Intraoperative analgesic effect of intrafunicular lidocaine injection during orchiectomy in isoflurane-anesthetized Martina Franca donkeys. J Equine Vet Sci 2014;34:793–8.

38. Shoukry M, Saleh M, Fouad K. Epidural anaesthesia in donkeys. Vet Rec 1975; 97:450–2.

39. Naeini AT, Rezakhani A, Ahmmadian M. Comparison of morphine, fentanyl, methadone, lidocaine and lidocaine epinephrine as caudal epidural analgesics in donkeys. J Appl Anim Res 1999;15:181–4.

40. Matthews NS. Anesthesia and analgesia for donkeys and mules. In: Muir W, Hubbell JA, editors. Equine anesthesia: monitoring and emergency therapy. 2nd edition. Milton, Ontario, Canada: Saunders Elsevier; 2009. p. 353–7.

41. Toutain PL, Ferran A, Bousquet-Melou A. Species differences in pharmacokinetics and pharmacodynamics. Handb Exp Pharmacol 2010;(199):19–48.

42. Wise LN, Kappmeyer LS, Mealey RH, et al. Review of equine piroplasmosis. J Vet Intern Med 2013;27:1334–46.

43. Abutarbush SM, Alfaqeeh SM, Mustafa G, et al. Evaluation of the use of atropine sulfate, a combination of butylscopolammonium bromide and metamizole

sodium, and flunixin meglumine to ameliorate clinical adverse effects of imido-carb dipropionate in horses. Am J Vet Res 2013;74:1404–8.

44. Donnellan CM, Page PC, Nurton JP, et al. Comparison of glycopyrrolate and atropine in ameliorating the adverse effects of imidocarb dipropionate in horses. Equine Vet J 2013;45:625–9.

45. Lawson E, Burden F, Elsheikha HM. Pyrantel resistance in two herds of donkey in the UK. Vet Parasitol 2015;207:346–9.

46. Corbett CJ, Love S, Moore A, et al. The effectiveness of faecal removal methods of pasture management to control the cyathostomin burden of donkeys. Parasit Vectors 2014;7:48.

47. Matthee S, Krecek RC, Milne SA, et al. Impact of management interventions on helminth levels, and body and blood measurements in working donkeys in South Africa. Vet Parasitol 2002;107:103–13.

48. Gokbulut C, Aksit D, Santoro M, et al. Plasma disposition, milk excretion and parasitological efficacy of mebendazole in donkeys naturally infected by Cya-thostominae. Vet Parasitol 2016;217:95–100.

49. Gokbulut C, Akar F, McKellar QA. Plasma disposition and faecal excretion of ox-fendazole, fenbendazole and albendazole following oral administration to don-keys. Vet J 2006;172:166–72.

50. Gokbulut C, Aksit D, Smaldone G, et al. Plasma pharmacokinetics, faecal excre-tion and efficacy of pyrantel pamoate paste and granule formulations following per os administration in donkeys naturally infected with intestinal strongylidae. Vet Parasitol 2014;205:186–92.

51. Clayton HM, Neave RM. Efficacy of mebendazole against Dictyocaulus arnfieldi in the donkey. Vet Rec 1979;104:571–2.

52. Urch DL, Allen WR. Studies on fenbendazole for treating lung and intestinal par-asites in horses and donkeys. Equine Vet J 1980;12:74–7.

53. Thiemann AK. Respiratory disease in the donkey. Equine Vet Educ 2012;24: 469–78.

54. Veneziano V, Di Loria A, Masucci R, et al. Efficacy of eprinomectin pour-on against Dictyocaulus arnfieldi infection in donkeys (Equus asinus). Vet J 2011; 190:414–5.

55. Getachew M, Trawford A, Feseha G, et al. Gastrointestinal parasites of working donkeys of Ethiopia. Trop Anim Health Prod 2010;42:27–33.

56. Mukbel RM, Torgerson PR, Abo-Shehada MN. Prevalence of hydatidosis among donkeys in northern Jordan. Vet Parasitol 2000;88:35–42.

57. Getachew MA, Innocent G, Reid SW, et al. A neglected and emerging helmin-thosis: a case equine fasciolosis. In: British Equine Veterinary Association Congress, Liverpool, UK, September 9-12, 2015. p. 21.

58. Kinabo LD, Bogan JA. Disposition of triclabendazole in horses, ponies and don-keys. Equine Vet J 1989;21:305–7.

59. Trawford AF, Tremlett JG. Efficacy of triclabendazole against Fasciola hepatica in the donkey (Equus asinus). Vet Rec 1996;139:142–3.

60. The Donkey Sanctuary. The clinical companion of the donkey. 1st edition. Matador Leicestershire, UK: Troubador Publishing ltd; 2018.

61. Khan A, Khan MS, Avais M, et al. Prevalence, hematology, and treatment of bal-antidiasis among donkeys in and around Lahore, Pakistan. Vet Parasitol 2013; 196:203–5.

62. Elsheikha HM, Mackenzie CD, Rosenthal BM, et al. An outbreak of besnoitiosis in miniature donkeys. J Parasitol 2005;91:877–81.

63. Lienard E, Nabuco A, Vandenabeele S, et al. First evidence of Besnoitia bennetti infection (Protozoa: Apicomplexa) in donkeys (Equus asinus) in Belgium. Parasit Vectors 2018;11:427.

64. Ness SL, Peters-Kennedy J, Schares G, et al. Investigation of an outbreak of besnoitiosis in donkeys in northeastern Pennsylvania. J Am Vet Med Assoc 2012;240:1329–37.

65. Veneziano V, Neglia G, Galietti A, et al. Efficacy of alphacypermetrin pour-on against natural Werneckiella equi infestation on donkeys (Equus asinus). Parasitol Res 2012;111:967–73.

66. Ellse L, Burden FA, Wall R. Seasonal infestation of donkeys by lice: phenology, risk factors and management. Vet Parasitol 2014;203:303–9.

67. Littlewood J. Chorioptic mange: successful treatment of a case with fipronil. Equine Vet Educ 2000;12:144–6.

68. Veneziano V, Galietti A, Mariani U, et al. Field efficacy of eprinomectin against the sucking louse Haematopinus asini on naturally infested donkeys. Vet J 2013;197:512–4.

69. Al-Mokaddem AK, Ahmed KA, Doghaim RE. Pathology of gastric lesions in donkeys: a preliminary study. Equine Vet J 2015;47:684–8.

70. Getachew AM, Innocent G, Trawford AF, et al. Gasterophilosis: a major cause of rectal prolapse in working donkeys in Ethiopia. Trop Anim Health Prod 2012;44: 757–62.

71. Kvaternick V, Pollmeier M, Fischer J, et al. Pharmacokinetics and metabolism of orally administered firocoxib, a novel second generation coxib, in horses. J Vet Pharmacol Ther 2007;30:208–17.

72. Anwer MN, Rasheed MA, Ashraf M. Pharmacokinetics of ketoprofen in healthy donkeys in Pakistan. J Anim Plant Sci 2012;22:966–9.

73. Rehman ZU, Ashraf M, Khan MA, et al. Pharmacokinetics of ketoprofen in healthy horses in Pakistan. J Anim Plant Sci 2012;22:584–7.

74. Sinclair MD, Mealey KL, Matthews NS, et al. Comparative pharmacokinetics of meloxicam in clinically normal horses and donkeys. Am J Vet Res 2006;67: 1082–5.

75. Cheng Z, McKellar QA, Nolan A, et al. Pharmacokinetics and pharmacodynamics of phenylbutazone and oxyphenbutazone in the donkey. J Vet Pharmacol Ther 1996;19:149–51.

76. Evangelista F, Tayari H, Degani M, et al. Sedative and respiratory effects of intramuscular detomidine and butorphanol in donkeys sedated for bronchoalveolar lavage. J Equine Vet Sci 2018;69:96–101.

77. Mostafa MB, Farag KA, Zomor E, et al. The sedative and analgesic effects of detomidine (Domosedan) in donkeys. Zentralbl Veterinarmed A 1995;42:351–6.

78. Naddaf H, Baniadam A, Rasekh A, et al. Cardiopulmonary effects during anaesthesia induced and maintained with propofol in acepromazine pre-medicated donkeys. Vet Anaesth Analg 2015;42:83–7.

79. Matthews NS, Taylor TS, Sullivan JA. A comparison of three combinations of injectable anesthetics in miniature donkeys. Vet Anaesth Analg 2002;29:36–42.

80. Matthews NS, Taylor TS. Anesthesia of donkeys and mules: how they differ from horses. In: Proceedings of the 48th Annual Convention of the American Association of Equine Practitioners, Orlando, Florida, USA, December 4-8, 2002.

81. Carmona JU, Giraldo CE, Aristizabal W, et al. Evaluation of the effects of the sedation with azaperone/acepromazine and immobilization with guaiphenesin/thiopentone in mules. Vet Res Commun 2007;31:125–32.

82. Matthews NS, Taylor TS, Skrobarcek CL, et al. A comparison of injectable anaesthetic regimens in mules. Equine Vet J Suppl 1992;(11):34–6.

83. Horspool LJI, Taylor DJ, McKellar QA. Plasma disposition of amikacin and interaction with gastrointestinal microflora in Equidae following intravenous and oral-administration. J Vet Pharmacol Ther 1994;17:291–8.

84. Horspool LJ, Sarasola P, McKellar QA. Disposition of ampicillin sodium in horses, ponies and donkeys after intravenous administration. Equine Vet J Suppl 1992;(11):59–61.

85. Lavy E, Ziv G, Aroch I, et al. Pharmacokinetics, intramuscular bio-availability, and bioequivalence of amoxycillin in donkeys. Zentralbl Veterinarmed B 1995; 42:284–92.

86. Oukessou M, Aissa M, Hmidouch A. Pharmacokinetics study of benzylpenicillin and amoxicillin in the donkey (Equus asinus). Indian Vet J 1994;71:1077–81.

87. Kum C, Gokbulut C, Sekkin S, et al. Pharmacokinetics of danofloxacin following intravenous and intramuscular administration in donkeys. J Vet Pharmacol Ther 2009;32:105–8.

88. Sekkin S, Gokbulut C, Kum C, et al. Plasma disposition of enrofloxacin following intravenous and intramuscular administration in donkeys. Vet Rec 2012; 171:447.

89. Kaartinen L, Panu S, Pyorala S. Pharmacokinetics of enrofloxacin in horses after single intravenous and intramuscular administration. Equine Vet J 1997;29: 378–81.

90. Miller SM, Matthews NS, Mealey KL, et al. Pharmacokinetics of gentamicin in Mammoth asses. J Vet Pharmacol Ther 1994;17:403–6.

91. Welfare RE, Mealey KL, Matthews NS, et al. Pharmacokinetics of gentamicin in donkeys. J Vet Pharmacol Ther 1996;19:167–9.

92. Whittem T, Firth EC, Hodge H, et al. Pharmacokinetic interactions between repeated dose phenylbutazone and gentamicin in the horse. J Vet Pharmacol Ther 1996;19:454–9.

93. Gonzalez F, Rodriguez C, De Lucas JJ, et al. Pharmacokinetics of a single intravenous dose of marbofloxacin in adult donkeys. Vet Rec 2007;161:133–6.

94. Carretero M, Rodriguez C, San Andres MI, et al. Pharmacokinetics of marbofloxacin in mature horses after single intravenous and intramuscular administration. Equine Vet J 2002;34:360–5.

95. Lavy E, Ziv G, Glickman A. Intravenous disposition kinetics, oral and intramuscular bioavailability and urinary excretion of norfloxacin nicotinate in donkeys. J Vet Pharmacol Ther 1995;18:101–7.

96. Park SC, Yun HI. Clinical pharmacokinetics of norfloxacin-glycine acetate after intravenous and intramuscular administration to horses. Res Vet Sci 2003;74: 79–83.

97. Horspool LJI, McKellar QA. Disposition of penicillin-G sodium following intravenous and oral-administration to equidae. Br Vet J 1995;151:401–12.

98. Lizarraga I, Sumano H, Brumbaugh GW. Pharmacological and pharmacokinetic differences between donkeys and horses. Equine Vet Educ 2004;16:102–12.

99. Oukessou M, Alsouss L. Pharmacokinetics of sulfonamides and trimethoprim in the donkey (Equus asinus). Zentralbl Veterinarmed A 1998;45:191–8.

100. Peck KE, Matthews NS, Taylor TS, et al. Pharmacokinetics of sulfamethoxazole and trimethoprim in donkeys, mules, and horses. Am J Vet Res 2002;63:349–53.

101. Gokbulut C, Boyacioglu M, Karademir U. Plasma pharmacokinetics and faecal excretion of ivermectin (Eqvalan paste) and doramectin (Dectomax, 1%) following oral administration in donkeys. Res Vet Sci 2005;79:233–8.

102. Kumar S, Kumar R, Sugimoto C. A perspective on Theileria equi infections in donkeys. Jpn J Vet Res 2009;56:171–80.

103. Trawford AF, Burden F, Hodgkinson JE. Suspected moxidectin resistance in cyathostomin in two donkey herds at the donkey sanctuary, UK. In: 20th International Conference of the World Association for the Advancement of Veterinary Parasitology. Christchurch (New Zealand), October 16-20, 2005.

104. Getachew AM, Innocent G, Proudman CJ, et al. Field efficacy of praziquantel oral paste against naturally acquired equine cestodes in Ethiopia. Parasitol Res 2013;112:141–6.

Key Aspects of Donkey and Mule Reproduction

Igor Federico Canisso, DVM, MSc, PhD[a],*, Duccio Panzani, DVM, PhD[b],
Jordi Miró, DVM, PhD[c], Robyn E. Ellerbrock, DVM, PhD[d]

KEYWORDS

- Asinine • Assisted reproductive techniques • Equid reproduction
- Reproductive physiology • Reproductive pathology • Mules • *Equus mulus*
- *Equus asinus*

KEY POINTS

- Donkeys are nonseasonal, polyestrous, territorial, and nonharem breeders. The jenny cervix is long and prone to laceration and adhesions after dystocia.
- Jacks have large testicles with a high spermatogenic efficiency, conversely, male hybrids have small testicles and typically do not produce sperm.
- Frozen donkey semen has better pregnancy rates in mares than jennies.
- Female mules display estrous cycle but are rarely fertile, but they can be used as embryo recipients for mule, horse or donkey embryos.

INTRODUCTION

Donkeys (*E asinus*) and their hybrids with horses (ie, *Equus mulus mulus*) have been used for centuries in agriculture, transport, and war. Although mechanization of agriculture and industrialization in the last century reduced the importance and number of both donkeys and their hybrids, these animals are still heavily used as pack animals and to pull carts in some African and Asian countries. In the Americas, donkeys are frequently crossed with mares to produce mules. Mules are used in mountainous regions for tourism purposes (eg, Grand Canyon), trail rides, territorial defense (eg, mountains of Argentina), and to herd cattle in large beef operations in Brazil. In North America and Western Europe, donkeys may also be kept as pets or as livestock guardians.

[a] Department of Veterinary Clinical Medicine, College of Veterinary Medicine, University of Illinois Urbana-Champaign, Urbana, IL 61802, USA; [b] Department of Veterinary Science, University of Pisa, Pisa 56122, Italy; [c] Department of Animal Medicine and Surgery, Faculty of Veterinary Medicine, Autonomous University of Barcelona, 08193 Bellaterra, Barcelona, Spain; [d] Department of Large Animal Medicine, College of Veterinary Medicine, University of Georgia, Athens, GA 30602, USA
* Corresponding author.
E-mail address: canisso@illinois.edu

Vet Clin Equine 35 (2019) 607–642
https://doi.org/10.1016/j.cveq.2019.08.014
0749-0739/19/© 2019 Elsevier Inc. All rights reserved.

Although industrialization almost led to the extinction of many European breeds, conservation programs recently developed by countries such as Spain, Italy, and Portugal are rescuing some of the endangered donkey breeds. The rediscovery of donkey milk for consumption, cheese, and cosmetics has also helped some threatened breeds, such as the Amiata rebound. In contrast, overpopulation of small-frame donkeys is a major concern in desert areas of the United States, some Caribbean Islands, and northeast Brazil. There, feral donkeys have no commercial value, and depend on governmental and nongovernmental agencies to develop contraceptives and population control programs. In the United States for instance, the Bureau of Land Management runs a program to control the population of feral donkeys on public lands.

Although there are similarities between donkeys and horses, which allow them to breed and produce hybrids, there are also many unique reproductive features of donkeys and mules. The objectives of this article are to review key aspects of donkey and mule reproductive physiology, reproductive medicine, and assisted reproductive techniques. This knowledge is useful for practitioners offering assisted reproductive techniques, but also for those advising the occasional client with a reproductive question.

KEY OVERVIEW OF THE FUNCTIONAL FEMALE GENITAL ANATOMY

The internal genitalia of jennies and mules are similar to mares; however, the jenny's internal genitalia is proportionally larger than in mares and mules.[1] The uterus is Y-shaped, with a uterine body of similar length to the uterine horns. The tips of the uterine horns reach the fifth lumbar vertebra cranially, and the ovaries are located more cranial than the ovaries of horses.[1] The mesometrium in the jenny is attached to the dorsal margin of the uterine horns and dorso-laterally to the body of the uterus excluding the cervix; this feature makes the 2 horns form a cranio-ventral convexity.[1] Jenny and mule ovaries have a similar bean-shape to the mare, with the ovarian cortex located inside the ovary, the medullar region located outside the ovary, and the ovulation fossa located at the free margin of the ovary. The broad ligament appendix and ovarian bursa are more prominent in jennies than mares.[1]

The caudal reproductive tract of jennies is more tilted dorsally than other farm animals, and the ventral commissure of the vulva is more concealed ventrally than the dorsal commissure. In normal mares, the vulvar length is two-thirds below the pelvic brim; in normal jennies, the vulvar length is entirely below the pelvic brim (**Fig. 1**). Subfertile jennies with abnormal vulvar conformation and pneumovagina or pneumouterus may benefit from a Caslick's operation or perineal body reconstruction (**Fig. 2**). Proportionally, jennies appear to have a larger clitoris than mares. The vulva of jennies have larger minor lips (visible inside the vestibule) than mares, and the vulva is slightly tilted ventrally, making contamination of the reproductive tract less likely in this species (see **Fig. 1**).[1]

The jenny cervix has a narrowed and tortuous lumen that represents a challenge for routine intrauterine procedures, particularly in small-frame maiden jennies. The prominent vaginal portion (1.5–3 cm) is connected to dorsal and ventral vaginal longitudinal folds that limit its lateral displacement. These features make the donkey cervix prone to lacerations during dystocias.[2,3] In addition, the vaginal portion of the cervix may have a straight conformation or various conformations that resemble the letters "L," "C," or "V" (**Fig. 3**). The clinical significance for these variations remains to be determined.

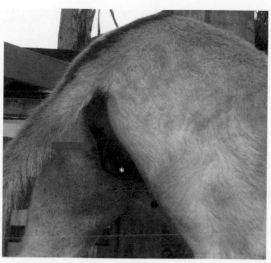

Fig. 1. Vulva of a jenny in estrus. The arrow denotes the level of the pelvic brim, and the asterisk denotes the clitoris glans.

The jenny cervix becomes longer, thinner, and well-toned during diestrus, and shorter, wider, softer, and relaxed during estrus.[4] The uterus becomes well-toned during diestrus and softer and relaxed during estrus.[4] In the large Poitou breed, the cervix varies from 4.5 to 8.0 cm in length, and 2.5 to 3 cm in width.[4]

PUBERTY AND SEASONALITY IN JENNIES

Puberty in healthy, well-fed jennies usually occurs between the first and second year of life,[2,3] but jennies should not be bred before age 3 years.[2] Studies performed before ultrasonography described donkeys as a long-day seasonal polyestrous species in temperate latitudes.[5] Further reports described the jenny as a nonseasonal annual polyestrous female even in temperate areas of the world.[6–8] A recent study from Portugal demonstrated that young jennies with a poor body condition score (≤4 out of 9) were likely to stop cycling during the fall and winter, whereas jennies with satisfactory scores ≥5 continued cycling throughout the year.[9] This is consistent with an Ethiopian study showing a positive association between body condition score and ovarian activity.[10] Silent estrus, prolonged luteal phase, and split estrus have also been described, but not in association with the anovulatory season.[5,7,11] Granulosa cell tumors and teratomas have also rarely been recorded in donkeys[12] and mules. However, it remains to be determined whether anti-Müllerian hormone and inhibin can be used as diagnostics markers for granulosa cell tumor in jennies and mules.

ESTROUS CYCLE

The duration of the donkey estrous cycle (~23–27 days) tends to be longer than mares (~21 days), whereas mules tend to be intermediary (22 days).[5,13,14] In donkeys, diestrus varies from 15 to 19 days, estrus varies from 4 to 10 days, and ovulation occurs the day before the end of estrus.[5,14,15] Mules have estrus lasting from 5 to 7 days. Variations occur according to the donkey breed and environment (**Table 1**). Estrus tends to be shorter during the spring and summer than in the fall and winter.[7,18,20,21]

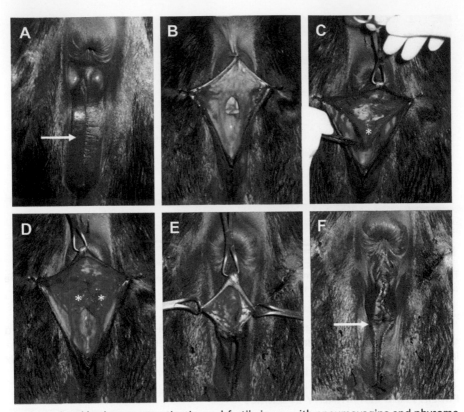

Fig. 2. Perineal body reconstruction in a subfertile jenny with pneumovagina and physometra. (*A*) The jenny's vulva is excessively long. The arrow points to the pelvic brim and the 2 bulging structures show the lidocaine block. (*B*) Two stay sutures have been placed and the dorsal aspect of the vulva exposed; (*C*) a flap (*asterisk*) was created by gentle dissection of the mucosa. (*D* and *E*) Both sides of the flap (*asterisk*) were sutured together in a simple continue pattern using absorbable suture (no. 2) to re-create a "roof" for the vestibule. (*F*) Final surgical reconstruction. After the "roof" was created, the space between the roof and the perineal body was closed with simple interrupted sutures (no. 2).

Progesterone concentration remains low up to the day after ovulation, slowly increases until 4 to 6 days post-ovulation, plateaus by days 14 to 16 post-ovulation and then starts to decline to reach baseline concentrations (<1 ng/mL) in 2 days.[17] In donkeys, 17β-estradiol increases from 10 pg/mL during early estrus to peak around 40 to 60 pg/mL at ovulation.[21] Follicle-stimulating hormone concentrations remain low throughout the estrous cycle, and peak 3 and 9 days post-ovulation.[15] Luteinizing hormone (LH) concentrations increase pre-ovulation, peak 2 days after ovulation, and then decrease to baseline throughout the remainder of the estrous cycle.[15]

Follicular deviation occurs 8 to 9 days before ovulation at approximately 19 to 20 mm follicular diameter.[15,22,23] In most donkeys the dominant follicle grows 2 to 3 mm/d from deviation to ovulation;[11,14] however, in the large breed Catalonian donkeys follicles grow up to ~4 mm/d.[8] Jennies have 1 follicular wave during the estrous cycle,[24] whereas no follicular waves were detected in mules.[13] Ovulatory diameter varies from 30 to 48 mm (**Table 2**), with a positive association between body frame

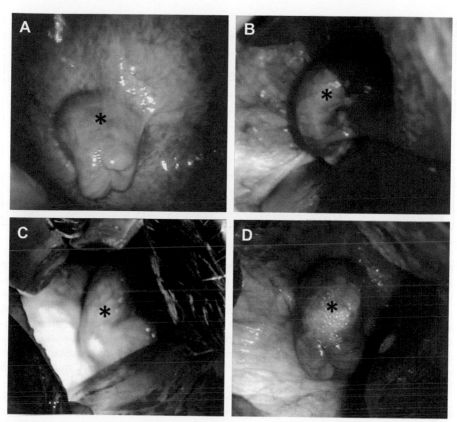

Fig. 3. Representative images of the vaginal portion of the jenny cervix (*asterisk*). (*A*) Straight type cervix; (*B*) C-like cervix; (*C*) L-like cervix; and (*D*) V-like cervix. ([*B–D*] Images kindly provided by Dr. Shenming Zeng, China Agricultural University.)

and follicular diameter.[8,14,25,29] In mules, the average follicular diameter the day before ovulation was 38.2 ± 2.2 mm.[13]

In estrus, the jenny displays signs, such as standing to be mounted by another female or male, mouth clapping, clitoral winking, urinating, and tail raising.[8,16,30–32]

Table 1					
Breed and regional variations in the donkey estrous cycle					
Breeds	**Location**	**Estrous Cycles (n)**	**Diestrus (d)**	**Estrus (d)**	**IOI (d)**
Mammoth[15]	United States	19	19 ± 0.6	6 ± 0.6	25 ± 0.7
Pega[5]	Brazil	13	18 ± 2.3	8 ± 2.5	26 ± 2.7
Pega[16]	Brazil	21	—	6 ± 2.1	—
Jegue norderstino[17]	Brazil	13	18 ± 2.0	6 ± 2.2	24 ± 3.2
Mammoth[18]	United States	33	17 ± 2.6	6 ± 2.1	23 ± 2.6
Amiata[19]	Italy	4	15 ± 2.0	8.5 ± 1.5	24 ± 1.8
Catalonian donkey[8]	Spain	10	20 ± 0.4	5.6 ± 0.2	25 ± 0.3

Abbreviation: IOI, interovulatory interval.

Table 2
Variation in follicular diameter at ovulation by donkey breed

Breeds	Location	Estrous Cycles (n)	Ovulatory Diameter (mm) Mean ± SD	Ranges	Daily Follicular Growth (mm)
Catalonian donkey[8]	Spain	36	44.9 ± 0.5	35–60	4
Martina-Franca[25]	Italy	20	42.9 ± 2.97	—	—
Martina-Franca[21]	Italy	120	43.7 ± 0.13	—	2.8
Poitou[26]	France	—	36.2 ± 3.0	—	2.0
Poitou[27]	India	9	41.1 ± 1.0	—	2.7
Mammoth[15]	United States	19	36	30–40	—
Pega and crosses[17]	Brazil	20	36.7 ± 3.6	28.5–46	—
Miranda[28]	Portugal	33	38.40 ± 0.68	30.29–47.86	3.18
Burro Mexicano[14]	Mexico	27	36.9 ± 0.7	—	2.0

Females may display the Flehmen response after smelling urogenital secretions from estrus jennies (**Fig. 4**). Jennies congregate into a sexually active group similar to cows, which is thought to help jacks identify females ready to be bred.[16,32] Mules show similar estrus signs with a more discreet clap mouth (I.F. Canisso, 2003–2008). Close to ovulation, estrus signs intensify and the follicle stops growing and becomes irregular and softer.[8,21] Occurrence of multiple ovulations is extremely variable (0%–50%) across breeds,[14,18,33,34] with the highest frequency in the Chinese Black donkey and Spanish and Portuguese breeds,[8,11,34] and around 33.3% in mules (15/45 cycles).[13]

Although the reproductive tract of jennies is proportionally larger than mares, assessment of the tract is challenging in small-frame animals. The use of lidocaine mixed with lubricant (20 mL of 2% lidocaine in 80 mL of carboxymethylcellulose) alone or in a combination with N-butylscopolammonium bromide (10–20 mg/animal, intravenously [IV]) may aid in transrectal examination. The ultrasonographic appearance of the reproductive tract of donkeys resembles the mare and mule,

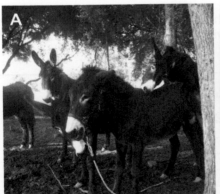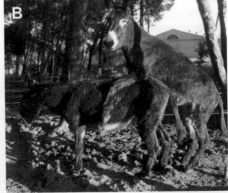

Fig. 4. (*A*) Group of jennies in estrus interacting in a sexually active group. One female is being mounted by an estrus jenny and teased by a third jenny. (*B*) Estrus jenny clap-mouthing and widening the pelvic limbs apart while being mounted by another estrus jenny.

with the exception that uterine edema is less pronounced in donkeys than in mares.[13,22] Whereas ovarian structures are similar in equids, the donkey corpus luteum often has a horizontal hyperechoic band or circular spot.[22,35,36] In some unusual cases, a central hypoechoic lacuna can also be seen.[22]

FUNCTIONAL AND REPRODUCTIVE ANATOMY AND PHYSIOLOGY OF DONKEY JACKS

The jack penis (root, shaft, and glans) and prepuce are anatomically similar to stallions; however, the donkey's penis is longer (**Fig. 5**A), and 2 nipples can be seen on each side of the sheath (**Fig. 5**B). The prepuce's internal lamina forms a structure identifiable externally as "preputial ring," although the ring is less pronounced than stallions. Whereas the gross anatomy of the scrotum is similar for all equids, jacks have a very pendulous scrotum. The scrotum's skin is soft and covered in sweat glands which plays a role in testicular thermal regulation.

Equids have ovoid testicles, with stallions having smaller testicles that are narrowed laterally, whereas the jacks' testicles are larger and more globular shaped (**Fig. 6**A). Mules have very small testicles with a shape intermediate to the stallion and jack. In the normal donkey, the testicles should be freely movable within the scrotum and may have a horizontal orientation or a slight

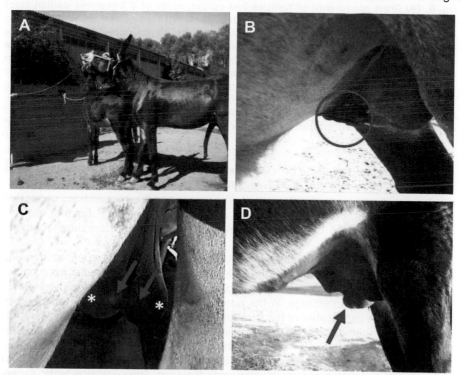

Fig. 5. External genitalia of donkey jacks. (*A*) Catalonian donkey with an erect penis. (*B*) Prepuce and scrotum from a mature jack. The circled area shows a prominent nipple. (*C*) Caudal view of the scrotum from a mature jack, note the pendulous scrotum with large testicles (*asterisk*) and prominent tail of the epididymis (⇓). (*D*) Donkey presenting unilateral rotation of the right testis. The arrow points to the epididymal tail pointing cranially rather than caudally.

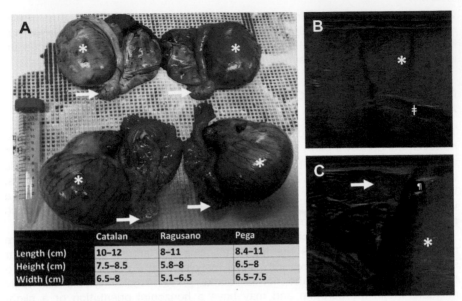

	Catalan	Ragusano	Pega
Length (cm)	10–12	8–11	8.4–11
Height (cm)	7.5–8.5	5.8–8	6.5–8
Width (cm)	6.5–8	5.1–6.5	6.5–7.5

Fig. 6. (*A*) Gross appearance of testicles and epididymides of a 2-year-old stallion (top) and a 2-year-old donkey (bottom). (*B*) B-mode ultrasonography (lateral view) of the testicular parenchyma (*asterisk*). Prominent central testicular vein (*double dagger*). (*C*) B-mode ultrasonography (lateral view) of the scrotum showing the testicular parenchyma (*asterisk*), testicular artery (*pilcrow*) and epididymal tail (⇒). The table displays mean testicular measurements for Catalan, Ragusano and Pega jacks. ([Table] *Data from* Canisso IF, Carvalho GR, Silva EC, et al. Some biometric aspects of the external genital tract from donkey Pega breed semen donors. *Ciencia Rural.* 2009; 39(9):2556-62; and Quartuccio M, Marino G, Taormina A, et al. Seminal characteristics and sexual behaviour in Ragusano donkeys (*Equus asinus*) during semen collection on the ground. *Large Anim Rev.* 2011; 17(4):151-55.)

inclination cranio-dorsally. The combined testicular volume in mature donkeys varies from 250 to 500 cm^3.[37,38] Testicular parenchyma consists of the seminiferous tubules in which spermatogenesis takes place, and the interstitium, constituted primarily of Leydig cells responsible for androgen production.[39] Each spermatogenic cycle lasts 10.5 days, and spermatogenesis duration is estimated to be 47.5 days.[39]

High spermatogenic efficiency and a relatively short length of spermatogenesis, coupled with large testicles make the jack the most efficient domestic mammal for sperm production.[39] This demands that donkeys have very large epididymides for sperm maturation and storage. In the normal jack the epididymal tail can be seen bulging from the caudal view of the scrotum, which helps differentiate testicular rotation (≤180°, nonpathological, no compromise of the blood flow) from the rare testicular torsion (>180°, pathologic, compromised blood flow) (**Fig. 5**).

The spermatic cord extends from the abdominal inguinal ring to the testis, and the cremaster muscle runs laterally alongside the cord. The very large testicular artery winds in association with testicular veins to form the pampiniform plexus (**Fig. 7**), which is responsible for maintaining the testis 4°C to 5°C cooler than body temperature. Donkeys have very prominent spermatic cords (23–28 mm diameter),[37] with unique histologic features (capsule rich in muscular tissue and veins with a thick muscular layer) that presumably facilitate venous blood flow

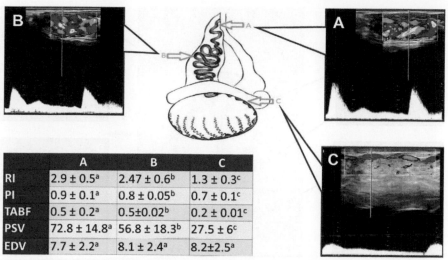

	A	B	C
RI	2.9 ± 0.5[a]	2.47 ± 0.6[b]	1.3 ± 0.3[c]
PI	0.9 ± 0.1[a]	0.8 ± 0.05[b]	0.7 ± 0.1[c]
TABF	0.5 ± 0.2[a]	0.5±0.02[b]	0.2 ± 0.01[c]
PSV	72.8 ± 14.8[a]	56.8 ± 18.3[b]	27.5 ± 6[c]
EDV	7.7 ± 2.2[a]	8.1 ± 2.4[a]	8.2±2.5[a]

Fig. 7. Blood flow in donkey testicles (n = 6). (*A*) Pampiniform plexus proximal; (*B*) pampiniform plexus supra-testicular; (*C*) testis periphery. EDV, end diastolic velocity (cm/s); PI, pulsatility index; PSV, peak systolic velocity (cm/s); RI, resistive index; TABF, total arterial blood flow. Different superscripts denote statistical differences. ([Table] *Data from* Rota A, Sgorbini M, Panzani D, et al. Effect of housing system on reproductive behaviour and on some endocrinological and seminal parameters of donkey stallions. *Reprod Dom Anim.* 2018; 53(1):40-47.)

from the testis and better testicular efficiency.[40] Cryptorchidism and testicular degeneration occur much less commonly in donkeys than stallions (I.F. Canisso, personal observations).

The testicular parenchyma has an echogenic granular homogeneous appearance on ultrasound (**Fig. 6**B, C), and a small amount (<5 mm) of anechoic fluid in the vaginal cavity is a normal finding. The central vein is visibly larger than in the stallion (see **Fig. 6**B). Interestingly, the donkey epididymal tail has a heterogeneous ultrasonographic appearance because of the convoluted epididymal duct (see **Fig. 6**C). A recent study concluded that donkeys have higher testicular artery flow than horses, and that pulsatility index was negatively correlated with sperm number and sperm velocity[41] (see **Fig. 7**).

The ductus deferens connect the tail of the epididymides to the urethra, and are easily palpable through the skin of the scrotum. The end of the duct entering the pelvic cavity, the ampulla, is more muscular and thicker in equids than other species, and is larger in donkeys than horses (25–35 mm vs 8–15 mm, respectively). The mucosa of the ampulla is more folded and glandular in donkeys[42] than stallions. Stallions are frequently affected with ampullary blockage; surprisingly, there is only 1 report of ampullary blockage in a 4-year-old jack. This jack responded to treatment with oxytocin, transrectal massage, and frequent semen collections.[43]

Although all 4 accessory sex glands contribute to the seminal plasma in jacks, their specific contributions are unknown. The bulbourethral glands are paired oval structures palpated off midline immediately after entering the anus, and the parenchyma has heterogeneous echogenicity on ultrasound (**Fig. 8**). Because of lumen collapse, small size, and proximity to the ampulla, the vesicular gland is the most challenging to appreciate on rectal palpation, but can be easily imaged

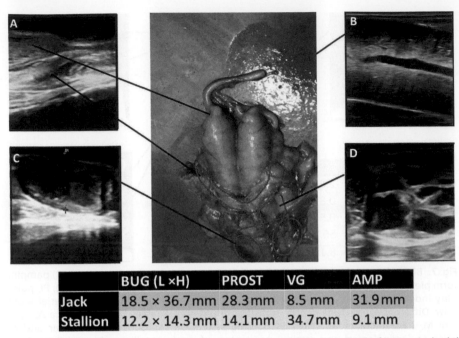

	BUG (L ×H)	PROST	VG	AMP
Jack	18.5 × 36.7 mm	28.3 mm	8.5 mm	31.9 mm
Stallion	12.2 × 14.3 mm	14.1 mm	34.7 mm	9.1 mm

Fig. 8. Ultrasonographic and gross images of the accessory sex glands from a jack. (*A*) Ampulla (AMP) and vesicular gland (VG); (*B*) longitudinal diameter of AMP; (*C*) longitudinal view of the bulbourethral gland (BUG); and (*D*) longitudinal prostate (PROST) view. The table displays measures for accessory sex glands in jacks (*top row*) and stallions (*bottom row*). H, height; L, length. ([Table] Data for stallions extracted from Pozor MA, McDonnell SM. Ultrasonographic measurements of accessory sex glands, ampullae, and urethra of normal stallions of various size types. *Theriogenology.* 2002; 58(7):1425-33.)

via transrectal ultrasound, particularly after teasing. The prostate gland can be felt as a bulging structure at midline caudal to the ampulla; it has heterogeneous parenchyma as it has intermingled anechoic areas of glandular tissue even before sexual stimulation (see **Fig. 8**).

Reproductive endocrinology is poorly understood in donkeys. One report involving 5 Amiata donkeys described the first appearance of sperm in the ejaculate at 18.7 months of age.[44] Another study involving 6 small-frame donkeys concluded that there were no apparent seasonal variations in semen quality;[45] however, these findings may differ in temperate climates. The authors' experience in the midwestern United States suggests that is an increase in semen volume and sperm morphologic defects and a reduction in sperm motility in the spring and summer in comparison with the fall (I.F. Canisso and R. Ellerbrock, 2014–2019).

Semen Collection and Evaluation

Jacks can be collected similarly to stallions; however, longer teasing times should be allowed for jacks.[32,46] It should be expected that a semen collection from a jack can take up to 30 to 60 minutes, with younger jacks slower than mature jacks.[46] Jacks can be trained to collect on a dummy mount, off a jenny, off a mare, or via ground collection (**Fig. 9**). Some jacks may allow multiple collections before losing interest. A previous review provides in-depth information on reproductive management of jacks.[32,47]

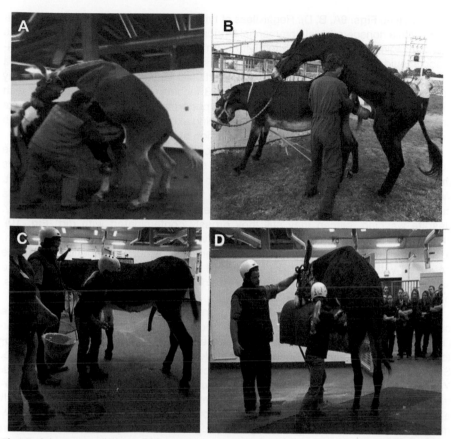

Fig. 9. (*A*) Mammoth jack collected with a Missouri artificial vagina mounting an estrus mare; (*B*) Catalan jack collected with a Hannover artificial vagina mounting an estrus jenny; (*C*) penis washing before semen collection; (*D*) jack collected with a Missouri artificial vagina while mounting the phantom.

In donkeys, chemical induction of ejaculation was unsuccessful using oral imipramine (3 mg/kg) followed by xylazine (0.66 mg/kg, IV), or a single dose of butorphanol (0.02 mg/kg, IV) and xylazine (0.33 mg/kg, IV).[48] A second study involving 55 donkeys evaluated combinations of imipramine (2 or 3 mg/kg, orally) followed by xylazine (0.44 , 0.66, or 0.7 mg/kg) 1 or 2 hours later and concluded that, although 74.5% of the animals presented arousal, only 1 animal ejaculated 38 minutes after xylazine injection.[49] Additional studies are needed to optimize dosages and protocols for donkeys.

The authors have used prostaglandin F2α (PGF2α) analogs (dinoprost [2.5–5 mg/ intramuscularly (IM) or sodium cloprostenol [125–250 µg/IM]) as an ancillary method to promote erection if thorough teasing fails.[32] Although donkeys may show side effects, such as sweating and leg trembling after PGF2α administration, this does not appear to affect the donkey's balance, ability to expose the penis, achieve an erection, or mount the female or phantom.

Donkey jacks can be collected with any type of artificial horse vagina. The authors typically use the Missouri type and rigid types such as the Hannover, Colorado, or

Botucatu (see **Figs. 9**A, B, D). Regardless of type, the artificial vagina should be lubricated with a nonspermicidal commercial lubricant. Missouri, Hannover, and Botucatu artificial vaginas are typically loaded with warm water at 51°C to 55°C, whereas Colorado should be filled at 55°C to 60°C. Whereas most donkeys can be collected with a "regular" length (45–50 cm, 18–22 inches) artificial vagina, miniature donkeys may need shorter artificial vaginas of ~30 cm (13 inches). Filters can be coupled with the collection bottle, or semen filtration can be performed after collection. Clean gauze can be used to filter semen in donkeys producing excessive amounts of gel, although the gel fraction is present in a smaller proportion of donkeys than stallions.[32,45,46]

The jack's penis should be washed before collection or natural cover to decrease contaminants, such as debris and bacteria in semen (see **Fig. 9**C). For shy donkeys that lose an erection easily, the penis can be washed after letting the jack mount. When training shy donkeys, it is best to wash the penis with wet cotton and avoid a cup or hose, as water splashing makes the donkey lose interest. Occasionally, despite washing, semen may still look grossly contaminated with dirt (**Fig. 10**). Normal gross appearance of donkey semen varies from slightly gray, to yellowish, to whitish, and the slightly yellow-tinged semen is a normal variation not to be confused with urospermia or pyospermia. If semen is heavily contaminated, the sample should be discarded, the jack washed again, and collected in 1 or 2 hours, or the next day when possible.

After collection, semen is processed similarly to stallions. Gel-free semen volume can be assessed by direct measurement, or more accurately by weighting the semen (1 mL = ~1 g). Sperm concentration is assessed with a hemocytometer, spectrophotometer, or nucleocounter (ChemoMetec, Lillerød, Denmark) using horse settings. Sperm concentration and the total number of cells are higher in donkeys than horses. Younger donkeys tend to produce ejaculates with lower volume and higher concentrations than older jacks.[46] Sperm motility parameters can be subjectively assessed with a standard optical microscope or with a computer-assisted sperm analyzer. Donkey motility parameters including velocity and progressive motility are also higher than stallions.[50,51] Jacks often have ejaculates containing 300 to 400 million sperm/mL, with 80% to 90% of total and progressive sperm motility. Young donkeys tend to produce gel-free ejaculates of ~30 to 50 mL, and older donkeys tend to produce gel-free ejaculates of ~60 to 90 mL.

Sperm morphology is typically assessed as part of a pre-purchase examination or infertility/subfertility evaluation.[50] Most donkeys have ≤15% morphologic defects, and although morphology is rarely linked with infertility in donkeys,[50] 1

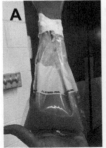
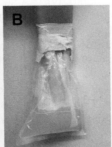
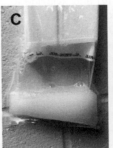
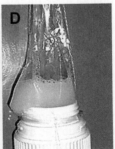

Fig. 10. Donkey semen gross appearance. (*A*) Grossly contaminated semen, despite extensive washing before collection in a sexually rested jack; (*B–D*) normal appearance of donkey semen.

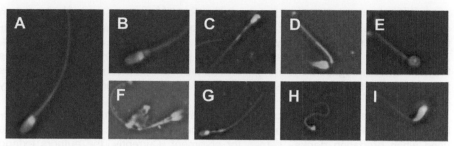

Fig. 11. Donkey sperm morphology. (*A*) Normal; (*B*) proximal protoplasmatic droplet; (*C–E*) abnormal sperm heads; (*F*) double sperm head; (*G*) distal protoplasmatic droplet; (*H, I*) malformed sperm heads.

infertile donkey was described to have oligospermia, and asthenozoospermia with proximal droplets.[52] Morphology can be performed with a wet-mount preparation with semen fixed in temperature-matched buffered formalin, or dry-mount preparation where smears are stained with eosin-nigrosin, Karras, or Romanoswsky methods.[50,52–54] In addition, a new system is available that heats sperms to 41°C, which immobilizes them so morphology can be assessed without staining using gentle pressure and a software (ISAS Trumoph Proiser, Valencia, Spain) (**Fig. 11**). The authors prefer to report sperm morphologic defects according to the type and region of the sperm; however, there are many ways to classify sperm abnormalities (eg, primary and secondary defects, major and minor defects, compensatory and noncompensatory).[50,53]

SEMEN COOLING AND SHIPPING

Donkey semen can be cooled and shipped in passive cooling semen containers, such as the Equitainer (Hamilton Thorne, Inc., Beverly, MA), Styrofoam semen boxes, and other devices (eg, Botubox, Botutainer Botupharma, Scottsdale, AZ). Equitainers and similar devices are preferred over Styrofoam boxes in regions with extreme weather conditions, because they provide good insolation and proper cooling. Many equine extenders successfully preserve donkey semen at 4°C, including ultra-high temperature pasteurized skimmed milk,[55] Kenney's extender,[56,57] INRA82

Table 3				
Pregnancy rates in jennies inseminated every 48 h until ovulation with fresh or cooled donkey semen				
	Breeding Dose			
Semen Type	**(Million/mL)**	**Vol. (mL)**	**Extenders**	**Fertility**
Fresh[55]	400[a]	10	Skimmed milk	6/7 (86%)
Cooled[55]	200[a]	10		9/20 (45%)
	460[a]	4		7/9 (78%)
	460[a]	4	INRA82 + 2% egg yolk	5/8 (64%)
Fresh[62]	500[b]	Extended 1:2	INRA96	30/60 (50%)
Fresh[61]	500[a]	15		6/15 (40%)
	1000[a]	15	Botusemen	11/15 (73%)
Fresh[60]	800[b]	15	INRA96	25/31 (81%)

[a] Denotes total sperm number regardless of motility.
[b] Denotes progressive motile sperms.

alone,[55,58] or with 2% of egg yolk added,[58] INRA96,[58–60] Botusemen,[61] and Baken extender (3% or 10% egg yolk)[57] (**Table 3**). Removal of seminal plasma by centrifugation can also increase the longevity of donkey semen on cooled storage;[63] however, adding 2% egg yolk to milk-based or to milk protein-based extenders eliminates the need for centrifugation. It is thought that donkey seminal plasma contains proteins that remove cholesterol from the plasma membrane, which reduces sperm longevity during cooling.

Until optimal extension practices for donkey semen are determined, horse guidelines (25–50 million sperm/mL and at least 1 part semen to 3 parts extender) are used when preparing donkey semen for shipment. Currently, the authors extend jack semen in INRA 96 containing 2% egg yolk to a concentration of 25 to 50 million/mL, and ship semen in an Equitainer or commercial Styrofoam equine semen container. Alternatively, semen be extended with a skim milk-based extender, centrifuged ($600g \times 15$ min if no cushion or $1000g \times 20$ min with 1 mL of cushion solution), and the pellet then resuspended in extender to 50 to 100 million/mL.

Although studies have used different breeding doses and volumes (see **Table 3**), it seems that better conception rates can be obtained when jennies are bred with at least 1 billion progressive motile sperm.[61] In the authors' practice, mares and jennies are bred with 2 billion progressive motile sperm, the uterus is flushed 6 hours post-breeding, and they are treated with ecbolics to aid uterine evacuation.[64] Barren mares or jennies with signs of endometritis (intrauterine fluid accumulation or infertility despite optimal breeding management with fertile semen) may require additional treatment. Artificial insemination of mares with fresh jack semen results in conception rates varying from 40% to 80%.[55,61,65]

SEMEN FREEZING

Protocols used to process donkey semen for freezing have been adapted from stallions. Egg yolk-based extenders such as lactose-EDTA (10%), sucrose-yolk (10%), lactose-EDTA (20%) and Botucrio (20%) have been widely used to freeze to donkey semen,[53,61,66] and milk-based or sodium caseinate milk-based extenders have also been used with some success.[55,67] For the University of Illinois Urbana-Champaign's donkey semen freezing program, semen is collected and processed as described above. The gel-free semen fraction is extended 1:1 when raw concentration is ≤200 million sperm/mL, 1:3 when raw semen concentration is >200 and ≤300 million sperm/mL, or 1:5 when sperm concentration is above 500 million sperm/mL. Raw semen is extended at 37°C (98.6°F) and then allowed to cool to room temperature at 20°C to 23°C. Lightly colored extenders are preferred (eg, BotuGold and Equi-Pro Cool Guard), as they allow for easy identification of the sperm pellet. After extension, semen is cushion-centrifuged (1 mL of cushion in 50 mL conical tube at $1000g$ for 20 min), the supernatant and cushion solutions are discarded, and the sperm pellet is resuspended in Botucrio.

Sperm concentration is determined with a nucleocounter and adjusted to 200 million sperm/mL. Extended semen is automatically loaded and sealed in 0.5-mL straws. Straws are cooled at 5°C for 20 minutes, then placed 4 to 6 cm above liquid nitrogen for 15 minutes or inserted into an automated freezing machine. Since optimal cooling and freezing curves have not been assessed for donkey semen, the authors use horse cooling and freezing curves (ie, 0.6°C–0.8°C/min and −30°C/min, respectively). A cooling curve of 0.25°C/min is successfully used by one of the authors at the Autonomous University of Barcelona (J.M.). Semen is thawed at 37°C for 30 to 60 seconds, or 42°C for 7 seconds, followed by 20 to 30 seconds at 37°C.

ENDOMETRIAL CULTURE, CYTOLOGY, AND BIOPSY IN JENNIES

Endometrial culture, cytology, and biopsy can be performed as pre-breeding and post-breeding screening tools, or as part of the workup following pregnancy loss. Cytologic findings may rule out false-positive or false-negative culture or indicate the presence and type of microorganisms involved (bacteria, presence of yeast, or hyphae). Culture and cytology can be performed with cotton-tip double-guarded swabs, cytobrushes, by small-volume uterine lavage, or by using endometrial biopsy for tissue-imprint culture and histology. Double-guarded swab and small-volume uterine lavage appear to be equivalent in jennies.[68]

Cytology of the healthy jenny estrus endometrium has a large amount of debris and the occasional presence of inflammatory cells. After insemination, jennies have a physiologic post-breeding inflammatory response marked by massive infiltration of neutrophils and eosinophils in the uterine lumen (**Fig. 12**), particularly with frozen semen.[67,68] Persistently high inflammatory cell counts in the uterine cytology are presumably associated with endometritis. Although cutoffs for physiologic versus persistent (pathologic) post-breeding inflammatory response in jennies have not been determined, the suggested cutoffs in mares are 48 to 96 hours.[64] In mares, eosinophils are released into the endometrium in response to fungal endometritis, pneumouterus, or during anaphylactic responses, but are rarely seen post-breeding.[69,70] The role of eosinophils in the jenny inflammatory response remains to be determined.

A recent study using 16S rRNA sequencing of samples collected from the clitoral fossa, vestibule, vagina, and uterus of fertile and subfertile jennies showed that bacterial families were similar between the different segments sampled; however, fertile animals had fewer bacterial counts in the vagina and uterus, and subfertile animals had richer diversity and counts of *Enterobacteriaceae* in the uterus and vagina.[71] Subfertile animals also had anatomic abnormalities of the reproductive tract, such as poor vulvar conformation and cervical damage.

Endometrial biopsy can be used to assess inflammation and degenerative changes (eg, periglandular fibrosis). One slaughterhouse specimen study demonstrated that jennies graded as category I had negative aerobic cultures, and jennies in the remaining categories had positive cultures with bacterial agents (**Table 4**),[72] similar to mares.[73] As *Enterobacteriaceae*, the main bacterial group identified in the 16S rRNA sequencing study,[71] was underrepresented and *Staphylococcus* species were

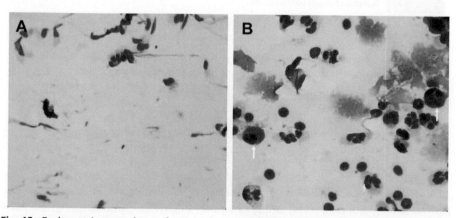

Fig. 12. Endometrium cytology of a jenny in estrus before (*A*) and after (*B*) artificial insemination. The arrows denote the eosinophils, and the symbol (⚡) a neutrophil.

Table 4
Aerobic culture of slaughterhouse specimens (n = 110) according to endometrial classification and isolated infectious agents

Isolates		Endometrial Categories vs Number of Isolates			
Types	n	I	IIA	IIB	III
Staphylococcus aureus	23	0	11	7	5
Coagulase-negative staphylococci	19	0	8	5	6
Streptococcus zooepidemicus	33	0	5	11	17
Non-hemolytic streptococci	4	0	3	1	—
Corynebacterium spp	20	0	7	5	8
Micrococcus spp	5	0	3	1	1
Proteus spp, *E. coli*, or *Candida albicans*	6	0	—	2	4

Data from Sokkar SM, Hamouda MA, El-Rahman SM. Endometritis in she donkeys in Egypt. *J Vet Med B Infect Dis Vet Public Health*. 2001; 48(7):529-36.

overrepresented in the slaughterhouse study, it is possible that contamination happened during sampling. *Staphylococcus* is a rare cause of chronic endometritis in mares.[73] In mares, *Streptococcus zooepidemicus*, the most common cause of endometritis,[73] was the second most prevalent group isolated from donkeys (see **Table 4**).[72]

The healthy donkey endometrium has more neutrophils, eosinophils, and highly branched uterine glands than mares.[74] Because these features by default render a higher category on the Kenney and Doig (1986) classification,[74] adjustments may be necessary to better reflect jenny endometrium (**Fig. 13**).[68] Biopsy specimens with many degenerative changes (19%–26%) have a high percent of polymorphonuclear leukocytes (PMNs) compared with healthy jennies in estrus (1.5%), but a lower percent

Category	Description
I	Healthy endometrium
IIA	Inflammation (↑PMNs-including eosinophils) ↓fibrosis. (<2 glandular nests). Normal stratum compactum
IIB	Moderate inflammation & fibrosis (2-4 glandular nests, ↓peri-glandular fibroblasts layers). Moderate endothelium changes. ↓ stratum compactum.
III	↑Fibrosis (>4 glandular nests, ↑peri-glandular fibroblasts layers). Significant endometrium damage. Absence or damaged stratum compactum.

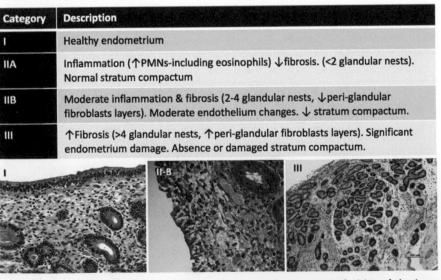

Fig. 13. Kenney and Doig (1986) biopsy categories adapted to particularities of the jenny. ([Table] *Data from* Silva JA, Papas M, Fernandes C, et al. Fibrosis in donkey endometrium: how can we interpret it? *Reprod Dom Anim* 2018; 53(52):84-99.)

of PMNs than jennies immediately after breeding (87.7%). Eosinophils increase during endometritis in jennies, and remain high in inflammatory and degenerative processes.[75]

In mares, endometrial degenerative changes are characterized by an increase in total collagen and collagen type 1 and a reduction in collagen type 3. In donkeys, such association does not seem to exist. In aged jennies with severely degenerated endometrium, the collagen remains under the basement membrane and surrounding endometrial glands.[76] The maintenance of collagen type 3 in aged jennies, despite large numbers of PMN infiltrating the endometrium, may explain why aged jennies are still able to conceive and carry pregnancies to term.

HORMONAL MANIPULATION OF THE ESTROUS CYCLE

PF2α and its analogs can be used to induce luteolysis and bring jennies or mules back into estrus (**Fig. 14**). There are minor to no adverse reactions (eg, colic-like, sweating, and loose manure) associated with dinoprost (5 mg), cloprostenol (0.075 mg), alphaprostol (3 mg), or luprostiol (7.5 mg). Dinoprost should be reduced to 2.5 mg when administered to very small jennies, because side effects have been noted in these animals with standard doses. Controversy exists regarding the earliest time-point that jennies can respond to a single PGF2α post-ovulation. Although it has been reported that jennies respond to cloprostenol administration 3 days post-ovulation by returning to estrus (**Table 5**),[35,77,78] clinical work seems to contradict these findings. In a preliminary study, 1 out of 6 jennies responded to alphaprostol administration 3 days post-ovulation.[36] These studies involved small numbers of jennies, and different types of PGF2α were used. In horses, the induction of luteolysis is not conducted before 5 days post-ovulation, and all jennies responded to a standard dose of PGF2α administered 5 or 10 days post-ovulation.[35]

Estrus duration in jennies varies based on time of the year, body condition score, and age. Induction of ovulation may be useful to narrow the ovulation window and facilitate breeding management or embryo transfer, and both human chorionic gonadotropin (hCG) and gonadotropin-releasing hormone (GnRH) agonists have been used to hasten ovulation (**Table 6**).[25,29,80]

The ideal follicular size for induction of ovulation follows a trend with body size, with small-frame jennies ovulating small follicles (28–32 mm), and larger frame jennies, such as the American Mammoth ovulating 40 to 44 mm follicles.[18] Jennies induced with either hCG or lecirelin with periovulatory follicles (36–40 mm) may also ovulate additional smaller follicles (30–35 mm).[25] In contrast, buserelin may not induce ovulation in jennies with periovulatory follicles averaging ∼33 mm.[29]

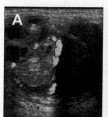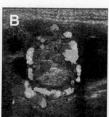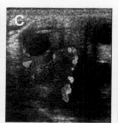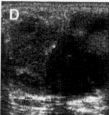

Fig. 14. Color Doppler of a 10-day-old donkey corpus luteum immediately before (*A*) and 1 h (*B*), 7 h (*C*), and 24 h (*D*) after administration of 5 mg of dinoprost.

Table 5
Induction of luteolysis in jennies using prostaglandin F2α analogs

Drug	Dose (IM, mg)	Cycles (n)	Days after Ovulation at PGF2α	Estrus	Interval to Estrus (d) or P4 Decline
Dinoprost[18]	5	58	Undefined	44/58 (76%)	4.4 ± 1.6
Cloprostenol[77]	0.075	10	3	10/10 (100%)	3.7 ± 1.2
		6	5	6/6 (100%)	3.5 ± 0.5
		5	7	5/5 (100%)	4.2 ± 1.3
		5	9	5/5 (100%)	4.6 ± 1.5
Cloprostenol[78]	0.075	22	3	21/22 (96%)	2.9 ± 0.5
Luprostiol[79]	7.5	169	Diestrus	NS	5 ca.
Alphaprostol[36]	3	6	3	1/6 (17%)	2[a]
		6	6	6/6 (100%)	4[a]

Abbreviations: IM, intramuscularly; NS, not specified.
[a] Progesterone declines to less than 1 ng/mL.

Whereas endometrial edema in the presence of at least 1 periovulatory follicle is a common criterion to induce ovulation in mares, endometrial edema is less pronounced in jennies. Waiting for a similar endometrial edema pattern in jennies may result in missed ovulations. Thus, teasing can be vital for determining when a jenny should be induced and bred. If no jack is available, jennies will show estrus to other jennies, horses, or male mules. Practical experience suggests that large donkeys should be induced with follicles ranging from 35 to 40 mm, the presence of mild endometrial edema, and positive teasing. Small-frame (ie, small standard) jennies will respond when follicles range from 32 to 35 mm. Very small (between mini- and small standard) jennies will respond when follicles are 28 to 32 mm in diameter.

ESTRUS SYNCHRONIZATION PROTOCOLS

Estrus synchronization reduces the number of reproductive examinations before breeding, and can be performed with PGF2α and its analogs alone,[18,81] in combination with sex steroid hormones,[18,82] and/or with GnRH[83] (**Fig. 15**, **Table 7**). The rationale for combining 2 injections of PGF2α is that jennies with a mature corpus luteum

Table 6
Induction of ovulation in jennies using hCG and GnRH agonists

Hormones	Number of Cycles	Dose (Route)	Ovulation Rates at 48 h after Induction	Induction-Ovulation Interval (h)
hCG[25]	27	2500 IU (IV)	23/25 (92%)	42.4 ± 13.0
Lecirelin[25]	43	100 µg (IV)	29/43 (67.4%)	42.8 ± 14.0
Control[25]	66	Control	6/66 (9.1%)	Not described
Buserelin[29]	103	3.3–0.4 mg (SC)	72/103 (69.9%)	49.1 ± 25.9
Control[29]	14	Control	2/14 (14.3%)	83.6 ± 31.9
Deslorelin[80]		0.8 mg (IM)	100% (30/30)	37.7 ± 2.3

Abbreviations: GnRH, gonadotropin-releasing hormone; hCG, human chorionic gonadotropin; IM, intramuscularly; IV, intravenously; SC, subcutaneously.

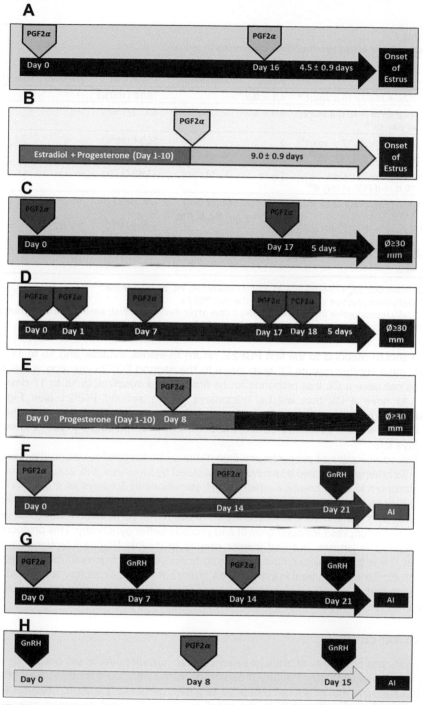

Fig. 15. Estrous synchronization protocols for jennies. (*A*) Double PGF2α 16 days apart[18]; (*B*) progesterone and 17β-estradiol followed by PGF2α on day 10[18]; (*C*) double PGF2α 17 days apart[18]; (*D*) multiple PGF2α administrations[81]; (*E*) progesterone for 10 days with PGF2α on day 8[81]; (*F*) double PGF2α-GnRH and timed artificial insemination (AI)[83]; (*G*) PGF2α-GnRH-PGF2α-GnRH and timed AI[83]; (*H*) GnRH-PGF2α-GnRH, and timed AI.[83]

Table 7
Summary of estrus synchronization protocols in jennies

Protocol	Days to Estrus	Induction of Ovulation	Jennies in Estrus (%)	Pregnancy Rate (%)
PGF2α + PGF2α 16 d apart[18]	4.5 ± 0.9	—	10/10 (100%)	—
P4+E2 daily × 10 d & PGF2α at day 10[18]	9.0 ± 0.9	—	8/11 (73%)	—
PGF2α + PGF2α 17 d apart[81]	5	—	56/81 (69%)	—
PGF2α: days 0, 1, 17, 18[81]	5	Ø≥30 mm[a]	21/74 (28%)	—
Intravaginal P4 device for 10 d and PGF at day 8[82]	12–16	Ø≥30 mm[b]	31/40 (77%)	—
PGF2α (day 0) + PGF2α (day 14)[83]	21	No CL and Ø≥28 mm[b]	6/9 (67%)	1/6 (17%)
PGF2α (day 0) + GnRH (day 7) + PGF2α (day 14)[83]			8/9 (89%)	5/8 (62%)
GnRH (day 0) +PGF2α (day 8)[83]			5/9 (55%)	3/5 (60%)

Abbreviations: E2, 17β-estradiol; Ø, follicle diameter; P4, progesterone.
[a] Daily reproductive ultrasound after the last PGF2α.
[b] Daily reproductive ultrasound starting 2 days after device removal; administration of buserelin acetate (0.4 mg, SC), and at 7 days the second PGF2α and AI with fresh extended semen.

(CL) should respond to the first PGF2α, return to estrus, ovulate, and 16 to 17 days later have another mature CL responsive to the second PGF2α injection. If the jenny does not have a CL that responds to the first PGF2α injection, in 16 to 17 days she should have a CL that will be responsive to the second PGF2α (see **Fig. 15**; **Table 7**). This protocol can be modified by administering GnRH 7 days after the first PGF2α to ensure ovulation, before the second PGF2α injection induces luteolysis 7 days later.[83]

The combination of progesterone (injectable or intravaginal releasing devices) and PGF2α attempts to mimic a luteal phase followed by luteolysis; this assumes that progesterone has a suppressive effect on LH secretions in donkeys as it does in cows (see **Fig. 15**; **Table 7**). In mares, progesterone alone does not inhibit LH and follicular growth, and progesterone is frequently administered in combination with estrogen for 10 days to suppress follicular growth and provide better synchrony. This protocol has been tried in jennies, but had inferior results to double PGF2α injections 16 days apart.[18] It is thus uncertain how sex steroid hormones affect gonadotropin secretions and follicular development in jennies. One study obtained satisfactory estrus synchronization with progesterone-releasing intravaginal devices; however, the presence of vaginitis and intrauterine fluid accumulation resulted in poor fertility.[84]

NATURAL COVER

Despite the popularity of artificial insemination, natural cover is still frequently used by the donkey industry. Pasture breeding of mares with jacks is often unsuccessful, because most mares are not receptive to jacks, particularly without previous exposure.[32,47,85] In-hand mating is the most suitable approach to breed mares with jacks. The mare can be physically restrained with a twitch, breeding hobbles, or restraining breeding stocks.[32,46,47] Chemical restraint may also be necessary to ensure safety of the jack and personnel involved. Regardless of restraint, the risks for accidents, such as the mare kicking the donkey or laying down during mounting is still of concern. Mares in-hand mated by donkeys typically have good fertility but may benefit from standard pre-breeding and post-breeding management with ecbolics and uterine lavage 6 hours post-breeding to reduce endometrium inflammation.[64]

Donkeys are nonharem territorial breeders, which is the opposite of stallions.[32,86] The jack delimits an area in the paddock, typically close to a water source and shade and food.[32] Jennies attracted to the jack's territory in pursuit for these essential elements are mated by the jack.[32] As estrus jennies are receptive to jacks, and less violent than mares, breeding accidents are extremely rare. Estrus jennies require minimal to no physical restraint during in-hand mating, or while being used as a mount during jack semen collection. Interestingly, jacks used to mate mares exclusively may refuse to breed jennies and may require training to mate jennies.[32]

Artificial Insemination

Jacks typically have excellent semen quality. Motility of fresh extended semen kept at room temperature (19°C–24°C) will only decrease ~10% over 24 hours.[56] Semen cooled at 4°C for 48 hours can have satisfactory fertility up to 48 hours after insemination[56,87] with motility decreasing to ~10% by 72 to 96 hours.[56]

Cryopreserved donkey semen has good post-thaw viability and motility,[53,67,88] and achieves conception rates of ~50% when used to inseminate mares,[53,65] but very poor conception rates (0%–28%)[53,55,65,89,90] when used to inseminate jennies. Authors have attempted to mitigate the deleterious effects of glycerol on donkey semen quality and jenny endometrial inflammatory response by re-diluting the semen after thawing with extender containing no glycerol, or by adding other cryoprotectants (glutamine, DMSO, dimethylformamide, and dimethylacetamide); however, conception rates remained poor.[65,90] The post-breeding inflammatory response is more pronounced in jennies than mares, and this acute endometrial inflammatory response may be responsible for poor conception rates when donkey frozen semen is used.[67,68]

Dexamethasone is used to modulate the post-breeding inflammatory response of susceptible mares.[64,91] As corticoids can induce laminitis, and many jennies are insulin-resistant and susceptible to laminitis, clinical use of dexamethasone in jennies is discouraged. Ketoprofen, a nonsteroidal selective COX-2 inhibitor, has also been administered in an attempt to modulate the endometrial inflammatory response with poor results.[68] Despite a downregulation in COX-2 expression, there was no decrease in PMN infiltration post-breeding in jennies treated with ketoprofen.[68] In contrast, in mares, ketoprofen, in combination with oxytocin, is reported to downregulate COX-2 and PMN infiltration.[92]

Removal of seminal plasma by centrifugation results in superior donkey semen quality for cooling and is required for semen freezing.[63] However, donkey seminal plasma reduces the inflammatory response of PMN after insemination by suppressing the PMN-sperm bound attachment in vitro,[63] decreases eosinophil numbers,[93] and seems to modulate the inflammatory response by inhibiting COX-2 gene expression in both the luminal epithelium and stratum compactum. Although no difference was seen in PMN proportion when post-thaw semen was resuspended in seminal plasma for artificial insemination, resuspension in seminal plasma tended to increase pregnancy rates in comparison with groups without seminal plasma.[67]

To maximize pregnancy rates it advised to perform deep horn inseminations with 1 billion total motile sperms,[94] or to resuspend frozen-thawed semen in seminal plasma to a final volume of 10 mL, and to flush the jenny's uterus 6 hours after breeding (**Table 8**).[67] Deep horn inseminations are appropriate for small breeding volumes of 2 to 4 mL. Larger volumes should be deposited into the uterine body.

Table 8
Pregnancy rates in jennies after insemination with fresh or cooled donkey semen

Type	Breeding Dose (Million Sperm)	Volume (mL)	Extender	Pregnancy Rate (%)
Fresh[55]	400	10	Skimmed milk	6/7 (86%)
Cooled[55]	200	10		9/20 (45%)
	460	4		7/9 (78%)
	460	4	INRA82 + 2% egg yolk	5/8 (64%)
Fresh[95]	500[a]	Extended 1:2	INRA96	30/60 (50%)
Fresh[61]	500	15	Botusemen	6/15 (40%)
	1 billion	15	Botusemen	11/15 (73%)
Fresh[60]	800[a]	15	INRA96	25/31 (81%)

Artificial insemination was performed every 48 h until ovulation.
[a] Progressively motile.

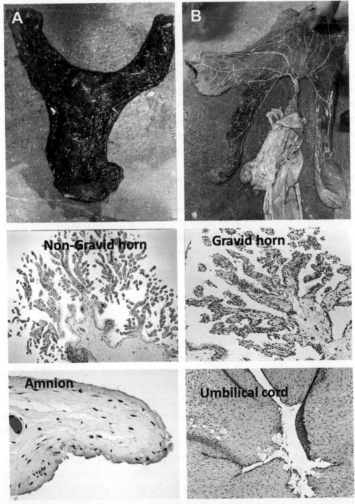

Fig. 16. Donkey fetal membranes. (*A*) Chorionic surface. (*B*) Allantoic surface of the chorioallantois.

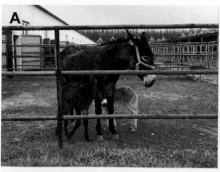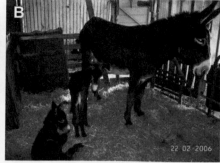

Fig. 17. Live twins without any complications in a Chinese Black jenny (*A*) and a Catalonian jenny (*B*).

Increasing the breeding dose perhaps saturates PMN and allows for more free sperm to enter the uterine tube. In addition, deep horn insemination may decrease the extent of PMN exposure *in utero*. However, these hypotheses have not been critically assessed.

Pregnancy

Gestation length is approximately 12 months (331–421 days).[2,19,34] As in all equids, donkey placentation is diffuse, epitheliochorial, and noninvasive (**Fig. 16**). The donkey chorioallantois has a higher concentration of microcotyledons per area when compared with the mare owing to extensive branching of the villi.[96] This feature makes the donkey placenta more efficient and may explain why it is relatively more common for jennies to deliver live twins than mares (**Fig. 17**).

Pregnancy diagnosis may be possible by transrectal ultrasonography starting 9 days after ovulation, although the chance of detecting a pregnancy so early is just

Table 9
First day of detection and diameter at first detection in 8 jenny conceptuses

Features	Days of Gestation (Range)	Diameter at First Detection (mm)
Detection of embryonic vesicle	10–14	4–8
Fixation of embryonic vesicle	13–21	16–29
Loss of spherical shape	17–23	26–31
Detection of embryo	18–24	3.5–5.5
Detection of heartbeat	20–26	—
Detection of allantoic sac	19–28	—
Detection of umbilical chord	31–47	—
Embryo at dorsal pole	21–44	—
Beginning descent of the embryo	31–42	—
Concluding descent of fetus	35–53	—
Detection of chest	54–64	14–20
Detection of stomach	60–71	—
Detection of eyeball	71–96	5.5–8
Detection of aorta	79–109	2.7–4.3

Data from Refs.[99–102]

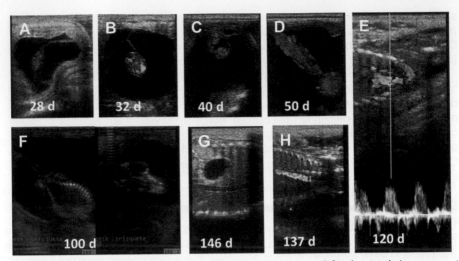

Fig. 18. Transrectal ultrasonographic images of embryonic and fetal growth in pregnant jennies. (*A* and *B*) The embryo is seen in the center of the embryonic vesicle (EV), with the B color Doppler showing a positive heartbeat. (*C*) The embryo is located dorsally in the EV. (*D*) A 50-day-old fetus with a positive blood flow in the umbilical cord. (*E*) Color Doppler identifying the fetal heart beat along with an M-mode ultrasound at the bottom of figure. (*F*) Cross-sectional images of the thorax (*left*) and the head (*right*); (*G*) fetal thorax and stomach; (*H*) aorta blood flow in a viable equine fetus.

9% to 33%. In clinical practice the first pregnancy diagnosis should be performed 12 to 15 days after ovulation. Maternal recognition of pregnancy in donkeys seems to be similar to horses, with the embryonic vesicle mobile in the uterine lumen until day 16 post-ovulation, at which point the embryonic vesicle fixes at the base of an uterine horn.[97–99] The embryonic vesicle starts losing its spherical shape around days 16 to 18, and the embryo proper appears at the ventral pole of the vesicle around days 19 to 21 (**Table 9**). Transrectal ultrasound features are summarized in **Table 9** for jenny conceptuses from pregnancy diagnosis until 110 days gestation and ultrasonographic images of pregnant jennies (from ~30 to ~150 days of gestation) are depicted in **Fig. 18**.

The embryonic vesicle grows approximately 3 mm/d from day 10 to day 18, 0.5 to 0.7 mm/d between days 17 and 31, and 1.6 to 2 mm/d until day 60.[98–100] This appearance of a growth plateau between 20 and 30 days gestation is due to developmental changes in the embryo and in its extraembryonic membranes during this period. A

Table 10 Monthly combined thickness of uterus and placenta in 17 Martina-Franca jennies		
Month	**Mean**	**Ranges**
6	8 ± 0.3	7.4–8
7	8.5 ± 0.3	7.9–8.9
8	8.9 ± 0.4	8.2–9.6
9	9.4 ± 0.4	8.8–10.1
10	10.3 ± 0.4	9.7–11
11	11 ± 0.4	10.5–11.9
12	11.7 ± 0.5	11–12.6

similar growth pattern in the horse has been attributed to an increasing uterine tone providing resistance to expansion of the vesicle in the cross-sectional plane.[103,104] Crown-rump growth of the embryo/fetus seems linear from its first appearance (3.5–5 mm) until day 90 (120 mm; last day it was possible to measure).[99,100]

While there have been no studies assessing the fetal heart rates in donkeys or hybrid fetuses under physiological and pathological conditions, one study reported a tendency for donkey fetal heart rate to increase the week before parturition.[99] Assessment of the caudal placental pole (eg, edema, intracervical fluid accumulation, and combined thickness of uterus and placenta [CTUP]) has been used to assess equine pregnancy for signs of ascending placentitis.[105] In the healthy pregnancy, the asinine CTUP grows linearly from the sixth month of pregnancy until foaling, with a substantial increase from the ninth to the twelfth month of pregnancy (**Table 10**).[106]

Progesterone and estradiol assays have been used as ancillary diagnostic tools to assess pregnancy well-being in mares;[105] however, in jennies such studies are lacking. Equine herpesviruses, donkey herpesviruses, equine viral arteritis, *Pseudomonas* spp, and *Salmonella* spp all have been described as cause of abortions in donkeys.[12] Although jennies are affected by similar horse pathogens, the true incidence of pregnancy loss in this species is currently unknown.

In the jenny, plasma progesterone concentrations increase between days 0 and 10 (from 0.9 to 19.9 ng/mL),[30] gradually decrease by day 30 (12–35 ng/mL), increase again between days 30 and 40, and then remain relatively constant (from 17 to 110 ng/mL) until a gradual decline from days 110 to 160.[30,107] Secretion of donkey chorionic gonadotrophin begins around the 40th day of pregnancy,[108] leading to secondary corpora lutea formation. From day 165 gestation until 15 days before parturition, mean progesterone concentrations range from approximately 4 to 7 ng/mL,[30,99] with an increase a few days before parturition.[30]

Plasma estrogen concentrations are higher than 100 ng/mL from day 90 until the month before parturition,[30] and concentrations are over 1000 ng/mL between weeks 21 and 33 of pregnancy.[99] Estrogens are excreted in high concentrations in the urine, and the Cuboni reaction, which is a fluorescent chemical reaction to detect estrogens in the urine, has been successfully used for pregnancy diagnosis in the jenny.[109] The reaction resulted in 83.87% true positives and 16.13% false negatives in pregnant jennies, and 86.96% true negatives and 13.04% false positives in nonpregnant jennies. Although the barium chloride test has also been used for pregnancy diagnosis, it is less reliable and is highly influenced by season.[109]

Although breeding mares to jacks results in good conception rates, there is a higher rate of early fetal loss in the first trimester of pregnancy when compared with mares bred by stallions. It has been suggested that this is a result of lower equine chorionic gonadotropin (eCG) production by mule pregnancies, thus decreasing the formation of accessory and secondary corpora lutea. The fetal genotype has a profound impact on eCG production, for instance, in mares carrying a mule conceptus, peak eCG concentrations are much lower and disappear much sooner from blood, than in a mare carrying a normal horse conceptus, conversely jennies carrying hinny pregnancies have much higher peak and prolonged duration of gonadotropin secretions than horse mares carrying horse pregnancies or donkeys carrying donkey pregnancies.[110] In contrast, jennies bred to stallions have much lower fertility than jennies or mares bred to jacks. It is unknown why there is such a discrepancy between these types of pregnancies.

While mules and hinnies are generally infertile, there have been reports in the literature of fertile female mules and hinnies producing and delivering fertile offspring when bred to stallions or jacks, resulting in mule foals or horse foals.[110] The haploid set of the horse (ie, 18 acrocentric autosomes) is so different to that of donkey (ie,

11 acrocentric autosomes), that meiosis by hybrid cells cannot proceed properly causing degeneration of germ cells. Interestingly, in 1 case of a fertile mule (diploid n = 63) carrying and delivering multiple offspring, the authors suggested that chromosome segregation during the proband meiosis favored the horse chromosomes to be present in the oocyte, that is, when the mule was sired by donkeys (diploid n = 62) the offspring were mules (diploid n = 63), whereas when the mule was bred by stallions (diploid n = 64), the offspring were normal fertile horses (diploid n = 64).[110] In contrast, there have been no reports of fertile male mules or hinnies, and generally they are known to not produce sperm owing to an inability to progress beyond meiosis I, but there is 1 report in the literature involving 1 male hinny capable of producing fully formed immotile sperm; however, it remains unknown whether male mules or hinnies are fertile.[111] Cyclic or acyclic mules can be excellent embryo recipients for donkey or horse embryos.[112] The authors administer 2 doses of PGF2α if the mule is cycling, followed by 3 to 4 consecutive days of 17β-estradiol (10 mg/animal), and then 1500 to 3000 mg of long-acting progesterone. After embryo transfer, the pregnancy can be maintained with weekly doses of long-acting progesterone. Cyclic mules can be administered PGF2α to induce luteolysis, and then have ovulation induced with hCG or GnRH agonists to be used as embryo recipients. Mules carrying horse or donkey embryos will foal similar to mares, and the placenta is grossly similar to mares and jennies.

PERIPARTUM

In the mare, mammary gland electrolytes and pH are used to predict imminent foaling.[113] In the days preceding parturition there are increased concentrations of calcium, magnesium, and potassium, and reduction in sodium and chloride, as well as a reduction in pH[113] In the jenny, calcium concentrations in mammary secretions increased starting 10 days before foaling, and reached 10.3 ± 0.65 mmol/L the day before foaling.[114]

First stage labor lasts between 20 and 135 minutes in jennies, and often goes undetected, although signs may include walking, frequent defecation and urination, flank

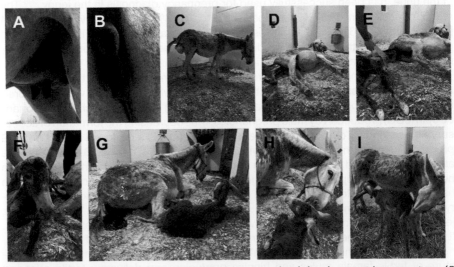

Fig. 19. Assisted parturition in a jenny. (A) Mammary gland development in prepartum. (B) Swollen vulva immediately before delivery. (C–G) Stage II of parturition. (H, I) Maternal-foal bounding.

watching, and the Flehmen response (**Fig. 19**). The second stage starts with allanto-chorion rupture, ends with foal expulsion, and generally lasts between 10 and 30 minutes. If no signs of a fetus are seen within 20 minutes of initiation of stage 2 labor, the jenny should be evaluated for a dystocia.

Mares carrying mule pregnancies display similar gestation length (~340 d), behavior, and duration of foaling stages to mares carrying and delivering horse pregnancies (I.F. Canisso, unpublished observations). However, 1 particularity, is that neonatal isoerythrolysis occurs in about 10% of the mule foals, which is significantly higher than horse foals.[115] Donkeys carry an antigen on their red blood cells denominated the donkey factor, and mules and hinnies as hybrids of donkeys also carry this antigen in their red blood cellsl.[115] Mares carrying and delivering mule pregnancies develop antibodies against this donkey factor.[115] During transfer of passive immunity, mule foals absorb these antibodies and can develop massive immune-mediated destruction of red blood cells as a consequence of attachment of specific antigen (the donkey factor) in their blood cells.[115] Thus, it is advisable that mule foals born from multiparous mares (which previously carried mule pregnancies) should be closely monitored for signs of neonatal isoerythrolysis in the first 3 days postpartum. In addition, mule foals born from mares with a history of having mule foals with neonatal isoerythrolysis should not be allowed to nurse in their dams for the first 48 hours postpartum to avoid transfer of passive immunity containing the antibodies against the donkey factor.

Donkeys are affected by similar causes observed in horses including lateral deviation of head and neck (**Fig. 20**), fetal monsters, and fetal malpostures;[12] however, the true incidence of the various causes of dystocias in donkeys is unknown. The general principles used to manage horse dystocias (assisted vaginal delivery, controlled vaginal delivery, fetotomy, and C-section) are applicable to donkeys. Donkeys are

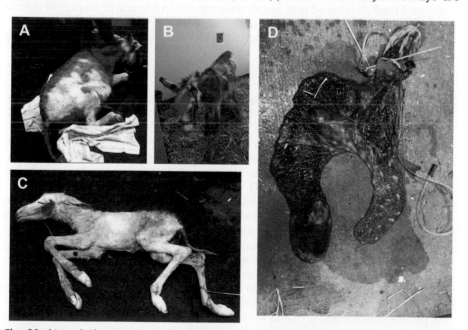

Fig. 20. (*A* and *B*) Jenny immediately before and after dystocia resolution. (*C*) Stillborn donkey foal immediately after delivery. (*D*) Placenta released with hydrocannulation of the umbilical cord.

prone to developing necrotic vaginitis after prolonged dystocias, and small amounts of topical ointment such as Quadritop (nystatin, neomycin sulfate, thiostrepton, and triamcinolone acetonide ointment) applied to the cervix and vagina may prevent cervical and vaginal adhesions (I.F. Canisso, personal observations).

The jenny usually passes the placenta 10 and 175 minutes after foaling.[116] Jennies are susceptible to the retained fetal membranes-metritis-laminitis complex similar to mares, and the condition can be exacerbated by the donkey's genetic predisposition to insulin resistance/metabolic syndrome. When faced with retained fetal membranes in donkeys, the authors use similar techniques to those used in horses,[117] including hydro-cannulation of the umbilical cord vessels (see **Fig. 20**), the Burns technique, and repeated doses of oxytocin. Uterine lavage can be performed with a large volume of tap water with added betadine and salt.[117] Ecbolics such as oxytocin (5–10 units, q 4–6 h, IM) and cloprostenol (125–250 μg q 12 h, IM), broad-spectrum antibiotics to control bacterial infection, and flunixin meglumine to prevent endotoxemia, are all recommended as part of the treatment of retained placenta and metritis (I.F. Canisso, personal observations).

Complete uterine involution in the jenny occurs around the 20th day postpartum.[27,60] The first ovulation postpartum occurs as early as day 9, with an average of 13 ± 2.5 days after parturition.[27,34,118] Up to 45.6% of Spanish jennies are acyclic during the first 20 days postpartum, probably owing to foal-heat suppression by unspecified environmental factors and by the newborn foal.[34] Silent postpartum estrus has been also described,[27] and seems to be more common during fall-winter foalings than spring-summer foalings (J. Miró, personal observations, 2014–2019). The first postpartum estrus results in lower pregnancy rates (45%–57%) compared with subsequent cycles (66%–81%).[34] Although parameters for foal-heat breeding have not been established for donkeys, the authors advise that jennies should not be bred on foal-heat if they: (1) retained fetal membranes more than 3 hours; (2) have poor uterine involution 7 days postpartum; (3) had dystocia; (4) developed metritis; (5) have urovagina and/or urometra; (6) have bruising in the vagina or vestibule; or (7) ovulate less than 10 days after foaling.

Embryo Transfer

Nonsurgical embryo flushing in donkeys is similar to the current technique in horses. The jenny uterus is flushed with 0.5 (maiden) to 1 L (multiparous) of medium at least 3 times for maximum embryo recovery.[33,62,95,119,120] Although not statistically significant, embryos recovered with lactated Ringer's solution and washed in equine holding media (EM Care Bodinco, the Netherlands) had pregnancy rates of 27.2% at 14 days, whereas embryos recovered in Dulbecco's phosphate solution resulted in only 7% pregnancies after embryo transfer (ET).

One main difference in the donkey transfer technique is that the vaginal part of the cervix is grabbed with 3 fingers and pulled backward, the tip of the gun blindly inserted in the cervical os, the sanitary sheath then broken, and the cervix manipulated to aid the transferring gun insertion and progression.[33] Manipulation of the cervix during donkey ET is necessary, because the jenny has a longer, smaller, and tighter cervix when compared with mares,[1,4] and administration of acepromazine (3.3 mg/100 kg/IV) to recipients before ET seems to aid in cervical relaxation.[33] Cervical manipulation is associated with PGF2α release, which may be followed by a decrease in progesterone plasma concentration,[119] and in turn affect luteal and embryonic survival after transfer. However, whereas sham transcervical ET 5 to 8 days after ovulation caused a transient PGF2α release in 2 of 4 jennies, there was no significant decrease in progesterone plasma concentration.[95]

Initial donkey ET attempts were disappointing when compared with those in mares. Despite recovery rates of 64%,[33,121] pregnancy rates 15 days after ET were extremely low, varying from 16.7% (with surgical transfer)[121] to 22.4% (nonsurgical transfer).[33] Studies exploring extra-specific pregnancies in the equid species by surgical transfers of horse embryos to donkey recipients and vice versa demonstrated that 63% and 67% were pregnant 40 days after ET, respectively, which was significantly better than previously reported with intraspecific ET. Concluding this "quest" investigating donkey embryo viability, embryos were nonsurgically transferred into synchronized recipients.[95] All 5 horse embryos transferred into donkey recipients resulted in 25-day pregnancies, whereas 50% of the donkey-in-horse (3/6) and donkey-in-donkey (6/12) ETs resulted in pregnancies at 25 days, a higher pregnancy rate than previously reported after donkey-in-donkey,[33] and comparable with donkey-in-horse[122] and horse-in-horse ET.[119] These findings were confirmed by others[123] who obtained a 45.4% pregnancy rate (5/11) transferring fresh 9-day-old donkey embryos to synchronized Pega donkey recipients.

These results suggest that the transcervical technique for ET was not the reason for the low pregnancy rates previously described in donkey recipients,[33,121] and that nonsurgical ET in donkeys can produce acceptable results, although increased pregnancy loss can occur when donkey embryos are transferred to mares.[122,124]

NUCLEAR TRANSFER

The first equid to be cloned was the first of the only 3 mules ever cloned. Clones were created using fibroblasts of a 45-day-old mule fetus and a mare's oocytes collected by ovary excision or transvaginal ultrasound-guided aspiration. Oocytes were then matured before the nuclear transfer. Metaphase II oocytes were denuded from the cumulus cells by hyaluronidase, the first polar body and metaphase plate were aspirated by an enucleation pipette, and then a disaggregated donor cell was aspirated and placed in the perivitelline space. Of 334 manipulated oocytes, 305 were transferred to recipient mares, resulting in 21 (6.9%) 14-day pregnancies. Only the embryos maintained and activated in the 3X/6X medium established pregnancies (5/113, 4.4%), only 3 of which resulted in the birth of live mules.[125–127]

REFERENCES

1. Renner-Martin TFP, Martin TFPR, Forstenpointner G, et al. Gross anatomy of the female genital organs of the domestic donkey (*Equus asinus* Linné, 1758). Anat Histol Embryol 2009;38:133–8.
2. Fielding D. Reproductive characteristics of the jenny donkey—*Equus asinus*: a review. Trop Anim Health Prod 1988;20:161–6.
3. Pugh DG. Donkey reproduction. AAEP Proceedings 2002;48:113–4.
4. Vendramini OM, Guintard C, Moreau J, et al. Cervix conformation: a first anatomical approach in Baudet du Poitou jenny asses. Anim Sci 1998;66:741–4.
5. Henry M, Figueiredo AE, Palhares MS, et al. Clinical and endocrine aspects of the oestrous cycle in donkeys (*Equus asinus*). J Reprod Fertil Suppl 1987;35: 297–303.
6. Fanti C. Il ciclo estrale nell'asina di Martina Franca: obsservazioni comportamentali ed ecografiche. Vet Prat Equina 2003;3:35–41.
7. Ginther OJ, Scraba ST, Bergfelt DR. Reproductive seasonality of the jenney. Theriogenology 1987;27:587–92.
8. Taberner E, Medrano A, Peña A, et al. Oestrus cycle characteristics and prediction of ovulation in Catalonian jennies. Theriogenology 2008;70:1489–97.

9. Quaresma M, Payan-Carreira R, Silva SR. Relationship between ultrasound measurements of body fat reserves and body condition score in female donkeys. Vet J 2013;197:329–34.

10. Lemma A, Bekana M, Schwartz HJ, et al. The effect of body condition on ovarian activity of free ranging tropical jennies (*Equus asinus*). J Vet Med A 2006;53:1–4.

11. Quaresma M, Payan-Carreira R. Characterization of the estrous cycle of asinina de Miranda jennies (*Equus asinus*). Theriogenology 2015;83:616–24.

12. Tibary A, Sghiri A, Bakkoury M. Reproductive patterns in donkeys. In: 9th World Equine Veterinary Congress Proceedings. Marrakech, Morocco, January 22–26, 2006. p. 311–9.

13. Gastal EL, Barros LO, Carneiro GF, et al. Follicular dynamics in mules. J Equine Vet Sci 2014;34:144 [abstract].

14. Díaz-Duran M, Zarco L, Boeta AM. Ovarian dynamics and estrous cycle length in the donkey (*Equus asinus*). Theriogenology 2017;103:1–8.

15. Vandeplassche GM, Wesson JA, Ginther OJ. Behavioral, follicular and gonadotropin changes during the estrous cycle in donkeys. Theriogenology 1981;16: 239–49.

16. Henry M, McDonnell SM, Lodi LD, et al. Pasture mating behaviour of donkeys (*Equus asinus*) at natural and induced oestrus. J Reprod Fertil Suppl 1991;44: 77–86.

17. Meira C, Ferreira JCP, Papa FO, et al. Study of the estrous cycle in donkeys (*Equus asinus*) using ultrasonography and plasma progesterone concentrations1. Biol Reprod 1995;52:403–10.

18. Blanchard TL, Taylor TS, Love CL. Estrous cycle characteristics and response to estrus synchronization in mammoth asses (*Equus asinus americanus*). Theriogenology 1999;52:827–34.

19. Crisci A, Panzani D, Rota A, et al. Ciclo ovarico dell"asina dell"Amiata: aspetti clinici e comportamentali. In: Secondo Convegno Nazionale sull'asino Proceedings. Palermo, Italy, September 21–24, 2006. p. 20–5.

20. Ginther OJ. Occurrence of anestrus, estrus, diestrus, and ovulation over a 12-month period in mares. Am J Vet Res 1974;35:1173–9.

21. Contri A, De Amicis I, Veronesi MC, et al. Effect of the season on some aspects of the estrous cycle in Martina Franca donkey. Theriogenology 2014;81:657–61.

22. Lemma A, Schwartz HJ, Bekana M. Application of ultrasonography in the study of the reproductive system of tropical jennies (shape *Equus asinus*). Trop Anim Health Prod 2006;38:267–74.

23. Quaresma M, Payan-Carreira R. Viability analyses of an endangered donkey breed: The case of the asinina de Miranda (*Equus asinus*). Anim Prod Sci 2015;55:1184–91.

24. Derar RI, Hussein HA. Ovarian follicular dynamics during the estrous cycle in jennies in upper Egypt. Vet Med Internet 2011;5:1–6.

25. Carluccio A, Panzani S, Tosi U, et al. Efficacy of hCG and GnRH for inducing ovulation in the jenny. Theriogenology 2007;68:914–9.

26. Trimeche A, Tainturier D. Echographic study of Poitou's jennies follicular kinetics during oestrus in spring and summer. Rev Med Vet (France) 1995;146:743–8.

27. Dadarwal D, Tandon SN, Purohit GN, et al. Ultrasonographic evaluation of uterine involution and postpartum follicular dynamics in French jennies (*Equus asinus*). Theriogenology 2004;62:257–64.

28. Quaresma M, Silva SR, Payan-Carreira R. Reproductive patterns in the non-breeding season in asinina de Miranda jennies. Reprod Domest Anim 2015; 50(5):784–92.

29. Camillo F, Vannozzi I, Tesi M, et al. Induction of ovulation with buserelin in jennies: in search of the minimum effective dose. Anim Reprod Sci 2014;151: 56–60.

30. Meira C, Ferreira JC, Papa FO, et al. Ovarian activity and plasma concentrations of progesterone and estradiol during pregnancy in jennies. Theriogenology 1998;49:1465–73.

31. Miragaya MH, Neild DM, Alonso AE. A review of reproductive biology and bio-technologies in donkeys. J Equine Vet Sci 2018;65:55–61.

32. Canisso IF, Davies Morel MCG, McDonnell S. Strategies for the management of donkey jacks in intensive breeding systems. Equine Vet Educ 2009;21:652–9.

33. Camillo F, Panzani D, Scollo C, et al. Embryo recovery rate and recipients' pregnancy rate after nonsurgical embryo transfer in donkeys. Theriogenology 2010; 73:959–65.

34. Galisteo J, Perez-Marin CC. Factors affecting gestation length and estrus cycle characteristics in Spanish donkey breeds reared in southern Spain. Theriogenology 2010;74:443–50.

35. Miró J, Vilés K, Anglada O, et al. Color Doppler provides a reliable and rapid means of monitoring luteolysis in female donkeys. Theriogenology 2015;83: 485–90.

36. Panzani D, Tardella M, Govoni N, et al. Effect of the administration of alfaprostol 3 or 6 days after ovulation in jennies: ultrasonographic characteristic of corpora lutea and serum progesterone concentration. Theriogenology 2018;121:175–80.

37. Canisso IF, Carvalho GR, Silva EC, et al. Some biometric aspects of the external genital tract from donkey Pêga breed semen donors. Ciencia Rural 2009;39: 2556–62.

38. Quartuccio M, Marino G, Taormina A, et al. Seminal characteristics and sexual behaviour in Ragusano donkeys (Equus asinus) during semen collection on the ground. Large Anim Rev 2011;17:151–5.

39. Neves ES, Chiarini-Garcia H, França LR. Comparative testis morphometry and seminiferous epithelium cycle length in donkeys and mules. Biol Reprod 2002;67:247–55.

40. Noronha PB, Neto JP, Borelli V. Aspectos morfológicos do funículo espermático de jumentos (Equus asinus—Linnaeus, 1758) da raça Pêga. Braz J Vet Res Anim Sci 2001;38:209–13.

41. Gacem S, Papas M, Catalan J, et al. Reproductive ultrasonography in Catalonian donkey. Reprod Domest Anim 2018;53:136 (abstract).

42. Abou-Elhamd AS, Salem AO, Selim AA. Histological and histochemical studies on the ampulla of the deferent duct of donkey (Equus asinus). J Adv Vet Res 2012;2:261–70.

43. Segabinazzi LG, Silva LF, Okada C, et al. Plugged ampullae in a donkey stallion (Equus asinus). J Equine Vet Sci 2018;63:24–6.

44. Rota A, Sgorbini M, Panzani D, et al. Effect of housing system on reproductive behaviour and on some endocrinological and seminal parameters of donkey stallions. Reprod Domest Anim 2018;53:40–7.

45. Gastal MO, Henry M, Beker AR, et al. Effect of ejaculation frequency and season on donkey jack semen. Theriogenology 1997;47:627–38.

46. Canisso IF, Carvalho GR, Morel MCGD, et al. Sexual behavior and ejaculate characteristics in Pêga donkeys (Equus asinus) mounting estrous horse mares (Equus caballus). Theriogenology 2010;73:56–63.

47. Canisso IF, Coutinho da Silva MA, Davies Morel MCG et al. How to manage jacks to breed mares. In: AAEP Proceedings. Las Vegas, Nevada, USA, December 5–9, 2009; 55:342–8.

48. Mráčková M, Hodinová K, Vyvial M, et al. Failure of pharmacologically-induced ejaculation in donkeys (Equus asinus) under field conditions: a test of two different treatment protocols. Israel J Vet Med 2017;72:35–8.

49. Sghiri A, AT, Idrissi El R. Behavioral response to imipramine/xylazine treatment in jackass. In: 9th World Equine Veterinary Congress Proceedings. Marrakech, Morocco, January 22–26, 2006. 348–50.

50. Canisso IF, Souza FA, de Carvalho GR, et al. Alguns aspectos fundamentais do exame clínico andrológico de jumentos (Equus asinus). Rev Bras Reprod Anim 2008;32:233–9.

51. Miró J, Lobo V, Quintero-Moreno A, et al. Sperm motility patterns and metabolism in Catalonian donkey semen. Theriogenology 2005;63:1706–16.

52. Crespilho AM, da Cruz Landim-Alvarenga F. Infertilidade associada a defeito microtubular dos espermatozóides de jumento (Equus asinus) avaliados por microscopia eletrônica de transmissão. Ciencia Rural 2006;36:1507–10.

53. Canisso IF, Carvalho GR, Morel MD, et al. Seminal parameters and field fertility of cryopreserved donkey jack semen after insemination of horse mares. Equine Vet J 2011;43:179–83.

54. Ortiz I, Dorado J, Acha D, et al. Colloid single-layer centrifugation improves post-thaw donkey (Equus asinus) sperm quality and is related to ejaculate freezability. Reprod Fertil Dev 2015;27:332–40.

55. Vidament M, Vincent P, Martin F-X, et al. Differences in ability of jennies and mares to conceive with cooled and frozen semen containing glycerol or not. Anim Reprod Sci 2009;112:22–35.

56. Santos GF, Henry M, Sampaio IBM, et al. Effect of cooling system and rate of cooling on sperm quality of donkey semen preserved at 5°C. Biol Reprod 1995;52:761–7.

57. Cottorello ACP, Amancio RC, Henry M, et al. Effect of storage temperature and extenders on "in vitro" activity of donkey spermatozoa. Theriogenology 2002;58: 325–8.

58. Rota A, Magelli C, Panzani D, et al. Effect of extender, centrifugation and removal of seminal plasma on cooled-preserved Amiata donkey spermatozoa. Theriogenology 2008;69:176–85.

59. Contri A, De Amicis I, Veronesi MC, et al. Efficiency of different extenders on cooled semen collected during long and short day length seasons in Martina Franca donkey. Anim Reprod Sci 2010;120:136–41.

60. Carluccio A, Gloria A, Robbe D, et al. Reproductive characteristics of foal heat in female donkeys. Animal 2017;11:461–5.

61. de Oliveira JV, Oliveira PV, Melo e Oña CM, et al. Strategies to improve the fertility of fresh and frozen donkey semen. Theriogenology 2016;85:1267–73.

62. Panzani D, Rota A, Romano C, et al. Birth of the first donkey foals after transfer of vitrified embryos. J Equine Vet Sci 2012;32:419 (abstract).

63. Miró J, Taberner E, Rivera M, et al. Effects of dilution and centrifugation on the survival of spermatozoa and the structure of motile sperm cell subpopulations in refrigerated Catalonian donkey semen. Theriogenology 2009;72:1017–22.

64. Canisso IF, Stewart J, Coutinho da Silva MA. Endometritis: managing persistent post-breeding endometritis. Vet Clin North Am Equine Pract 2016;32:465–80.

65. Oliveira JV, Alvarenga MAU, Melo CM, et al. Effect of cryoprotectant on donkey semen freezability and fertility. Anim Reprod Sci 2006;94:82–4.

66. Canisso IF, Souza FA, Escobar JMO, et al. Freezing of donkey semen (*Equus asinus*). Rev Invest Vet Peru 2008;19:113–25.

67. Rota A, Panzani D, Sabatini C, et al. Donkey jack (*Equus asinus*) semen cryo-preservation: studies of seminal parameters, post breeding inflammatory response, and fertility in donkey jennies. Theriogenology 2012;78:1846–54.

68. Vilés K, Rabanal R, Rodríguez-Prado M, et al. Effect of ketoprofen treatment on the uterine inflammatory response after AI of jennies with frozen semen. Theriogenology 2013;79:1019–26.

69. Slusher SH, Freeman KP, Roszel JF. Eosinophils in equine uterine cytology and histology specimens. J Am Vet Med Assoc 1984;184:665–70.

70. Snider TA, Sepoy C, Holyoak GR. Equine endometrial biopsy reviewed: observation, interpretation, and application of histopathologic data. Theriogenology 2011;75:1567–81.

71. Maschio C, Busalleu E, Mirò J. Preliminary study on the microbiota of the reproductive tract of Catalan jennies. Reprod Domest Anim 2017;52:95 (abstract).

72. Sokkar SM, Hamouda MA, El-Rahman SM. Endometritis in she donkeys in Egypt. J Vet Med B Infect Dis Vet Public Health 2001;48:529–36.

73. Canisso IF, Coutinho da Silva MA. Bacterial endometritis. In: Sprayberry KA, Robinson NE, editors. Robinsons current therapy in equine medicine. 7th edition. Philadelphia: Elsevier; 2015. p. p683–8.

74. Abd-Elnaeim MM. Morphological characteristics of the donkey (*Equus asinus*) uterus during estrus: light, scanning and transmission electron microscopic study. J Agric Vet Sci 2008;2:47–57.

75. Papas M, Noto F, Bonilla S, et al. Histological findings from endometrium biopsies. Reprod Domest Anim 2001;52:121 (abstract).

76. Silva JA, Papas M, Fernandes C, et al. Fibrosis in donkey endometrium: how can we interpret it? Reprod Domest Anim 2018;53:84 (abstract).

77. Carluccio A, Tosi U, Contri A, et al. Corpus luteum sensitivity to PGF2α administration in the Martina Franca jenny. Vet Res 2006;30:171–3.

78. Carluccio A, Panzani S, Contri A, et al. Luteal function in jennies following PGF2α treatment 3 days after ovulation. Theriogenology 2008;70:121–5.

79. Perez-Marin CC, Galisteo I, Perez-Rico A, et al. Effects of breed, age, season, and multiple ovulations on cyclic, PGF2α-induced, and postpartum estrus characteristics in Spanish jennies. Theriogenology 2016;85.1045–52.

80. Yang F, Ma J, Yang W, et al. Precise ovulation control using slow-releasing GnRH analog in jennies. In: First International Symposium on Donkey Science, proceedings. Donge, Shandong, China: 2017. p. 221–4.

81. Zeng S, Weigang Y, Shuaishuai W, et al. Technological protocol in reproductive management of intensive raising donkeys. In: First International Symposium on Donkey Science Proceedings. 2017. p. 159–70.

82. Zhou J, Cui D, Liu Q, et al. Preliminary results of synchronization of estrus and ovulation in jennies. J Equine Vet Sci 2018;66 (abstract).

83. Fanelli D, Tesi M, Rota A, et al. Studies on the use of prostaglandin F2α and gonadotropin-releasing hormone analogs for timed artificial insemination in jennies. J Equine Vet Sci 2019;74:36–41.

84. Miró J, Torrens M, Gimenez S, et al. Oestrus induction and synchronization by PRID™ in Balear jennies. Reprod Domest Anim 2010;45:94 (abstract).

85. Lodi LD, Henry M, Paranhos da Costa MJR. Behavior of donkey jacks (*Equus asinus*) breeding horse mares (*Equus caballus*) at pasture. Biol Reprod 1995;52:591–8.

86. Canisso IF, McDonnell SM. Donkey breeding behavior with an emphasis on the Pega breed. In: Matthews NS, Taylor ML, editors. Veterinary care of donkeys. Ithaca (NY). Available at: http://www.ivis.org/advances/Matthews/canisso/chapter.asp. Accessed June 15, 2019.

87. Rota A, Magelli C, Impeduglia R, et al. Effect of extender and method of preservation on motility of cooled stallion spermatozoa. Anim Reprod Sci 2005;89:281–3.

88. Flores E, Taberner E, Rivera MM, et al. Effects of freezing/thawing on motile sperm subpopulations of boar and donkey ejaculates. Theriogenology 2008;70:936–45.

89. Glatzel P, Houssain El K, Tibary A. Stallions and jackasses of Moroccan horse and mule breeds. Initial results using fluid and frozen semen in mule breeding. Berl Munch Tierarztl Wochenschr 1981;94:445–8.

90. Trimeche A, Renard P, Le Lannou D, et al. Improvement of motility of post-thaw Poitou jackass sperm using glutamine. Theriogenology 1996;45:1015–27.

91. Bucca S, Carli A, Buckley T, et al. The use of dexamethasone administered to mares at breeding time in the modulation of persistent mating induced endometritis. Theriogenology 2008;70:1093–100.

92. Aurich C, Rojer H, Walter I. Treatment of estrous mares with the non-steroidal anti-inflammatory drug vedaprofen reduces the inflammatory response of the endometrium to insemination. Anim Reprod Sci 2010;121:104.

93. Vilés K, Rabanal R, Rodríguez-Prado M, et al. Influence of seminal plasma on leucocyte migration and amount of COX-2 protein in the jenny endometrium after insemination with frozen-thawed semen. Anim Reprod Sci 2013;143:57–63.

94. Oliveira J, Papa F, Melo-Oña C, et al. New procedures to freeze donkey semen and its influence on mares and jennies fertility. J Equine Vet Sci 2012;32:503–4.

95. Panzani D, Rota A, Crisci A, et al. Embryo quality and transcervical technique are not the limiting factors in donkey embryo transfer outcome. Theriogenology 2012;77:563–9.

96. Veronesi MC, Villani M, Wilsher S, et al. A comparative stereological study of the term placenta in the donkey, pony and thoroughbred. Theriogenology 2010;74:627–31.

97. Bessent C, Ginther OJ. Comparison of early conceptus mobility between mares and jennies. Theriogenology 1988;29:913–20.

98. Meira C, Ferreira JCP, Papa FO, et al. Ultrasonographic evaluation of the conceptus from days 10 to 60 of pregnancy in jennies. Theriogenology 1998;49:1475–82.

99. Crisci A, Rota A, Panzani D, et al. Clinical, ultrasonographic, and endocrinological studies on donkey pregnancy. Theriogenology 2014;81:275–83.

100. Gastal EL, Santos GF, Henry M, et al. Embryonic and early foetal development in donkeys. Equine Vet J 1993;25:10–3.

101. Carluccio A, Villani M, Contri A, et al. Rilievi ecografici della gravidanza precoce nell' asina di Martina Franca. Pract Equina 2005;16:31–5.

102. Roberts BN, Gilbert RO, Bergfelt DR, et al. The early conceptus in Caribbean jennies. J Equine Vet Sci 2018;66:208–9.

103. Ginther OJ. Fixation and orientation of the early equine conceptus. Theriogenology 1983;19:613–23.

104. Palmer E, Driancourt MA. Use of ultrasonic echography in equine gynecology. Theriogenology 1980;13:203–16.

105. Canisso IF, Ball BA, Erol E et al. Comprehensive review on equine placentitis. In: AAEP Proceedings. Las Vegas Nevada, USA, December 5–9, 2015; 61. p. 490–509.

106. Carluccio A, Noto F, Parrillo S, et al. Transrectal ultrasonographic evaluation of combined utero-placental thickness during the last half of pregnancy in Martina Franca donkeys. Theriogenology 2016;86:2296–301.

107. Hoffmann B, Bernhardt AW, Failing K, et al. Profiles of estrone, estrone sulfate and progesterone in donkey (*Equus asinus*) mares during pregnancy. Tierarztl Prax Ausg G Grosstiere Nutztiere 2014;42:32–9 [in German].

108. Urwin VE, Allen WR. Pituitary and chorionic gonadotrophic control of ovarian function during early pregnancy in equids. J Reprod Fertil Suppl 1982;32: 371–81.

109. Kubátová A, Fedorova T, Skálová I, et al. Non-invasive pregnancy diagnosis from urine by the Cuboni reaction and the barium chloride test in donkeys (*Equus asinus*) and alpacas (*Vicugna pacos*). Pol J Vet Sci 2016;19:477–84.

110. Henry M, Gastal EL, Pinheiro LEL, et al. Mating pattern and chromosome analysis of a mule and her offspring. Biol Reprod 1995;52:273–9.

111. Trujillo JM, Ohno S, Jardine JH, et al. Spermatogeneis in a male hinny: histological and cytological studies. J Hered 1969;60:79–84.

112. Camillo F, Vannozzi I, Rota A, et al. Successful non-surgical transfer of horse embryos to mule recipients. Reprod Domest Anim 2003;38:380–5.

113. Ellerbrock RE, Canisso IF. How to interpret pH profiles of mammary gland secretions to predict imminent parturition in mares. In: AAEP Proceedings Orlando, Florida, December 3–7, 2016; 62. p. 187–92.

114. Carluccio A, De Amicis I, Panzani S, et al. Electrolytes changes in mammary secretions before foaling in jennies. Reprod Domest Anim 2008;43:162–5.

115. McClure JJ, Koch C, Traub-Dargatz JT. Characterization of a red blood cell antigen in donkeys and mules associated with neonatal isoerythrolysis. Anim Genet 1994;25:119–20.

116. Carluccio A, Gloria A, Veronesi MC, et al. Factors affecting pregnancy length and phases of parturition in Martina Franca jennies. Theriogenology 2015;84: 650–5.

117. Canisso IF, Rodriguez JS, Macarena S, et al. A clinical approach to the diagnosis and treatment of retained fetal membranes with an emphasis placed on the critically ill mare. J Equine Vet Sci 2013;33:570–9.

118. Carluccio A, Tosi U, Contri A, et al. Correlation between follicular size and ovulation induction in Martina Franca jennies. Reprod Domest Anim 2006; 41:245–6.

119. Panzani D, Vannozzi I, Marmorini P, et al. Factors affecting recipients' pregnancy, pregnancy loss, and foaling rates in a commercial equine embryo transfer program. J Equine Vet Sci 2016;37:17–23.

120. Koblischke P, Kindahl H, Budik S, et al. Embryo transfer induces a subclinical endometritis in recipient mares which can be prevented by treatment with non-steroid anti-inflammatory drugs. Theriogenology 2008;70:1147–58.

121. Vendramini OM, Bruyas J-F, Fieni F, et al. Embryo transfer in Poitou donkeys, preliminary results. Theriogenology 1997;47:409 (abstract).

122. Allen WR, Boyle MS, Antczak DF. Between-species transfer of horse and donkey embryos: a valuable research tool. Equine Vet J 1985;17:53–62.

123. Peña-Alfaro CE, Barros LO, Carneiro GF, et al. Embryo transfer in Pega donkeys (*Equus asinus*) in Brazil. J Equine Vet Sci 2014;34:185.

124. Allen WR. Immunological aspects of the endometrial cup reaction and the effect of xenogeneic pregnancy in horses and donkeys. J Reprod Fertil Suppl 1982; 31:57–94.
125. Woods GL, White KL, Vanderwall DK, et al. Cloned mule pregnancies produced using nuclear transfer. Theriogenology 2002;58:779–82.
126. Woods GL, White KL, Vanderwall DK, et al. A mule cloned from fetal cells by nuclear transfer. Science 2003;301:1063–73.
127. Vanderwall DK, Woods GL, Sellon DC, et al. Present status of equine cloning and clinical characterization of embryonic, fetal, and neonatal development of three cloned mules. J Am Vet Med Assoc 2004;225:1694–9.

Hoof Disorders and Farriery in the Donkey

Alexandra K. Thiemann, MA, Vet MB, Cert EP, MSc, AFHEA, MRCVS[a,b,*],
Luke A. Poore, MSc, MA, Vet MB, Cert ES (Orth), MRCVS[c]

KEYWORDS

- Donkey • Mule • Hoof • Farriery • Lameness • Laminitis

KEY POINTS

- Hoof disease and hoof related lameness is very common in donkey populations throughout the world.
- Hoof disease is seen in working and companion animals and contributes significantly to poor welfare, morbidity, and mortality.
- There are anatomic and radiologic differences between donkey and horse hooves. Donkeys have more upright and oval feet. The mule hoof has components of both the donkey and horse.
- Donkeys often present with severe end-stage lameness and laminitis owing to their stoical behavioral traits, which can lead to delayed detection of disease.
- Donkeys hooves are often neglected, becoming overgrown and unbalanced. Good collaboration between the farrier and veterinarian is necessary to resolve these issues.

INTRODUCTION

The prevalence of hoof diseases is extremely high in donkey populations globally and In many cases these problems are preventable with improved management and working practices. Good hoof care relies on close collaboration and communication between the veterinarian, farrier, and owner. There are anatomic differences between the hooves of donkeys and horses. Understanding these differences improves the ability of professionals to provide optimal hoof care for these animals. Laminitis and white line disease are major clinical issues when the diet is inappropriate and underfoot conditions are too wet. Flexural deformities and neglect are common in working donkeys. The detection of lameness in donkeys may be delayed owing to their stoical nature.

Disclosure Statement: The authors have nothing to disclose.
[a] Education, The Veterinary Department, The Donkey Sanctuary, Brookfield Farm, Offwell, Honiton, Devon EX14 9SU, UK; [b] The Veterinary Hospital, Brookfield, Honiton, Devon EX14 9SU, UK; [c] The Veterinary Department, The Donkey Sanctuary, Brookfield Farm, Offwell, Honiton, Devon EX14 9SU, UK
* Corresponding author.
E-mail address: Alex.thiemann@thedonkeysanctuary.org.uk

EPIDEMIOLOGY OF FOOT DISEASE

Recent studies have shown that hoof disease and lameness are highly prevalent in donkeys in a variety of situations, and are responsible for poor welfare. Post mortem data from 1444 aged donkeys in a UK sanctuary over a 7-year period found that foot disorders were present in 44.8% of cases.[1]

An assessment of 2500 donkeys kept on farms at The Donkey Sanctuary, UK, found that 27.2% presented with foot lameness. The main cause of the lameness was foot abscesses 10.7%, the majority of which originated at the white line. Other causes of foot lameness included keratoma-like lesions (2.8%), acute laminitis (2.7%), and chronic laminitis (2.8%). These findings highlight the importance of foot disease as a cause of morbidity in donkeys and the need for good foot care and management to decrease the risk of developing any of these conditions. When looking at possible risk factors for the development of foot lameness, it is interesting to note that in the same population 26% of the donkeys had evidence of white line disease. Poor quality hoof associated with this condition is likely to predispose to the development of white line abscesses with purulent discharge and abscess tracts often evident in dorsal areas of the foot. In 2018, 27.2% of all mortalities at The Donkey Sanctuary were associated with foot disease. This equated to 2.6% of the sanctuary population being euthanized for foot-related lameness (unpublished data from animal welfare indicators assessments, Karen Rickards, The Donkey Sanctuary 2019).

An assessment of 12 donkey dairy farms in Europe reported that 18.7% of the donkey herds showed evidence of hoof neglect.[2]

Lameness evaluation of working draught donkeys in Pakistan found 100% of donkeys to be lame, with conditions directly related to the hoof.[3] These included white line infection, sheared heels, poor hoof balance, abnormal conformation, and a broken forward hoof pastern axis (HPA).

Specific hoof problems have been associated with climate, management, and work undertaken. High incidences of subsolar abscesses and seedy toe are found in countries with wet ground conditions, and working donkeys are noted to have a high prevalence of severe multilimb lameness.

ANATOMY AND CONFORMATION OF THE DONKEY HOOF

The donkey hoof has a distinctive oval shape compared with the horse and generally has a dorsal hoof wall that is, 5° to 10° more upright (**Fig. 1**). In the healthy donkey foot, the frog is well-developed, especially at the palmar aspect, but the apex does not extend under the pedal bone as in the horse (**Fig. 2**). It is for this reason that heart bar shoes are not usually considered appropriate for donkeys when support for the pedal bone is required. The sole is thick and the wall thickness remains constant from toe to heel. The narrow conical shape of the hoof has allowed the donkey to be used on narrow tracks and be sure footed on difficult terrain.

Donkeys are often narrow chested and many suffer from congenital conformational defects owing to indiscriminate breeding practices. These undesirable conformation types can cause lateromedial hoof imbalances, and subsequent limb deformities.

The extensor process of the distal phalanx is located on average 1 cm below the coronary band, so that the distal aspect of the second phalanx is located within the upper part of the hoof capsule.[4]

Radiographic parameters of the donkey hoof are given in **Table 1**,[4] and illustrated in **Fig. 3**. Studies of donkey hoof capsules show that there are differences in the distribution and density of the horn tubules compared with horses. If the underfoot environment is wet, the donkey hoof will absorb excessive moisture, resulting in a weaker

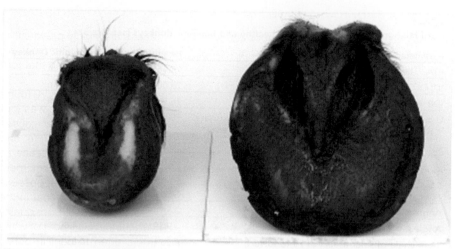

Fig. 1. Donkey hoof (*left*) compared with a horse hoof (*right*) from solar surface, showing differences in shape between the species.

mechanical structure prone to infection that predisposes to white line disease, thrush, and deformation. Although it may be useful to maintain good hoof moisture content in arid conditions, excess moisture such as found in much of the UK is detrimental to the health of the donkey's hoof capsule.

The donkey hoof has a 5-point loading pattern with pressure taken at each quarter, heel, and toe. This pattern, together with the thick sole, enables substantial resections of the hoof wall without affecting the integrity of the interface between the pedal bone and hoof capsule.

HANDLING AND BEHAVIORAL ISSUES TO CONSIDER

The donkey's behavior differs from horses and a lack of understanding of these differences has led donkeys to be mislabeled as stubborn or aggressive animals. In their

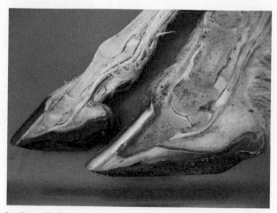

Fig. 2. Split hoof donkey (*left*) compared with a horse (*right*) showing increased distance from the top of the pedal bone to the coronary band in the donkey, and difference in position of the frog relative to P3.

Table 1 Hoof radiographic parameters from healthy and laminitic donkeys (see Fig. 3)		
Parameter	**Healthy Donkey**	**Laminitic Donkey**
IDA = hoof wall depth proximal	15.46 mm	17.76 mm
IDM = hoof wall depth middle	15.60 mm	20.36 mm
IDB = hoof wall depth distal	16.20 mm	20.18 mm
D = distance from extensor process of P3 to coronary band	10 mm	13.02 mm
Solar depth	10 mm	Variable
U = angle of pastern to P3 to surface	59.83°	59.10°
S = angle of hoof wall to surface	61.61°	59.03°
TS = angle of P3 to surface	64.11°	71.55°
Angle H = TS-S (capsular rotation)	2.5°	12.52°
Angle R = U-TS	−9.39°	−14.80°
SA = angle of solar aspect of P3 to surface	8.26°	10.89°

Data from Collins SN, Dyson SJ, Murray RC, et al. Radiological anatomy of the donkey's foot: Objective characterisation of the normal and laminitic donkey foot. Equine Vet J 2011;43(4):478-486.

natural habitat, they have to defend small groups in resource-poor areas and are less able to outrun predators than the horse. They have subsequently developed a more marked freeze and fight response than horses, with a subtler flight response and concomitant stoicism in the face of pain and disease.

Recognition of subtle behavioral signs such as turning the head away or stepping sideways can allow identification of fear in a donkey at an early stage. Development of these fear responses in a donkey that cannot avoid a perceived negative experience, for instance a veterinary or farriery interaction, can lead to attempts by the donkey to squash the examiner against a solid object, which can be dangerous. A further escalation of these fear-related behavioral traits can lead to the donkey

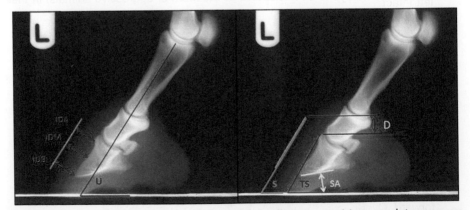

Fig. 3. Lateral radiographs of a donkey hoof to illustrate positions used to measure different parameters (see **Table 1**). D, distance from extensor process of P3 to coronary band; IDA, hoof wall depth proximal; IDB, hoof wall depth distal; IDM, hoof wall depth middle; S, hoof wall angle to surface; SA, angle of solar aspect of P3 to surface; TS, angle of P3 to surface; U, angle of pastern to P3.

demonstrating fight behaviors, including striking out with a front limb and/or kicking forward or backward with their hind limbs.[5]

To avoid fear-related behavior, donkeys are best handled in the presence of a bonded companion, which decreases their general stress level.

Mules exhibit a complex combination of behavioral traits from both the horse and donkey. If subtle signs of fear are missed, mules can show explosive behavior with violent defensive reactions.

Many donkeys and mules are not well-handled and it can be hard for the farrier or veterinarian to work on them. It is extremely helpful if owners are encouraged to pick out their donkey or mules feet daily and if such animals will accept being led on a head collar or halter and tied up safely. Donkeys and mules have a very good memory of aversive events, so it is preferable to sedate difficult animals rather than enter a prolonged conflict.

Owners can be taught basic shaping behaviors using positive reinforcement techniques that over time will allow safe handling of donkeys and mules.

TRIMMING THE NORMAL DONKEY HOOF

The farrier and veterinarian involved donkey care should be aware of basic differences in the anatomy of the donkey hoof compared with the horse. Reported differences and techniques have been reported,[6] with the following points providing practical guidance.

- Assess the donkey before and after trimming to evaluate gait and lameness.
- Aim to trim every 6 to 10 weeks depending on underfoot conditions and workload.
- Keep the donkey limb low during trimming to avoid pain, especially in geriatric or arthritic donkeys.
- Avoid abducting the limbs or unbalancing the donkey.
- Trim the sole first because the sole of the donkey's hoof capsule does not flake away naturally and requires paring to maintain concavity. In animals with chronic laminitis, the sole may never regain concavity. The raised area just inside the hoof wall at the toe region is the sole callous and should be left intact
- Overgrown or infected frog tissue should be pared back, loose degenerate tissue removed, and the frog sulci and grooves cleaned. The frog is an important weight-bearing structure that aids circulation within the hoof and should not be overtrimmed.
- The walls should be weight bearing rather than the sole. The trimming angles are guided by the HPA and frequently require the heels to be lowered to avoid a broken forward HPA. The wall is rasped or trimmed with nippers and the toe is trimmed last. In general, the angle of hoof growth just distal to the coronary band should be used as a guide.
- Assess the lateromedial balance and trim to enable equal weight distribution.
- Donkeys frequently have conformational defects such that an ideal hoof shape is not achievable, and the trim is then aimed for comfort and functionality.
- The outer hoof wall can be rasped gently and can be rounded off with the leg held forward. Over-rasping weakens the structure.
- In arid conditions, it can be extremely hard to trim feet and soaking the hooves can be helpful before trimming.
- In most cases, donkey feet are too moist and there are several areas of white line disease and poor hoof quality. Excess trimming can cause bruising and bleeding.

Donkeys are rarely shod because their hooves are hard wearing; however, in some countries there is a custom of fitting shoes poorly, which leads to lameness and foot disease.

Plastic or acrylic shoes are used extensively in donkeys in the Donkey Sanctuary, UK, for donkeys with thin soles or chronic foot disease. They are relatively easy to make into the correct shape and, if used with a flexible solar support gel, can provide comfort to donkeys with ongoing hoof issues (**Fig. 4**).

TRIMMING THE OVERLONG HOOF

It is common to find donkeys with neglected hooves that have continued to grow without being worn away or trimmed and begin to turn up at the toe and lead to a "Turkish slipper" appearance. The overgrowth can be extreme, resulting in hyperextension of the tendons and joints (**Fig. 5**). Before these hooves are trimmed, ideally, lateral radiographs should be obtained to monitor the position of the pedal bone and to determine whether remodeling or damage have occurred. If there is no underlying bone damage, in most instances these hooves can be returned to normal conformation with few trims from a skilled farrier (**Fig. 6**), using the following guidelines.

- Remove the frog and sole overgrowth and then reduce the heels first. This allows the bearing surface to sit correctly on the ground.
- Remove toe overgrowth, stop paring when thumb pressure on sole reveals slight give.
- Dress back the dorsal wall of the hoof with a rasp once the toe has been removed; be guided by the angle of the proximal hoof wall adjacent to the coronary band.
- Remove the degenerate hoof wall and white line.
- Analgesia may be needed for a short period of time owing to alteration in the hoof angles.

PREVENTION OF HOOF DISEASE
Diet

Nutritional requirements of donkeys are discussed elsewhere in detail (see Faith A. Burden and Nicola Bell's article, "Donkey Nutrition and Malnutrition," in this issue). For the purpose of considering hoof health, the diet should:

- Supply sufficient micronutrients to support good hoof development

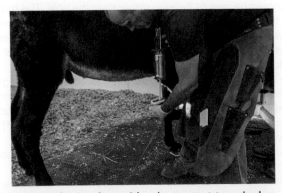

Fig. 4. Farrier fitting an acrylic rim shoe with solar support to a donkey.

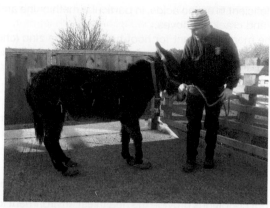

Fig. 5. Donkey with neglected overlong hooves.

- Be low in nonstructural carbohydrates (starches and sugars) to avoid inducing hyperglycemia and excessive insulin secretion
- Contain sufficient calories to maintain a body condition score of 3
- Be provided in clean and dry underfoot conditions and associated with physical activity.

Most diets for donkeys are inadequate, having excessive calories leading to obesity or fewer calories resulting in a poor body condition score and associated problems. There is no information on the nutritional requirements for proper hoof health in donkeys, but in horses the following components are required.

- *Energy* – severe energy restriction decreases hoof growth, shifting protein and fat to be used a source of energy. Excess energy results in fat accumulation, promotes hyperinsulinemia, and increases the risk of equine metabolic syndrome (EMS), endocrinopathic laminitis, and hyperlipidemia.
- *Proteins and amino acids* – sulfur-containing amino acids such as methionine and cysteine are found in high levels in keratinized tissue like the epidermis of the

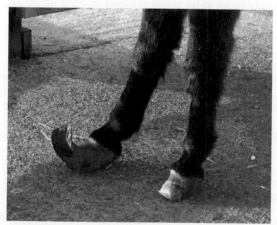

Fig. 6. Donkey hoof after trimming overlong hoof.

hoof. Diets deficient in amino acids, in particular methionine and cysteine, lead to poor quality and cracked hooves.

- *Minerals* – the most important for hoof health include zinc (chelated to proteins increases intestinal absorption), copper, and calcium. Selenium has a narrow safety margin and excess supplementation can lead to damage to the integument (hoof, epidermis, and hair).
- *Vitamins* - in particular biotin and vitamin A.

The Donkey Sanctuary recommends providing a nutritionally balanced feed supplement to donkeys on calorie-restricted diets, young stock, pregnant jennies, and whenever undernutrition needs to be rectified.[7]

MANAGEMENT

Clean, dry underfoot conditions provide the healthiest environment for good hoof care. Excess moisture in deep bedding or wet fields lead to increased sole and horn moisture in the hoof and a weakened structure prone to secondary damage and infections.[8] These conditions can be difficult to provide in some geographic locations, depending on season, and donkeys will benefit from being on dry concrete standing for much of the day.

Ideally, regular hoof care should include daily hoof picking to remove stones/dirt and inspect the solar surface.

The interval between farriery depends on the rate of hoof growth, workload, and underfoot conditions. In general, 6 to 10 weeks are acceptable normal trimming intervals.

Many donkeys that are kept as companion animals suffer from obesity and lack of exercise that contribute to foot disease, so some method to encourage walking and diet restriction while avoiding boredom is required. The Donkey Sanctuary has produced a resource detailing methods of environmental enrichment that will help with weight control and well-being with donkeys needing to loose weight.[8]

Vaccination

Donkeys should be routinely vaccinated against tetanus. Penetrating wounds to the hoof are common when hooves are moist, allowing *Clostridium tetani* to enter, proliferate, and release toxins. Donkeys are frequently left out of vaccination programs, and tetanus antitoxin may need to be given in cases of hoof penetration, in particular in animals with an unknown vaccination history.

Routine Testing

Testing for pituitary pars intermedia dysfunction (PPID) is recommended for donkeys over 15 years old. Increased adrenocorticotropic hormone (ACTH) concentrations, considering season, can be diagnostic and associated with increased risk of endocrinopathic laminitis. Animals with a positive diagnosis of PPID require treatment with pergolide.

Testing for EMS is recommended for donkeys with a body condition score of 4 to 5, and positive results can be used to guide dietary and physical activity management. See **Table 2** for normal seasonal ACTH and insulin values.

LAMENESS EXAMINATION AND DIAGNOSTIC ANESTHESIA

The lameness examination of donkeys has similarities to the evaluation of horses and ponies. The examination should commence with a general clinical evaluation and

Table 2 Normal seasonal ACTH and insulin concentrations in donkeys		
Insulin (μIU/mL)	0–15.1	Any season
ACTH (pg/mL)	2.7–30.4	November to June
	9.0–49.1	July to October

assessment of conformation. In donkeys, conformation is especially important with both carpal and tarsal valgus being commonly seen. Abnormal HPA and both latero-medial and dorsopalmar/dorsoplantar foot imbalances are also common.

Careful evaluation of the solar surface in donkeys and mules with consistent and systemic application of hoof testers often yields useful clinical information with seedy toe, bruising, keratomas, and subsolar abscessation often found.

Gait analysis is an essential component of the lameness examination in donkeys and mules, but can be challenging owing to behavioral constraints. A systematic approach and an experienced handler are essential. Gait analysis in a straight line can give important information and allow recording of baseline lameness values, but also information about dynamic and static foot balance.

Lameness evaluations on a circle with a lunge are often not possible in donkeys and mules because they are often not used to this training modality. Evaluation in a circle can, however, be performed in hand and will often, as in horses, exacerbate lameness detected in a straight line.

Proximal and distal flexion tests performed separately can also exacerbate lameness evident from an initial gait analysis and provide important information regarding range of motion of joints, which may be restricted in donkeys owing to fibrosis or soft tissue injury.

Diagnostic anesthesia can be performed as in other equids and is extremely useful to localize lameness to the foot. Regional nerve blocks, the palmar digital and abaxial sesamoid nerve blocks, and intrasynovial anesthesia, including distal interphalangeal and navicular bursa blocks, are feasible. The anatomic location of the distal interphalangeal joint in donkeys makes a dorsal approach challenging, although a palmar approach allows arthrocentesis.

RADIOGRAPHY

Radiographs of the donkey foot can be obtained with low output portable machines (minimum 15 mA). Preparation of the foot before obtaining radiographs includes cleaning the sole and hoof wall and removal of loose horn or sole. Appropriate sedation protocols may improve the quality of foot radiographs in painful or anxious donkeys and keeping a bonded companion in close proximity can increase compliance. The main radiographic projections of the foot are similar to the horse and outlined with reference to the donkey.

Lateromedial View

Lateromedial views of the distal phalanx require the foot to be raised on a block of sufficient height to bring the level of solar surface to the center of the beam. Because laminitis is a common problem in donkeys, correctly labeling lateromedial radiographs with a radiopaque marker on the dorsal hoof wall provides valuable clinical information. This includes the alignment of the third phalanx in relation to the hoof capsule, modeling of the dorsodistal aspect of the third phalanx and separation of the hoof wall. The lateromedial view is also important to assess dorsopalmar (and plantar) balance of the foot and to identify degenerative joint disease of the distal interphalangeal joint.

Dorsopalmar Weight-Bearing View

A dorsopalmar weight bearing view is particularly useful to assess lateromedial foot balance.

Palmaroproximal–Palmarodistal (and Plantarodistal) Oblique View

This view is useful for evaluation of the palmar and plantar processes of the third phalanx and to identify pathology associated with septic osteitis.

Dorsoproximal–Palmarodistal (and Plantarodistal) Oblique View

The dorsoproximal–palmarodistal oblique view centered on the third phalanx is useful to assess focal demineralization of the third phalanx consistent with septic osteitis. In comparison with horses, septic osteitis is common in donkeys. Resorption of the third phalanx owing to pressure from a keratoma is also common in donkeys compared with horses and can be identified with this view.

COMMON CONDITIONS OF DONKEY HOOVES
White Line Abscess

White line abscesses are often associated with stretched or damaged white lines, or gravel penetration, and can be difficult to drain owing to the thick wall and sole in donkeys. As in the horse, treatment requires poulticing, analgesia, and tetanus protection. Any donkey with severe lameness not responding to treatment requires a foot radiograph to ensure the infection is not tracking into the pedal bone. Any painful condition that limits access to food and water can result in hyperlipidemia.

Seedy Toe or White Line Disease

This condition is very common in donkeys kept in the Northern hemisphere, where conditions underfoot are often moist. Etiology and treatment are similar to the horse[9]; however, extensive hoof resections may be required. In cases of severe white line disease, the diet, general health, underfoot conditions, and workload may need to be modified.

LAMINITIS

Laminitis is a serious problem in companion donkeys, who often have several risk factors for this condition, including obesity, EMS, hyperinsulinemia, access to grazing, inappropriate feeding, and PPID[10] (**Fig. 7**). Donkeys can also develop sepsis-associated and supporting limb laminitis.

Clinical signs in donkeys include recumbency, short stride, increased digital pulses, and in severe cases, weight shifting and altered weight distribution. The main problem for these animals is delayed recognition owing to their stoicism to pain and tendency to lie down and walk slowly. Some owners, especially in nonridden animals, do not recognize these behaviors as a problem.

Endocrinopathic laminitis develops secondary to insulin dysregulation from EMS or PPID. Epidemiologic information for this condition in donkeys is lacking, but experience suggests that it is highly prevalent and underdiagnosed.

PPID is suspected in animals with resting ACTH concentrations above the reference range (see **Table 2**). In animals with inconclusive values, a dynamic test with thyrotropin-releasing hormone (thyrotropin-releasing hormone stimulation test) is

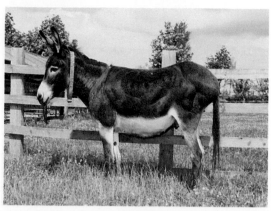

Fig. 7. Obese donkey; note the extensive fat pads.

highly recommended. The dexamethasone-suppression and the combined dexamethasone thyrotropin-releasing hormone tests do not seem to be useful to diagnose PPID in donkeys.[11]

The hoof capsule of affected donkeys may show laminitic rings; however, radiographs are useful to determine the extent and severity of any damage to the third phalanx. It is important to note that radiographs need to be interpreted using donkey-specific values. In severe cases, farriery and hoof care can improve the long-term welfare of the donkey, but full recovery may not be possible (**Figs. 8** and **9**).

Treatment regimes for pain control are similar to horses, mainly based on the use of nonsteroidal anti-inflammatory drugs at donkey-appropriate doses. When additional analgesia is required, drugs such as acetaminophen (paracetamol) at 20 mg/kg 2 times per day or opioids should be considered. In our experience, analgesia needs to be provided based on donkey composite pain scores rather than by timed intervals. The Donkey Sanctuary is currently trialing the use of donkey-specific composite and facial pain scores similar to those available for horses.[12] Regular use in the clinic is a valuable tool in deciding when to modify analgesia. As mentioned, donkeys with

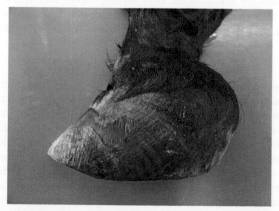

Fig. 8. External appearance of laminitic donkey hoof. Note the ringed appearance to hoof and previous attempts to rasp back the toe.

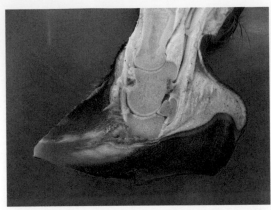

Fig. 9. Split section of same hoof as in **Fig. 8,** showing extensive destruction of P3 and severe pathology.

severe pain can rapidly develop anorexia and hyperlipidemia, so nursing care and assessment of blood triglyceride concentrations are central to their treatment.

Heart bar shoes are not advised owing to the more caudal frog position in donkeys, but supportive bandages, Styrofoam support, and deep bedding are useful to redistribute weight away from the tip of the third phalanx. Oral or parenteral acepromazine may encourage rest and decrease distress.

Treatment for underlying endocrinopathies is similar to the horse. Pergolide is the treatment of choice for PPID. In some animals, this drug causes a decreased appetite, which can lead to hyperlipidemia. In these cases, reducing the dose and close monitoring during initial therapy are recommended.

Treatment for insulin dysregulation is aimed at reducing weight, limiting carbohydrate-rich diets, and increasing physical activity, if possible. In donkeys, it is contraindicated to have sudden decreases caloric intake or changes in feed, but there should be a long-term plan to transition to a low calorie and high fiber diet. Metformin (20 mg/kg, 2 times per day) may be used to decrease intestinal glucose uptake and promote insulin sensitivity, and is best used as an adjunct to correct grazing management for short periods.

Weight loss can be encouraged with levothyroxine (0.1 mg/kg once per day) because this drug increases the metabolic rate, appetite, and insulin sensitivity; however, its use may have welfare implications in donkey subjected to dietary restrictions.

FRACTURES

Although fractures of the third phalanx are seen in donkey populations, they are not as common as in horses. Hoof casts are an effective means of stabilizing third phalanx fractures and are easy to apply in standing donkeys. Foot casts can also treat other conditions, including heel bulb and pastern lacerations, hoof wall avulsions, and collateral ligament injuries. Advantages of foot casts over traditional bandaging include increased durability and immobilization, decreased expense, and decreased treatment time when faced with multiple bandage changes. Before applying the cast, the hoof and surrounding structures should be prepared by removing the shoe (if applicable) and trimming the hoof to prevent pressure points along the edges of the cast. Any lacerations that will be covered with the cast should be treated and lightly bandaged. A 7.5-cm orthopedic casting tape works well for donkey hooves (**Fig. 10**).

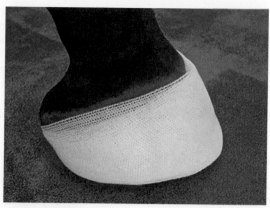

Fig. 10. Donkey hoof with cast.

KERATOMA

Keratomas are recognized in donkey hooves. They are benign rare growths of the keratin producing epidermal cells of the coronary band and solar corium, and in horses are thought to arise owing to irritation or pressure. There are few studies on possible risk factors and etiology in donkeys.[13] Diagnosis is usually made on clinical suspicion and confirmed by radiography and histology. There may be abnormal deviation of the white line, usually inward, that may show separation and caseous or abnormal pale disorganized tissue instead of normal white laminae. This finding can be associated with a convex overlying hoof capsule and in some cases there could be recurrent abscessation of the white line at the site of the keratoma (**Fig. 11**).

Radiographs show lysis of the third phalanx underneath the lesion. Typically, the third phalanx shows smooth pressure necrosis in a semicircle, which distinguishes keratomas from aggressive pedal bone infections.

In suitable cases, the keratoma can be removed surgically. Because the lesions can occur in more than 1 hoof, all feet should be carefully inspected and if necessary radiographed before surgery. Concurrent disease such as laminitis, dropped sole, and osteoarthritis affect the decision to perform surgery, especially in the aged donkey.

Surgery can be performed standing or under general anesthesia, after a very thorough cleaning and disinfection of the hoof a day before operating. A tourniquet is needed to prevent hemorrhage obscuring the site. Regional antibiotic perfusion is

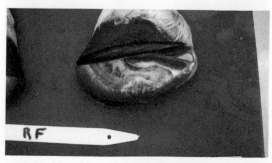

Fig. 11. Transverse section of hoof showing site of keratoma lesion damaging pedal bone.

useful as in the horse, but technically challenging owing to the smaller size of the blood vessels. The surgical site is kept clean and dry until new laminae are formed and hardened; a support shoe may be needed to prevent movement either side of the defect.

Histologically, the keratoma shows laminar hyperplasia and dyskeratosis with loss of the tubular structure in the stratum medium and atrophy of the stratum internum.

Recurrence can be a problem and feet must be monitored until the defect has grown out.

FLEXURAL DEFORMITIES

Acquired flexural deformities are recognized in donkeys and can become severe through neglect. In young animals, overfeeding and imbalanced diets are usually the cause. Initially the heel will be non-weight bearing, with an increased HPA angle. If untreated, the dorsal hoof wall can reach a vertical line (**Fig. 12**), a stage 1 contracture of the deep flexor tendon develops, and can progress to the stage 2, where the hoof wall tips beyond the vertical line. Treatment, as in the horse, relies on farriery and corrective shoeing for selected cases.[14] Affected donkeys need to be radiographed to determine the extent of any damage to the bone or joints, and analgesia during correction. Severe cases may require inferior check ligament desmotomy or deep digital flexure tenotomy for resolution or improvement.[15]

This condition has also been seen in working donkeys where they are pulling carts with extreme weights, and in geriatric nonworking donkeys. In these cases the etiology is thought likely owing to pain in the upper limbs and joints, leading to abnormal weight bearing and tendon shortening. **Fig. 13** demonstrates successful treatment of a geriatric donkey with severe contracture through a multimodal approach involving hoof expansion and farriery.[16]

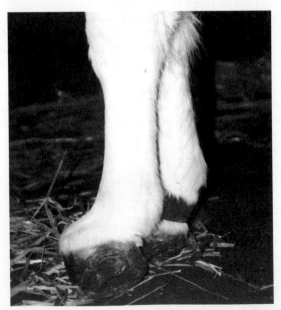

Fig. 12. Stage 1 contracture of deep digital flexor showing hoof wall approaching vertical.

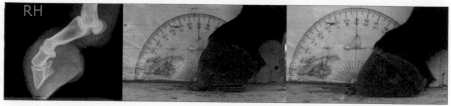

Fig. 13. Treatment of severe deep digital flexor contracture using hoof expansion and farriery.

SUMMARY

This review covers many of the conditions associated with hoof disease in the donkey. Preventive care is the key to avoiding many of the serious conditions that can occur. Foot disease and poor farriery are major welfare concerns of donkeys throughout the world and are associated with pain, mortality, and loss of production.

REFERENCES

1. Morrow LD, Smith KC, Piercy RJ, et al. Retrospective analysis of post-mortem findings in 1,444 aged donkeys. J Comp Pathol 2011;144(2–3):145–56.
2. Francesca D, Segati G, Brascic M, et al. Effects of management practices on the welfare of dairy donkeys and risk factors associated with signs of hoof neglect. J Dairy Res 2018;85(1):30–8.
3. Burn RCE, Pritchard JC, Barr ARS, et al. The range and prevalence of clinical signs and conformation associated with lameness in working draught donkeys in Pakistan. Equine Vet J 2014;46(6):771–7.
4. Collins SN, Dyson SJ, Murray RC, et al. Radiological anatomy of the donkey's foot: objective characterisation of the normal and laminitic donkey foot. Equine Vet J 2011;43(4):478–86.
5. Haines A, Goliszek J. Donkey and mule behaviour for the veterinary team. UK-Vet Equine 2019;3(1):27–32.
6. Evans L, Crane M. The musculoskeletal system [Chapter 9]. In: Linda E, Michael C, editors. The clinical companion of the donkey. Leicestershire (England): Troubador Publishing Ltd; 2018. p. 113–30.
7. Available at: https://www.thedonkeysanctuary.org.uk/what-we-do/knowledge-and-advice/for-owners/what-to-feed-your-donkey. Accessed April 15, 2019.
8. Available at: https://view.pagetiger.com/EnvironmentalEnrichmentforDonkeys/EnvironmentEnrichmentfordonkeys. Accessed April 15, 2019.
9. O'Grady SE. A fresh look at white line disease. Equine Vet Educ 2011;23(10): 517–22.
10. Menzies- Gow N. Laminitis in horses. Practice 2018;40(9):411–9.
11. Mejia-Pereira S, Perez-Ecija A, Buchanan BR, et al. Evaluation of dynamic testing for pituitary pars intermedia dysfunction diagnosis in donkey. Equine Vet J 2018. https://doi.org/10.1111/evj.13034.
12. Gleerup KB, Lindegaard C. Recognition and quantification of pain in horses: a tutorial review. Equine Vet Educ 2015;1:47–57.
13. Paraschou G. Keratoma like lesions in donkeys. Manchester (United Kingdom): British Veterinary Dermatology Study Group; 2017. 11/12.

14. Walmsley JP. Flexural deformities of distal interphalangeal joints in a group of young donkeys. Equine Vet Educ 1998;7:4–6.
15. Thiemann AK, Rickards K. Donkey hoof disorders and their treatment. Practice 2013;35:134–40.
16. Buil J. Deformidade flexural em burros: cuatro casos clinicos. [II congresso internacional de medicina de asininos]. Patologias do casco: deformidade flexural em asininos. Vila real (Portugal): University of Tras-os-montes e Alto Douro; 2014.

Moving?

Make sure your subscription moves with you!

To notify us of your new address, find your **Clinics Account Number** (located on your mailing label above your name), and contact customer service at:

Email: **journalscustomerservice-usa@elsevier.com**

800-654-2452 (subscribers in the U.S. & Canada)
314-447-8871 (subscribers outside of the U.S. & Canada)

Fax number: **314-447-8029**

**Elsevier Health Sciences Division
Subscription Customer Service
3251 Riverport Lane
Maryland Heights, MO 63043**

*To ensure uninterrupted delivery of your subscription, please notify us at least 4 weeks in advance of move.

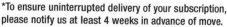

Printed and bound by CPI Group (UK) Ltd, Croydon, CR0 4YY

24/10/2024

01778553-0007